ONCOGENOMICS AND CANCER PROTEOMICS – NOVEL APPROACHES IN BIOMARKERS DISCOVERY AND THERAPEUTIC TARGETS IN CANCER

Edited by **César López-Camarillo**
and **Elena Aréchaga-Ocampo**

Oncogenomics and Cancer Proteomics – Novel Approaches in Biomarkers Discovery and Therapeutic Targets in Cancer

http://dx.doi.org/10.5772/1745
Edited by César López-Camarillo and Elena Aréchaga-Ocampo

Contributors

Norfilza M. Mokhtar, Nor Azian Murad, Then Sue Mian, Rahman Jamal, Elena Aréchaga-Ocampo, Nicolas Villegas-Sepulveda, Eduardo Lopez-Urrutia, Mayra Ramos-Suzarte, César López-Camarillo, Carlos Perez-Plasencia, Claudia H. Gonzalez-de la Rosa, Cesar Cortes-Gonzalez, Luis A. Herrera, Laurence A. Marchat, Elisa Azuara-Liceaga, Carlos Pérez-Plasencia, Lizeth Fuentes-Mera, Miguel A. Fonseca-Sánchez, Ali Flores-Pérez, Pouya Jamshidi, Clark C. Chen, Lili Jiang, Xueshan Qiu, Daniela Ferreira, Filomena Adega, Raquel Chaves, Mª Dolores Pastor, Ana Nogal, Sonia Molina-Pinelo, Luis Paz-Ares, Amancio Carnero, Hiroko Kozuka-Hata, Yumi Goto, Masaaki Oyama, Olga Villamar-Cruz, Luis E. Arias-Romero

Published by InTech

Janeza Trdine 9, 51000 Rijeka, Croatia

Publishing Process Manager Dimitri Jelovcan

Typesetting InTech Prepress, Novi Sad

Cover InTech Design Team

Additional hard copies can be obtained from orders@intechopen.com

Oncogenomics and Cancer Proteomics –
Novel Approaches in Biomarkers Discovery and Therapeutic Targets in Cancer,
Edited by César López-Camarillo and Elena Aréchaga-Ocampo
p. cm.
ISBN 978-953-51-1041-5

For EU product safety concerns:
IN TECH d.o.o., Prolaz Marije Krucifikse Kozulić 3, 51000 Rijeka, Croatia,
info@intechopen.com or visit our website at intechopen.com.

Meet the editors

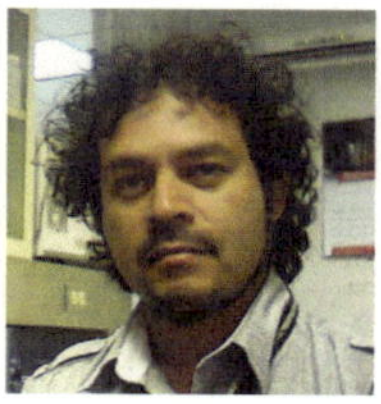

César López-Camarillo received his BS from Autonomous University of Chihuahua in 1988, MS from Center for Research and Advanced Studies (CINVESTAV-IPN) in 1994, and his PhD from National School of Medicine and Homeopathy-IPN in 2003. He is a professor researcher at the Genomics Sciences Program of Autonomous University of Mexico City. Dr. Camarillo´s research is directed to the identification of novel biomarkers in breast cancer through the use of genomics and proteomics technologies, and the microRNAs profiling in cancer. Dr. Camarillo is the recipient of Lola e Iggo Flisser-OUIS-UNAM award, XIX National Biomedical Research Prize, Capital City Heberto Castillo Award, and Breast Cancer Research Bristol Award.

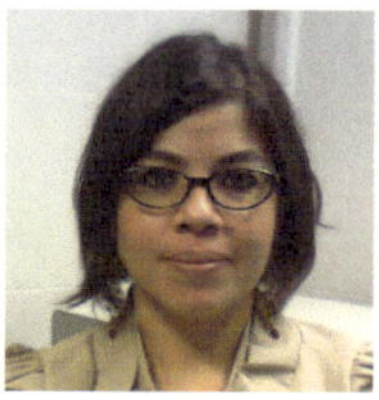

Dr. Elena Aréchaga received her BS in Biology from the Faculty of Biological Sciences at the Autonomous University of the State of Morelos in 2000. During her studies in biology, Dr. Aréchaga began research in plant molecular biology at the Center for Research on Nitrogen Fixation of the National Autonomous University of Mexico in 1998. Subsequently, she obtained her MS in Molecular Biomedicine in 2003, and PhD in Molecular Biomedicine in 2007, from Center for Research and Advanced Studies (CINVESTAV-IPN). She joined the National Cancer Institute in Mexico Research Associate in 2008. Dr. Aréchaga is interested in genomics cancer research. And her studies are directed to the identification of microRNAs and proteins associated with radiotherapy resistance in lung cancer.

Contents

Preface

Today, cancer research is focused on determining how genome and proteome level information may be useful as tools in prevention, diagnosis, and prognosis. The development of "omics" technologies, such as proteomics and transcriptomics has opened new research areas for scientists working on cancer research. This book presents the latest advances in cancer genomics and proteomics focused on identification of tumoral biomarkers and potential therapeutic targets in the most common human neoplasias including glioblastoma, oral squamous cell carcinoma, and breast, lung, prostate, and colorectal cancers. In addition, critical reviews of the relevant roles of microRNAs, animal models and the application of gene regulatory networks to validate potential therapeutic targets in cancer are also included.

Chapters in "Oncogenomics and Cancer Proteomics - Novel Approaches in Biomarkers Discovery and Therapeutic Targets in Cancer" present comprehensive and expert perspectives on the most common cancers from bench to bedside applications by an international team of experts in the field. This edited collection is subdivided into two sections titled: I) Genomic expression profiling in cancer, and II) Proteomic expression profiling in cancer. Proteomic technologies based on two-dimensional electrophoresis (2DPAGE and 2D-DIGE), or on isotope labeling methods followed by mass spectrometry (MS) analysis applied to the identification of differential protein expression in cancer are also discussed. This book will contribute greatly to the scientific and medical community by providing up-to-date discoveries of oncogenomics and their important roles in cancer translational research. It is intended for students, scientists, clinicians, oncologists and other health professionals working in the field of cancer research.

Dr. César López-Camarillo
Genomics Sciences Program, Autonomous University of Mexico City, Mexico

Dr. Elena Aréchaga-Ocampo
Cancer Biomedical Research Unit, National Institute of Cancerology, Mexico

Section 1

Genomic Expression Profiling in Cancer

Chapter 1

Genomic Expression Profiles: From Molecular Signatures to Clinical Oncology Translation

Norfilza M. Mokhtar, Nor Azian Murad, Then Sue Mian and Rahman Jamal

Additional information is available at the end of the chapter

http://dx.doi.org/10.5772/53766

1. Introduction

Study related to diseases such as cancer has changed tremendously for a decade. For many years, the study was restricted largely to a single gene or a few genes in cancer cells. The studies have uncovered the roles of individual genes in the uncontrolled behavior of cancer cells. Studying the functional roles of genes in cancer cells has deepened our understanding not only the cancer cells as well as normal cells. Since 2003 onwards, the trend of publications was focusing on the analysis of thousands of genes with related molecular pathways. Steps taken from this analysis is then translated to clinical practice for the biological markers for an early detection, monitoring, prognosis of the disease and response to therapy.

The completion of the Human Genome Project in 2003 enabled a new era in biological sciences, in particular molecular medicine. The availability of the database of full sequences of approximately 3 billion base pairs and approximately 30,000 genes in human DNA will lead to a better understanding of physiological and pathophysiological changes in human body. Genome-wide expression technology allows the simultenous analysis of thousands of genes in a single experiment. The availability of the technology alters the way biological experiments can be designed. This has resulted of so called 'discovery biology'. The large amount of data produced by microarray resulted to new and unexpected features of cellular functions.

Since it was first introduced, microarrays are widely used for basic research, the development of prognostic tests, target discovery or toxicology researchs. The new form of cancer screening utilizes the molecular data generated from microarray studies. We will discuss the application of gene profiling data in the clinical screening of cancer. It is hopefully will give a broad picture the pipeline required to discover biomarkers of cancer.

The chapter is subdivided into a series of sections; each will discuss the scientific evidence on the molecular and cellular studies in selected cancers. We will try to critically assess the evidence upon which the theory on the cancer was built. The conversion of normal cells into cancer cells is a complex process and multistep processes. Scientists for many years tried to uncover the causes of cancer and emphasize certain oncogenes, or tumor suppressor genes or other groups of genes. Further information on how these findings were translated to the clinical settings will be provided. To date, with the massive gene expression profile data available to the researchers, there are still major hurdles in validating and reproducing the results. We will discuss the major drawbacks associated with the use of molecular signatures as the biomarkers or response to treatment.

2. Molecular signatures in colorectal carcinoma

Colorectal cancer (CRC) is a type of cancers that develops in the colon or the rectum of the human digestive system or gastrointestinal tract (1).Colorectal cancer is the third leading cause of death in both men and women in the US with 141,210 new cases and 49,380 death expected in 2011 (2). CRC progresses slowly over a period of time usually between 10 to 15 years (3, 4). The tumor begins with noncancerous polyps where the tissues that form the lining of the colon or rectum differentiate into cancerous tissues (5). Approximately, 96% of colorectal cancers are adenocarcinomas, which arise from the glandular tissue (6). It can grow along the lining of the epithelium into the wall of the colon and rectum and invade the digestive system (7). In addition, the cancerous cells can also penetrate into the circulating systems, the blood and lymphatic systems which known as metastasis (7). Typically, the cancerous cells will first spread into the nearby lymph nodes and subsequently penetrate into other organs such as liver, lungs and ovary through blood vessels (8, 9). Colorectal cancer can be classified as tumors/nodes/metastasis (TMN) staging and Dukes classification (12). The TMN assigns the number based on three categories, T, M and N, which are the degree of invasion of the intestinal wall, lymph node involvement and the degree of metastasis, respectively (10). The higher number of TNM system indicates the advanced stage of colorectal cancer (10).

Unhealthy lifestyles such as alcohol consumption, high intake of red meat, obesity, smoking and lack of physical activities are among the risk factors for CRC (1, 11). Age and gender also play significant role in the development of CRC as the risk is higher in male and elderly(7). People with inflammatory bowel disease such as ulcerative colitis and Crohn's disease are also at high risk of getting CRC (12). Among the patients with Crohn's disease, approximately, 2%, 8% and 18% of the patients will develop CRC after 10, 20 and 30 years, respectively (12). About 20% of patients with ulcerative colitis develop CRC within the first 10 years (13). Mutations in genes such as *KRAS, APC,* and *MMR* are the well-documented genetic factor that contributes to colorectal cancer (3, 14, 15). Individual with family history of CRC in two or more first degree relatives have 2 or 3-fold greater risk of getting CRC and this has accounted for 20% of all cases (7). Examples of CRC involving genetic mutations are hereditary nonpolyposis colorectal cancer (HNPCC or Lynch Syndrome), Gardner syndrome and Familial adenomatous polyposis (16).

Diagnosis of CRC is based on tumor biopsy performed during the sigmoidoscopy or colonoscopy (7). CT scan of chest, abdomen and pelvis could be performed to determine the metastasis state and in certain cases, PET or MRI may be used to assist in the diagnosis (7).Molecular testing for patients with a strong family history can be performed to identify mutation, thus initiate early diagnosis and screening in family members. In addition, molecular characterization of mutations involved in CRC may help doctors to plan a better treatment strategy for the patients. Managing our lifestyles can help us to reduce our risk of getting CRC, for example by improving lifestyle through regular exercise, increasing the consumption of whole grains, fruits and vegetables and reducing the red meat intake (17). The treatments for CRC include surgery, chemotherapy and radiotherapy.

2.1. Molecular biology of colorectal cancer

Colorectal cancer is a multistep process that includes accumulation of several genetic and epigenetic alterations (18, 19). It is well characterized that the adenoma to carcinoma sequence is due to accumulation of the genomic alteration, which is induced by genomic instability (4, 20). Genomic instability is an event, which will increase tendency of the genome to acquire mutations when several important processes in maintaining and replicating the genome are malfunction. It is a hallmark of many human cancers (20). There are three well-reported genomic instability pathways that could lead to colorectal cancer, which will be discussed in details below.

a. **Chromosomal instability (CIN)**

Chromosomal instability lead to increase rate of losing or gaining chromosomes during cell division and accounts for 15% to 20% of sporadic CRC as well as Lynch Syndrome (Hereditary Non-Polyposis Colorectal Cancer) (21).There are three mechanisms involved in this process that includes structural chromosome instability, the chromosome breakage-fusion-bridge (BFB) cycles and numerical instability (22). Structural chromosome instability is caused by high incidences of DNA double-strand breaks, which may lead to abnormalities in chromosomal segregation during mitosis. Chromosomal damage may result in mitotically unstable chromosome, which may promote an event known as breakage-fusion-bridge (BFB) (22). An abnormal number of centrosome may be caused by abnormal mitotic polarity as well as unequal segregation of chromosomes during the anaphase stage (23). CIN promotes cancer progression by increasing clonal diversity (21). In the clinical perspective, large meta-analysis has shown that CIN is a marker of poor prognosis in colorectal cancer (20).

b. **Microsatelite instability (MIN)**

Microsatellites are repetitive sequences of DNA, which is highly varied between individuals (24). The most common microsatellites in human is a dinucleotide repeat of CA (25). MIN is a condition, which is manifested by damaged DNA due to defective in the DNA repair mechanism. CRC with the presence of MIN have a better prognosis compared to CRC with CIN (26). MIN involves the inactivation of the DNA Mismatch

Repair (MMR) genes via aberrant methylation or somatic mutation (26). HNPCC or Lynch Syndrome is an example of CRC, which is caused by MIN with 15% occurrence (27). MIN could cause CRC in 2 mechanisms; 1) mutations in the MMR genes where error in the microsatellite repeat replication is unfixed. This leads to the inactivation of tumor suppressor genes (TSG), a group of genes which is crucial in maintaining cell cycle progression and apoptosis induction (20). Inactivation of these genes may lead to tumorigenesis through uncontrolled cell division 2) epigenetic changes that silence the MMR genes (20).

c. **CpG Island Methylation and CpG Island Methylator Phenotype (CIMP)**

Hypermethylation of the promoter region of a gene that contains CpG Island (CGI) and global DNA hypomethylation are associated with epigenetic instability in colorectal cancer (20). CGIs are short sequences rich in the CpG dinucleotides and are observed in the 5′ region of almost half of all human genes (28). *In-vitro* study of BRAF in CRC cell lines showed no correlation between BRAF and CIMP (29).

2.2. Genome Wide Association Study (GWAS) in colorectal cancer

The completion of Human Genome Project in 2003 and the International HapMap Project in 2005 have opened up a new era in genetic and phenotype correlation study (30). The completion of these two projects has made the Genome wide association study (GWAS) possible. GWAS is considered as the most powerful tool to study the association between phenotypes and genotypes and also to identify common, low-penetrance susceptibility loci in a particular disease. In addition, GWAS can also be employed to investigate gene-environment interactions and the pooled analyses may also lead to the identification of novel modifying genes. Several GWAS studies have been performed in colorectal cancer and several loci were identified to be associated with CRC such as 8q24 (128.1-128.7 Mb, rs6983267) (31, 32). The *C-MYC (MYC)* oncogene is located approximately 300 kb from this region and is often over-expressed in CRC (33). Validation studies have confirmed that rs6983267 loci as the most promising variant in CRC, which has increased the chance of getting CRC by approximately 1.2 fold (33, 34). Recent publication has suggested that this variant is involved in enhancing the Wnt signaling and MYC regulation, which are known pathways in carcinogenesis (35). However, further functional analyses are still needed in order to determine the function of this variant. In the Japanese population, this variant leads to an increase risk of CRC with an allelic OR=1.22. Even after the adjustment for confounders, the OR remains significant (OR = 1.25). In the ARCTIC report, a locus at 9p24 was identified to be associated with CRC and was confirmed in the Colorectal Cancer Family Registry. Several numbers of loci that include 18q21:*SMAD7*; 15q13.3:*CRAC1*; 8q23.3: *E1F3H*; 14q22.2:*BMP4*; 16q22.1: *CDH1* and 19q13.1:*RHPN2* were also found to be associated with CRC. These genes have been shown to be involved in CRC progression. Studies conducted in Korean and Japanese patients with CRC have identified a novel susceptible locus in *SLC22A3*, which was significantly associated with distal colon cancer (36). The variant, rs7758229, was located on 6q26-q27 with OR=1.28. Three variants, rs7758229, rs6983267 and rs4939827, in *SMAD7* together with alcohol consumption may increase the risk of CRC by approximately two-fold. Several variants including rs6983267, rs6695584, rs11986063, rs3087967, rs2059254 and rs72268855 showed evidence of association with CRC in Singaporean Chinese (31). sSNP rs3087967 at 11q23.1 was associated with increased risk of CRC in men (OR=1.34) compared to women (OR=1.07). The rs 10318 at locus 15q13 (GREM1) was also associated with CRC with OD =1.19 (37).

Almost half of the susceptibility loci in CRC are located nearby the transforming growth factor beta gene (*TGF-β1*), which is important in the carcinogenesis (38). An elevated level of *TGF-β1* was linked to tumor progression and recurrence in CRC. Germline mutations in components of *TGF-β1* signaling pathway such as SMAD4 is responsible for the high-penetrance juvenile polyposis syndrome. Other genes are *SMAD4, RHPN2, BMP4, BMP2* and *GREM1*.

2.3. Gene expression profiling in colorectal cancer

Gene expression profiling was performed to compare between colorectal adenomas and CRCs and the result showed that the level of six cancer-related gene sets were increased in CRCs compared to adenomas (FDR<0.05). These include genes that involved in chromosomal instability, proliferation, differentiation, angiogenesis, stroma activation and invasion. Changes in the activity of the chromosomal instability were the most significant gene set (FDR=0.004) (39). The key genes that are associated with colorectal adenoma to carcinoma progression are AURKA, TPX2 (Chromosomal instability), PLK1 (Proliferation), ADRM1 (Differentiation), SSCA1 (Stroma activation), SPARC and PDGFRB (Invasion). The expression levels of these genes were significantly higher in CRC compared to adenoma (p<1e-5). Overexpression of AURKA induces centrosome amplification, aneupploidy and cellular transformation *in vitro* (40). AURKA interacts with TPX2 and plays a role in centrosome maturation and spindle formation (41). The polo-like kinase 1 (PLK1) is important in spindle formation and cell cycle progression during the G2 and M phase (42).

Wu and colleagues showed that the extracellular matrix and metabolic pathways were activated and the genes related to cell homeostatsis were downregulated. In this study, they compared cancer transcriptome using massive parallel paired-end cDNA sequencing in 3 different tissues, CRC tissue (stage III), adjacent non-tumor tissue and normal tissue from a 57 years old female patient. They detected 1660, 1528 and 941 significant differential genes (DEGs) between the CRC and adjacent tissue, the CRC and normal tissue; and the adjacent and normal tissue respectively. 15-prostaglandin dehydrogenase (*15-PGDH*) was downregulated in cancer compared to normal tisssue, which is common oncogenic event in approximately 80% of CRC cases. The transition between adenoma and carcinoma processes involved inactivation of *TGFBR2*, thus progressive inactivation of this gene from cancer-adjacent and normal tissue was expected. In addition, *APC, MYH, CD133, IDH1* and *MINT2* were also dysregulated in CRC. They also identified many genes involved in extracellular matrix (ECM) receptor interactions were highly dysregulated in cancer. The findings showed that all collagen type proteins were overexpressed up to 1000-fold in cancer tissue.

In addition, members of MMP family, which degraded the ECM structures, were also induced significantly in tumor. These include MMP1, MMP3, MMP14 and MMP7. Other cell-cell adhesion-related molecules for examples laminins (LAMA4, LAMA5, LAMB1, LAMB2 and LAMC2) and integrins (ITGA5, ITGB5, ITGA11 and ITGBL1) were elevated in cancer tissues. It was suggested that "angiogenesis switch" was activated in tumor tissues since vascular endothelial growth factor (VEGF) was found to be upregulated. In conclusion, up-regulation of the ECM pathway and the angiogenic growth factors may lead to remodelling of the ECM pathways as well as expansion of the new vessel networks, which subsequently resulted in CRC progression. Since their results in concordance with previous studies that showed the ECM pathway was subjected to intensive epigenetic modification, therefore this ECM may be a good candidate as prognostic biomarkers in CRC (43).

3. Molecular signatures in ovarian cancer

Ovarian cancer is among the top ten leading cancers among women the United States. In this country alone, there are approximately 22,280 new cases and 15,500 estimated death in 2012 (44). At our local population, approximately 1627 women were diagnosed in 2003 to 2005 and the figure showed increasing trend in 2007(45).In Japan and Sweeden, the incidence of ovarian cancer per 100,000 women is 3.1 cases and 21 cases respectively (Green et al., 2012). Due to vague or absence of early signs and symptoms, patients suffer from this cancer seek late treatment (46). Therefore, the cancer is normally diagnosed late when the disease is not longer confined to the ovary. Based on different morphological characterisitcs of the cancer, it is divided into epithelial and nonepithelial types. The epithelial type is further subdivided into serous, mucinous, endometrioid and clear cells. On the other hand, the nonepithelial is granulosa cells, mixed germ cells tumour, immature teratoma, dysgerminoma and teratoma. The risk factor for this cancer is unclear, however the **E**uropean **P**rospective **I**nvestigation into **C**ancer and Nutrition (EPIC) cohort study has recently documented that women who smoke more than 10 cigarettes a day had doubled the risk to develop mucinous ovarian cancer (47). This has suggested that the effect of smoking differs based on different histological subtypes of ovarian cancer(47). On the other hand, a study has shown that long period of breastfeeding seems to have reduced risk of ovarian cancer (OR = 0.986, 95% CI 0.978-0.994 per month of breastfeeding) (48).This effect of breastfeeding was also varies between histological subtypes as there was no association between breastfeeding and borderline serous or mucinous cancer (48).

Ovarian cancer was initially divided based on molecular pathways involved in the development and progression of the subtypes (49). Type I is low-grade serous, low-grade endometrioid, mucinous and clear cells. They are believed to arise from benign lesions such as ovarian inclusion cyst or endometriotic lesions. These lesions follow the stepwise pattern, whereby it evolved from the benign adenoma to borderline and finally to malignant tumours (table 1).

Type II ovarian cancer is high-grade serous, high-grade endometrioid and undifferentiated. The common mutations that are found in these subtypes are p53, BRCA1/2, PIK3CA with chromosomal instability. They normally involve the peritoneum and grow rapidly.

Characteristics of tumour	Type I	Type II
Type of tumor	Low-grade serous	High-grade serous
	Low-grade endometrioid	High-grade endometrioid
	Mucinous	Undifferentiated
	Clear cell	
Common mutations and genetic modifications	KRAS	p53
	BRAF	BRCA1
	PTEN	BRCA2
	CTNNB1	PIK3CA
	Microsatellite instability	Chromosome instability

Table 1. Ovarian subtypes based on common mutations and genetic modifications

In clinical practice, the gyneoncologist still use CA125 as the biomarker to monitor treatment of this cancer. However, it is not sensitive and specific to detect the cancer in its early stage (46). It is of great demand to find new molecular marker for the ovarian cancer.

Ovarian cancer is treated by surgery, radiation or platinum-taxane based chemotherapy depending on the subtypes and extent of the cancer (50). Patients at stage I and II will undergo bilateral salphingo-oophorectomy. While for advanced cases, adjuvant chemotherapy combined with surgery is highly recommended. With the latest understanding on the mutational types of ovarian cancer, mitogen activated protein kinase (MEK) inhibitor such as CI-1040 was used to test the potential therapeutic agent in *in vitro* ovarian cancer cell line (51). This cell lines containing KRAS or BRAF mutations, which are known mutations for type I ovarian cancer. The targeted therapy for type II ovarian cancer encounters difficulty due to lack of common molecular pathways. In two cohort studies involving 16 international centers, women with BRCA1 or BRCA2 mutation were treated with two different doses of Olaparib (52). This drug is orally active poly(ADP-ribose) polymerase (PARP) inhibitor. The result showed a promising therapeutic indexin ovarian cancer patients with mutation of BRCA1 or BRCA2 (52).Based on this study, Olaparib has possible as therapeutic agent in type II ovarian cancer.

3.1. Molecular biology of ovarian cancer

Ovarian cancer is a heterogenous disease and thus, there is no clear molecular genetics involved in the transition of normal ovarian epithelial cells into cancer cells. Approximately 10 to 15% of ovarian cancer is thought to run in the families (53). It is closely related to BRCA1 and BRCA2 mutation (53). It was recently published that suggested screening of BRCA1/2 mutation in patients with ovarian cancer prior to chemotherapy treatment (54). This is because presence of such mutations may influence the treatment outcomes (54). Human DNA repair mismatch genes for example MLH1 and MSH2 accounts for 10% of patients with hereditary nonpolyposis colon cancer syndrome (55). Other related genes include glutathione S-transferase M1 (GSTM1) is associated with endometrioid or clear cells ovarian cancer.

Approximately 85% of ovarian cancer is regard as sporadic with no apparent hereditary factors. Accumulation of mutagenic genes and deregulation of signaling pathway frequently lead to the development of cancer. Different subtypes of ovarian cancer reveal different molecular pathways. Coagulation pathway was reported to be disturbed in clear cell ovarian carcinoma (56). Genes that stimulate or inhibit coagulation were noted to be dysregulated. Angiogenesis and glycolysis are two major activated pathways in clear cell ovarian carcinoma (56). Vascular endothelial growth factor (VEGF) and its receptor FLT1 were upregulated in this type of cancer and involved in angiogenesis. Earlier study by Yamaguchi et al 2010, reported molecular pathway related to clear cell ovarian cancer was related to hypoxia-inducible factor 1 (HIF1α) (57). HIF1α regulates ADM, which is related to angiogenesis. It also regulates genes that are linked to glucose metabolism including SLC2A1 in glucose transport and HK1/HK2 and ENO1/ENO2 in glycolysis. Both pathways could act as potential therapeutic target based on the small interfering RNA of genes related to these pathways combined with antiangiogenic drug, Sunitinib(56).

3.2. Gene expression profiling in ovarian cancer

In ovarian cancer study, microarray was used to classify 113 samples from five different histopathological subtypes; endometrioid, serous, mucinous, clear cell and mixed type according to the gene expression pattern (58). The results showed 95% of all samples were clustered within their expected groups. Gene expression profile in this study failed to distinguish between high-grade endometrioid and serous ovarian cancer. The result derived from the principal component analysis demonstrated the separation of celar cell, mucinous and endometrioid with serous ovarian cancer. This can be explained through the origin of these types of cancer, which is Mullerian epithelium. In contrast to serous ovarian cancer, which most likely arise directly from ovarian surface epithelium (58). Microarray was also used to distinguish between various grades of clear cells ovarian cancer from other subtypes of ovarian cancer including serous papillary (59). Among genes identified were E-cadherin and osteonidogen were detected at high level in clear cells. While discoidin domain receptor family member (DDR1), estrogen receptor 1 and cytochrome P450 4B1 were at a low level in clear cells ovarian cancer compared to other ovarian cancers (59).

A separate microarray study was done on 285 of various grades of endometrioid and serous ovarian cancer samples that were analysed together with low-grade serous and endometroid ovarian cancer (60). The result showed high-grade serous subtype was related to overexpression of Wnt/βcatenin and cadherin pathway genes including N-cadherin and P-cadherin but low E-cadherin protein expression. This finding demonstrated the high-grade serous ovarian cancer contained messenchymal expression pattern. Also it has suggested there is epithelium-mesenchymal transition in this subtype of ovarian cancer. High expression of genes related to proliferation and extracellular matrix-related genes such as COL4A5, COL9A1 and CLDN6. Immune cell markers such as CD45, PTPRC and lymphocyte markers, CD2, CD3D and CD8A were expressed low in the high-grade serous subtype (60).

Gene expression profiling was also performed to detect genes that were differentially expressed in primary ovarian cells as compared to the neighboring metastatic tissue omentum (61). Among significant genes include hepsin (HPN), which is related to epithelial cells. Using immunohistochemistry technique, HPN protein was localised in epithelial cells, suggestive that it can be a marker of epithelia cells and not cancer (61). In advanced stage of ovarian cancer, predictive markers were suggested to be different. For example EZH2, PTTN and Lamin-B, were positively detected in primary as well as metastatic omental tissue. MGB2 is another biomarker that significantly overexpressed in primary as well as ovarian metastatic tissue. To characterize two different cancers; breast and ovarian cancers that involve serosal cavities, gene expression profiling was carried out (62). About 288 differentially expressed genes with at least 3.5-fold up-regulated in breast and ovarian/peritoneal serous cancers (62). These groups of genes may potentially used to distinguish both cancers for better therapeutic intervention.

Microarray of the nonepithelial ovarian cancer or type II ovarian cancer is still limited. Despite its rare incidence of this subtype of ovarian cancer, we have performed microarray assay on the formalin-fixed paraffin embedded tissues (63). About 804 differentially expressed genes with at least 2-fold change ($P<0.005$) (63). Among the significant genes were EEF1A2 and E2F2; which were up-regulated in nonepithelial ovarian cancer as compared to the normal ovarian cells. EEF1A2 may act as oncogene and play an important role in the progression of cancer (64). E2F2 plays a role in cell cycle and positive immunostaining in all subtypes of nonepithelial ovarian cancer may suggest its role as an oncogene (63).

4. Molecular signatures in endometrial cancer

Cancer of endometrium is cancer arises from the inner lining of the uterus. The cancer appears in multiple histologic subtypes as a result of műllerian differentiation. They are divided into two broad groups that include endometrioid and non-endometrioid (65). The recent surgical staging of endometrial cancer is based on the International Federation of Gynecology and Obstetrics in 2008 (66). Endometrial cancer is divided into two types based on the underlying pathogical findings and clinical observations. There are endometrioid (type I) and nonendometrioid carcinoma (type II). The former is the commonest type (85% of total cancer) with history of estrogen exposure with underlying endometrial hyperplasia (67).Also the cancer cells expressed estrogen and progesterone receptor and typically of low histopathological grade (68). The majority of patients are relatively young with good prognosis. While the second type is less common and it is not related to estrogen. It presents with high histopathological grade with poor prognosis. The cancer has an underlying atrophic endometrium (69). Apart from this classification, there are still cancers that do not fit into these two categories, in particular endometrioid carcinoma with high histopathological grade (67).

Endometrial cancer is the most common malignancy of gynecological tract in the United States (44). The incidence is relatively high compared with Southeast countries such as

Malaysia where the cancer affects approximately 3.3% of women between the year 2003 to 2005 (70) and the figure increases to 4.6% in 2007 (45) . Among the main races in Malaysia, Chinese has the highest age-standardized incidence rate with 4.5 per 100,000 population, followed by Indians and Malays (45). Failure to control overweight problem, manage chronic anovulation and increased usage of estrogen, are most likely the reason for continued high incidence for this cancer.

Risk factors associated with endometrioid endometrial cancer include old age, unoppossed exposure of estrogen as in estrogen replacement therapy, nulliparity and obesity. Also it is seen in diseases associated with high estrogen level, such as polycystic ovarian syndrome and estrogen-secreting ovarian cancer (71). Presence of estrogen increases the proliferative activity of endometrial cells, therefore causing higher chance to cause coding errors and somatic mutations (72). For nonendometrioid type, the risk factors are slightly different, which include additional history of primary cancers such as breast, colorectal and ovarian cancer (73). Combined oral contraceptives can interruptwith the menstrual cycle seems to have good benefits in reducing the risk of endometrial cancer (74). The current treatment for the disease is a combination of surgery with or without an adjuvant chemotherapy consisting of intravenous cisplatin, doxorubicin and cyclophosphamide (75). Diagnosis of this cancer is based on the clinical symptoms with underlying risk factors for endometrial cancer. Postmenopausal women under 50 years old presented with vaginal bleeding were reported to be free from endometrial cancer (76). This was based on the initial screening using transvaginal ultrasound scanning and endometrial biopsy procedure. The patients were follow-up between one to five years (76).

4.1. Molecular basis of endometrial cancer

Endometrial cancer can be divided based on its molecular change. Type 1 or endometrioid endometrial cancer was documented to have PTEN mutation(67).However, a recentcase control study investigating on the single nucleotide polymorphism in several cancer-related genes include PTEN, PIK3CA, AKT1, MLH1 and MSH2 failed to show any association with endometrial cancer (77).Approximately 20 to 40% of this type displayed mircosatellite instability or β-catenin mutations. Additionally, K-ras mutations occur in 15 to 30% of this cancer. Mutations in p53 and E-cadherin were detected in about 10 to 20% of cases and the lowest percentage of genetic alteration is in p16 inactivation. The genetic pattern in type II or nonendometrioid endometrial cancer is slightly different from the endometrioid type. This small percentage tumour comes from mesenchymal cells.The majority of this cancer (80 to 90%) has p53 mutations or E-cadherin alterations (78, 79). The type of cancer rarely contains mircosatellite instability, β-catenin or K-ras mutations (67).Sporadic endometrial cancer with positive microsatellite instability (MIN) was not associated with somatic mutations of mismatch repair genes such as MSH2 and MLH1 (80). Poor association was also observed between positive MIN with mutations in genes with coding region microsatellites repeats (80).

Genetic alterations	Endometrioid or type I	Nonendometrioid or type II
Microsatellite instability	20 - 40%	0 – 5%
K-ras mutations	15 - 30%	0 – 5%
p53 mutations	10 – 20%	90%
PTEN inactivation	35 – 50%	10%
β-catenin mutations	25 – 40 %	0 – 5%
p16 inactivations	10%	40%
E-cadherin alterations	10 – 20%	80 – 90%

Table 2. Molecular changes in both subtypes of endometrial cancer (67)

4.2. Molecular carcinogenesis of endometrial cancer

Endometrial cancer cells has the ability to proliferate without control or able to spread throughout the body following multistep processes.

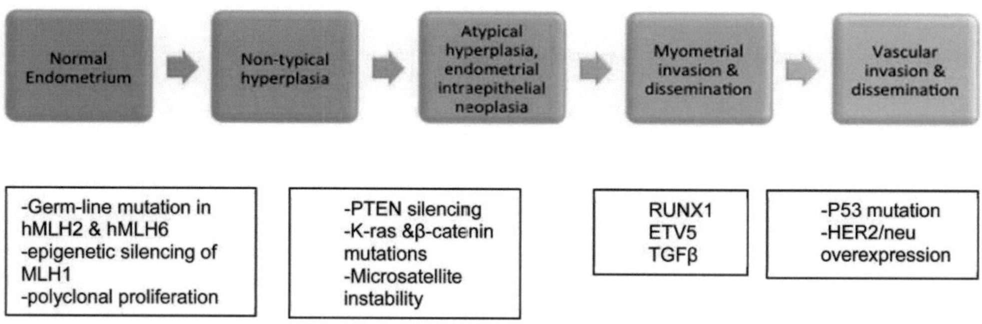

Figure 1. Figure 1: A model of endometrial cancer development. The genetic alterations at the early stage are different from the late stage of endometrial cancer (72).

4.3. Gene expression profiling in endometrial cancer

Earlier studies on the microarray in endometrial cancer tried to discriminate between different histologic types of endometrial cancer using the genomic expression profiling (81). The study analysed 119 endometrial cancer consisted of endometrioid, papillary serous, mixed mullerian tumor and normal cells. The result showed 151 genes that were significantly expressed with at least 2-fold change among endometrioid as compared to papillary serous cancer (P<0.001). Among the genes detected were BUB1, CCNB2 and Myc) (81). Comparing between mixed mullerian tumors and endometrioid revealed 1,132 genes that were significantly different with at least 2-fold change (81). High expression of IGF2 (somatomedin A) was reported in mixed mullerian tumor as compared to endometrioid and papillary serous tumour (81). Our local data showed low expression of IGF2 in endometrioid endometrial cancer compared with normal endometrium (82). Low expression of IGF2 was corresponds to an early stage of endometrial cancer (83). All reported results from these expression profiling studies have concluded that different histologic types of endometrial cancer displayed different expression profiles.

The use of microarray when combined with laser capture microdissection (LCM) tissues has presented reliable results (84). However, the decision whether to use the LCM technique is still relied on the ratio of stromal cells to the surrounding cancer cells. Pathways that are closely related to endometrial cancer were identified after isolation of microdissected cancerous cells was used (82). Among the significant pathways comprise of Wnt-β catenin, insulin action, cell cycle and NOTCH and B-cell pathways (82). The malignant potential of endometrial cancer cells was studied to identify gene signatures of vascular invasion (85). Total of 18-gene signatures were differentially expressed with at least fold change of 2. Among the genes were IL8, MMP3, COL8A1 and ANGPTL4, which were closely related to invasiveness, vascular biology and matrix remodelling (85). Microarray was also used to discrimate between different genetic backgrounds. As an example, molecular profiling was used to differentiate between self-described African-American with self-described Caucasian women (86). The result failed to differentiate the racial group using molecular background. This was probably due to limited sample size to represent the whole population.

5. Molecular signatures in breast cancer

Breast cancer is the most frequent cancer in women in most parts of the world (87). Approximately 1.1 million of women in the world were diagnosed with breast cancer every year and 410,100 died from the disease. Breast cancer can be divided into two main types; ductal carcinoma and lobularcarcinoma (88). The most common type is ductal carcinoma, which starts in the tubes or ducts that move milk from the breast to the nipple. Lobular carcinoma originates from lobules in the breast that produce milk. Breast cancer could become invasive where the cancerous cells may acquire the properties to escape from its primary sites into other tissues in the breast. Noninvasive or also known as 'in situ' indicates that the cancerous cells have not yet invaded other tissues within the breast. There are several grading systems used to classify breast cancer, which include histopathology, grade, stage and receptor status (89). Breast cancer staging uses TNM system, which is based on the size, the spreading and metastatic properties of the tumor to the other organs. There are 3 receptors on the surface as well as in the cytoplasm and nucleus of the breast cancer cells (90). The receptors are estrogen receptor (ER), progesteron receptor (PR) and HER2 receptor (90). Immunohistochemistry technique may be employed to differentiate whether the tumor has positive or negative ER, PR and HER2 receptors (90).

Risk factors of getting breast cancer in women include age and gender. The risk of getting breast cancer is increased in elderly (88). Women are 100 times more likely to get breast cancer compared to men. Genetic factors may also play a role in the development of breast cancer, although it is estimated that only 5-6% of breast cancer are hereditary (91). Mutations in the BRCA1 and BRCA2 genes account for 80% of hereditary breast cancer (92). Patient's positive for BRCA1 and/or BRCA2 may have 50% to 80% lifetime risk of developing breast cancer and 15% to 65% risk of developing ovarian cancer (92, 93). Other risk factors are high-fat-diet, alcohol intake, environmental factors such as tobacco smoking and radiation (94).

The diagnosis of breast cancer is based on the microscopic analysis of breast biopsy, mammography and clinical breast exam (95). However, if the test is inconclusive, then Fine Needle Aspiration and Cytology (FNAC) may be used (96).Stage 1 breast cancer is treated with lumpectomy to remove a small part in the breast and usually have high prognosis. Stage 2 and 3 cancers are treated with lumpectomy or mastectomy, chemotherapy and radiation and usually have poor prognosis and high risk of recurrence. Stage 4 has poor prognosis and is treated by various combination of all treatments. Drugs used to treat breast cancer include hormone-blocking therapy for ER+ patients (tamoxifen, aromatase inhibitors), chemotherapy (cyclophosphamide and doxorubicin) and monoclonal antibodies (trastuzumab) for HER2+ breast patients (97).

5.1. Genome wide association study (GWAS) in breast cancer

A single nucleotide polymorphism (rs2046210, A/G allele) at 6q25.1 was identified in Chinese women. In a pooled analysis study performed in the East Asian, European, and African ancestries, this variant was also found to be associated with breast cancer risk in Chinese women (OR=1.3), Japanese women (OR=1.31), European (OR=1.07), and American women (OR=1.18) (98). However, there was no association observed in African American women (OR=0.81). This variant was found to be associated with increased breast cancer risk in all Chinese in Tianjin, Nanjing, Taiwan and Hong Kong. This was also in agreement with three studies conducted in Japanese women (Nagoya, MEC and Nagano) as well as studies performed in European women (NBHS, CBCS and LIBCSP). A putative functional variant, rs6913578 was identified at 1,440 downstream of rs2046210, which was associated with breast cancer risk in Chinese (r^2=0.91) and European ancestry (r^2=0.83), but not in Africans (r^2=0.57). Genes located at rs2046210 are *PLEKHG1, MTHFD1L, AKAP12, ZBTB2, RMND1, C6Orf211, C6orf97, ESR1, C6orf98, SYNE1* and *NANOGP11. In vitro* functional analysis on rs6913578 altered luciferase reporter activity hence may influence the DNA binding protein interactions, which subsequently lead to alteration of their neighboring genes expression. Electrophoretic mobility shift assay confirmed that the C allele of rs6913578 alter the DNA-nuclear protein interaction and could modify the expression of neighboring genes.

There was an association between an increased breast cancer risk with rs9397435 at the 6q25.1 locus in European, Chinese and African populations. This variant was located at 2,854 bp downstream of rs2046210 and 1,414 downstream of rs6913578. However, this variant was weakly correlated with rs2046210 in Europeans (r^2=0.087) and African (r^2=0.039) (99). Turnbull and colleagues conducted a GWAS in 3,659 European ancestry cases and 4,897 controls. They found that SNP rs3757318, which was located at 200kb upstream of ESR1 and 34,253bp of upstream of rs2046210 has the most significant association with breast cancer risk (OR=1.21). It was strongly correlated with rs2046210 in Chinese populations (r^2=0.48) but weakly correlated in Europeans (r^2=0.181) (100).

In Ashkenazi Jews population, Gold and colleagues performed three phases of GWAS in 249 familial breast cancer cases and 299 controls. In the first phase, they compared the allele frequencies of 150,080 SNPs in 249 high-risk, BRCA1-BRCA2 mutation-negative AJ familial cases with control cases. In phase II, 343 SNPs were genotyped from 123 regions, which were most significantly associated with breast cancer including 4 SNPs in *FGFR2* region in other sets of 950 consecutive breast cancer cases. Major associations were replicated in third independent set of 243 breast cancer cases and 187 controls. The results showed a significant association at rs1078806 in the *FGFR2* region of chromosome 6q22.33 with OD=1.26 for all cases combined. Candidate genes in this locus such as *ECHDC1* and *RNF146*, which encode for mitochondrial fatty acid oxidation and ubiquitin protein ligase were among the known pathways in the pathogenesis of breast cancer (101). It is well known that results reported from GWAS could not be applied across all ethnicities. This is not surprising since most all variants are tagging SNPs, therefore they exist differently in the genetic make-up of different ethnic groups. Hence, it is important to determine the SNPs in breast cancer or any particular diseases in different populations to identify the risk of developing the disease in an individual.

5.2. Gene expression profiling in breast cancer

A research done to study bimodal gene expression profiles in breast cancer using 5 studies that used different microarray platforms including cDNA arrays, Affymetrix and Agilent (102). Bimodality is a conditional expression property of a particular gene and is associated with certain physiological conditions such as disease state and normal. They found 866 bimodal genes shared across all platforms. These genes were enriched in breast cancer-associated genes and involved in pathways related to carcinogenesis for example: *ERBB2, ESR1, CEACAM5* and *AR*. They also examined the close neighbor group and the analysis showed that 15 out of 23 bimodal genes were known and have been reported as breast cancer associated genes. These include *TCAP, PSMD3, GRB7 and CXCL10* (PMC2822536).

Microarray was also used to classify the differential gene expression in ER+ve and ER-ve breast cancer patients. A study showed that 67 genes were overexpressed in ER+ve tumors while 17 were overexpressed in ER-ve breast cancer. *ADCY1, ACOT4 AR, ATP2A3, DNAJA4* were examples of genes that overexpressed in ER+ve breast cancer. An example of genes that were overexpressed in ER –ve were *ACN9, EGFR, LYN* and *MALL* (103).

Gene expression profiling of tumor-associated stroma in breast cancer showed large changes during cancer progression (104). In this study, laser capture microdissection was used to dissect the normal epithelium, stroma, tumor epithelium and tumor-associated stroma samples followed by microarray and gene ontology analyses. Tumor-associated stroma undergoes massive changes in the expression profile of genes composed of the extracellular matrix, matrix metalloproteases and cell cycle-related protein. An increased in the mitochondrial ribosomal proteins and decreased in cytoplasmic ribosomal proteins were also observed in both, the tumor epithelium and stroma. The changes in expression profiles of the tumor-associated stroma were somewhat similar to tumor epithelium, which indicated that the tumorigenesis occured even before the tumor cells invaded into the stroma.

Gene expression profiling using whole genome oligonucleotide microarrays to catalog molecular variation in 52 widely used breast cancer cell lines. The cell lines were divided into different categories including luminal with ER positive, basal and ER-ve, which subdivided into basal A (established at UT Southwestern including 2 BRCA1 mutant lines) and basal B (non-tumorigenic lines and several highly invasive cell lines). They identified 80 loci of high level of amplification in 35 different cell lines. These include increased expression of known oncogenes involved in breast cancer, for example *MYC* (8q24), *CCND1* (11q13) and *ERBB2* (17q12). Gain or losses resulting in increased or decreased expression of oncogenes or tumor supressor genes, which subsequently led to breast cancer. Using DR-Correlate, 3,511 genes were differentially expressed and correlated significantly with altered gene copy number (FDR<0.05). In total, 487 genes were resided in loci of high-amplitude CNA including known breast cancer genes such as *EGFR, FGFR1, ERBB2, PPMID* and *ZNF217*. In addition, several genes involved in oncogenesis such as cell proliferation, survival, migration/invasion, ER-signaling, maintenance of genome integrity were also upregulated in cancer cell lines. These include *E1F3H, CDC6, GAB2* (cell proliferation), *MCL1, APIP, MAP3K3* (survival), *ADAM9, CDD4* (migration/invasion), *MUC1, NCOA3* (ER-signaling), *RAD21, RAD9A* and *RAD51C* (maintanence of genome integrity) (105).

Gene expression profiling study was carried out on peripheral blood cells for an early detection of breast cancer in 121 females referred for mammography. Genome Survey Microarrays v2.0 that contains 32,878 probes representing 29,098 genes was used to determine the differentially expressed genes in breast cancer compared to normal. Genes that expressed higher in blood of breast cancer patients were *EEF1G, RPL14, RPLL15* (translation), *ATP5E, ETF1, ATP6V0B* (cellular biosynthetic process), *TIRAP, DEFA3* and *ANXA1* (response to external stimulus). Several genes involved in cellular lipid metabolic process, steroid metabolic process, catecholamine metabolic process and phenole metabolic processes were downregulated in breast cancer compared to normal control. These include *HDC, PEMT, HEXA, ACAT* and *SULT1A4* (106).

6. From lab to bedside: FDA approval

Advances in genomic research resulting in new molecular tools that serves as prognostic and predictive markers in cancer treatment. Particularly in breast cancer, surgeons know that early detection is one of the keys to successful treatment. If breast cancer is caught early, the tumor can be surgically removed and with an appropriate treatment, most patients can recover. However, within 5 to 10 years, 30% increase number of patients with early stage breast cancer develops metastases. The identification of patients with high risk of distant recurrence is essential for systematic adjuvant therapy to be most effective. At the same time, adjuvant therapies such as chemotherapy and hormonal therapy (e.g. Tamoxifen or aromatase inhibitors) may reduce the risk of distant metastases by approximately one-third for some patients. It is estimated that more than 70% of patients receiving such therapy may have survived without it –and may have safely avoided the harmful side effects (107-109).

Commercially available multigene molecular tests such as Oncotype DX® (Genomic Health, USA) and MammaPrint® (Agendia, Netherlands) have revolutionized the predictive and prognostic tools in clinic. Using the patients' own genetic expression patterns, it can provide clinicians with more information on the treatment outcomes of using chemotherapy, endocrine therapy or combination therapies by stratifying the risk of recurrence for patients. Oncotype DX® and MammaPrint® provide clinical judgment as opposed to laboratory results that requireinterpretation by a clinician. Moreover, the algorithm used to reach this judgment is proprietary and thus inaccessible to the clinician. Therefore the arrival of the first generation of multigene molecular test involved a need for a paradigm shift in the configurations of persons and tools that marry genomic techniques to market, legal, and regulatory strategies in ways that reframe conceptions of risk, diagnosis, prognosis, therapy, discovery, utility, and validity. In addition, regulatory bodies need to handle these new advances without sacrificing patient's safety. These first generation multigene molecular tests are considered the first regulatory-scientific hybrid products (110).

The Oncotype DX® is a multigene panel which has been clinically validated to predict the risk of recurrence for those women with early stage (I, II, IIIa) invasive breast cancer that are estrogen-receptor positive (ER^+), human epidermal growth factor receptor negative ($Her2^-$), lymph node negative or positive, and predict who may or may not significantly benefit from adjuvant chemotherapy. While MammaPrint® analyzes 70 genes from an early-stage breast cancer tissue sample to determine if the cancer has a low or high risk of recurrence within 10 years after diagnosis. They claimed to be the first and only FDA-cleared IVDMIA breast cancer recurrence assay in their official website, http://www.agendia.com/pages/mammaprint/21.php (110). The researchers at the Netherlands Cancer Institute (NKI) who discovered it, established a company to commercialize it as a test (111). Oncotype DXbegan as a commercial platform; the company (Genomics Health) that produced it did not discover a signature but rather constructed it by asking users at every step what clinical question they wanted the signature to answer and what data would be credible in that regard. The test has been designed to minimally disrupt existing clinical workflows (110, 112). MammaPrint requires a change in pathologists' and clinicians' routines in terms of specimen storage. MammaPrint requires specimen to be stored in RNARetain®, a proprietary RNA storage liquid instead of the standard FFPE block. Breast cancer classification was based on genomic signature instead of histopathology diagnosis as well as clinical judgement on the decision for chemotherapy treatment (113). Thus, while these two trials signify a new departure for clinical cancer trials on a number of levels – they both incorporate new models of interaction between biotech companies and public research. They also aim to establish the clinical relevance of genomic markers and also embody a different socio-technical direction. One attempts to accommodate established routines, while the other openly challenges prevailing evidential hierarchies and existing biomedical configurations (110).

The legal statute of the USA gives the US Food and Drug Administration (FDA) the power to regulate drugs and devices, with the multigene molecular tests fall under the less rigorous medical devices statute. The FDA has traditionally exercised 'enforcement discretion' by leaving the actual performance of 'in-house' tests to be regulated by a different mechanism defined by the Clinical Laboratory Improvement Amendments (CLIA). It is a set of federal regulatory standards that falls under the authority of the Centers for Medicare and Medicaid Services (114). The intention was to ensure the reliability and accuracy of clinical laboratory testing. FDA regulators have suggested the development of translational medicine tests such as Oncotype DXand MammaPrint might constitute an entirely new regulatory category. In 2006 and 2007, the FDA published two versions of 'Draft Guidance', signaling the Agency's inclination to step in and take direct responsibility for the novel test category. In 2007, MammaPrint was submitted to the FDA and successfully obtained FDA clearance after only 30 days. An 'FDA cleared' button promptly appeared on all commercial MammaPrint material (http://www.agendia.com/pages/mammaprint/ 21.php). Given the non-binding nature of the FDA draft guidance, Genomic Health chose not to pursue this regulatory route. Instead they try to gain 'official' recognition from the clinicians via inclusion in the clinical practice guidelines of professional oncology organizations. The company viewed the pursuit of FDA clearance as much more costly and time-consuming than simply lobbying professional organizations of clinicians – many of whom the founders already knew through their previous works at Genentech (110). The American Society of Clinical Oncology (ASCO) included Onco*type* in its 2007 guidelines and the US National Comprehensive Cancer Network (NCCN) followed suit in its 2008 guidelines.

6.1. Study design of the multigenes panel

In cancer epidemiology, both retrospective case – control studies and prospective cohort studies are observational, rather than experimental, studies. Neither type of study involves random assignment of exposure hence; observed associations between exposures and disease do not provide as strong a basis for claims of causality as in experimental studies. The most serious limitation of epidemiological studies is their non-experimental nature, not whether they are retrospective or prospective. In therapeutics, many retrospective analyses are also non-experimental, with treatment selection based on patient factors and referral pattern rather than on randomization. Such studies are also often conducted without a written protocol and are unfocused, with numerous patient subsets and endpoints compared without control for the overall chance of a false-positive conclusion. In contrast, prospective randomized clinical trials contain internal control of treatment assignment, careful and proscribed data collection (including outcomes and endpoints), and a focused analysis plan that is developed before the data are examined (112).

Many biomarker studies are conducted with convenience samples of specimens, which just happen to be available and are assayed for the marker. They have not prospectively determined subject eligibility, power calculations, marker cut-point specification, or analytical plans. Such studies are more likely resulting in highly biased conclusions and truly deserved to be pejoratively labeled as "retrospective." However, if a "retrospective" study is designed to use archived specimens from a previously conducted prospective trial, and if certain conditions are prospectively delineated in a written protocol before the marker study is performed, it might be considered as a "prospective – retrospective" study. Such a study should carry considerably more weight toward determination of clinical utility of the marker than a simple study of convenience, in which specimens and assays were happened to be available. Multiple studies of different candidate biomarkers based on archived tissues from the same prospective trial would present a greater opportunity for false-positive conclusions than a single fully prospective trial focused on a specific biomarker. Consequently, independent confirmation of findings for specific biomarkers in multiple prospective – retrospective study (115).

6.2. Oncotype DX breast cancer assay

The Oncotype DX® analyzes the expression of 21 genes (16 cancer-related and 5 reference genes) within a tumor to determine a recurrence score (RS) using reverse transcription PCR (RT-PCR) in formalin-fixed, paraffin-embedded (FFPE) breast cancer tissue samples. In the earlier stage, the researchers has to show that RNA extracted from FFPE tissues could match fresh tissue results in terms of producing a high concordance in the RT-PCR results (116, 117).To interpret the result, Oncotype DX test results assign a Recurrence Score (RS) – a number between 0 and 100 – to the early-stage breast cancer or DCIS as stated below:

- RS lower than 18: The cancer or DCIS has a low risk of recurrence. The benefit of chemotherapy for early-stage breast cancer or radiation therapy for DCIS is likely to be small and will not outweigh the risks of side effects.
- RS between 18 and 31: The cancer or DCIS has an intermediate risk of recurrence. It's unclear whether the benefits of chemotherapy for early-stage breast cancer or radiation therapy for DCIS outweigh the risks of side effects.
- RS greater than 31: The cancer or DCIS has a high risk of recurrence, and the benefits of chemotherapy for early-stage breast cancer or radiation therapy for DCIS are likely to be greater than the risks of side effects.

The RS corresponds to a specific likelihood of breast cancer recurrence within 10 years of the initial diagnosis, as well as response to adjuvant treatment. Using recurrence score, it may be possible for healthcare providers and patients to determine whether adjuvant chemotherapy is needed following primary therapy for breast cancer (118, 119).

i. **NSABP Study B-14**

The Oncotype *DX* was developed and clinically validated on the basis of a retrospective analysis of the existing material from two randomized clinical trials (NSABP-B-20 and NSABP-B-14). The signature is based on the expression of genes that are associated with proliferation, ER signaling, HER2, and invasion (118). The 21 multigene chosen were always at the top of the list in published literature. The developers used the samples from 447 patients as the 'discovery' or 'training' set to select the 21 genes eventually included in the Onco*type* test. Company researchers then applied an algorithm to the results of the tests and developed the aforementioned RS score. They believe the score is one of the strengths of the Onco*type* test: as a single number on a continuous 0–100 scale and not a category (that is, yes/no, good/poor). It is supposed to provide clinicians with 'useful' information as a basis on which to act, while preserving clinical decision-making as a clinician's prerogative, since by not providing a categorical answer it does not entail a specific intervention (110). Results from this study demonstrated that Onco*type DX* is an accurate and reliable predictor of breast cancer recurrence. (120). The study also concluded that the RS has been validated as quantifying the likelihood of distant recurrence in tamoxifen-treated patients with node-negative, estrogen receptor-positive breast cancer (118).

ii. NSABP Study B-20

About 668 samples of cancer tissue from a clinical trial called NSABP B-20 ("A Clinical Trial to Assess Tamoxifen in Patients with Primary Breast Cancer and Negative Axillary Nodes Whose Tumors Are Positive for Estrogen Receptors) were used to show that Onco*type DX* can predict chemotherapy benefit (119). The study concluded that the RS of the assay not only quantifies the likelihood of breast cancer recurrence in women with node-negative, estrogen receptor-positive breast cancer, but also predicts the magnitude of chemotherapy benefit (118).

iii. Kaiser Permanente study

A large clinical study of 234 cases and 631 controls available for pathology studies (after screening of 4964 patients) conducted by Kaiser Permanente confirmed in a community setting that Onco*type DX* helps to predict the likelihood of breast cancer survival at 10 years (121). The primary objective of this study was to determine whether the proportion of patients who were free of a distant recurrence for more than 10 years after surgery was significantly greater in the low-risk group than in the high-risk group. The second primary objective was to determine whether there was a statistically significant relation between the RS and the risk of distant recurrence. The cutoff points were prespecified to classify patients into the following categories: low risk, intermediate risk and high risk. The cutoff points were chosen on the basis of the results of NSABP trial B-20. The study concluded that in a large, population-based study of lymph node-negative patients not treated with chemotherapy, the RS value was strongly associated with risk of breast cancer death among ER-positive, tamoxifen-treated and -untreated patients.

iv. SWOG 8814 study

SWOG-8814 was a randomized phase III clinical trial of 1,477 postmenopausal women, all of whom had estrogen receptor-positive (ER+) breast cancer that had spread to the axillary lymph nodes. All women in the trial got daily tamoxifen for up to five years, longer than the standard therapy for treating ER+ breast cancer. One arm of 361 patients got only tamoxifen. The rest got tamoxifen plus a three-drug chemotherapy regimen of cyclophosphamide, Adriamycin®, and 5-fluorouracil, a combination known as CAF. Investigators retrospectively analyzed tumor specimens from this trial using the Oncotype *DX*® in 367 women with ER-positive, mainly tamoxifen-treated lymph node-positive, the RS assay quantified the likelihood of breast cancer recurrence and also predicted the magnitude of chemotherapy benefit (122).

v. Oncotype DX TAILORx Trial

Following the development of the specialized translational research program from National Cancer Institute (NCI), the Program for the Assessment of Clinical Cancer

Tests (PACCT) launched the TAILORx trial (123).Since the validation of the Oncotype DX Breast Cancer Assay Recurrence Score were able to clearly show that the multigene panel were able to predict chemotherapy with hormonal treatment benefit for patients with high Recurrence Score while patients with low Recurrence Score do not benefit from chemotherapy. However as high as 37% of patients fall into the intermediate range, which do not show a clear outcome of the benefit of chemotherapy (122). A randomized prospective clinical trial is currently ongoing to further validate a group of node-negative, ER+ breast cancer patients with a RS in the intermediate range, which is known as **T**rial **A**ssigning **I**ndividua**L**ized **O**ptions for Treatment (**Rx**) TAILORx conducted by the North American Breast Cancer Group (http://www.cancer.gov/clinicaltrials/noteworthy-trials/tailorx). Since 2006, the trial enrolled 10,000 patients (of which 4500 were to be in the randomized arm) in 900 participating centers (110). Patients with mid-range RS will be randomized for chemotherapy while patients with low and high RS will not be randomized as the outcome has been clearly defined in previous studies.

6.3. Recommendation of use as tumor marker

Because Oncotype *DX* was able to achieve level II evidence to support it's prognostic role, Oncotype DX has received approval from the American Society of Clinical Oncology (ASCO) in the2007 guidelines (124). It was included in the National Comprehensive Cancer Network (NCCN) 2008 guidelines (Breast Cancer version 1.2011 [http://www.nccn.org].) as an option to evaluate prognosis and as a complement to clinicopathological features to predict response to chemotherapy for patients with ER-positive, node-negative breast cancer. None of the microarray-based prognostic signatures has been endorsed by these professional bodies.

6.4. MammaPrint

MammaPrint (initially known as the 70 Gene Amsterdam Signature) was originally developed as an academic/scientific endeavor using whole genome microarray technology. The objective was to develop a gene expression signature that could accurately identify early stage breast cancer patients who were either at high risk or at low risk of recurrence and, therefore, enable more individualized treatment. The MammaPrint investigators from the NKI-AVL in collaboration with the Rosetta Inpharmatics (a Seattle company) procured and analyzed 78 tumors with the whole-genome microarray. Out of the 25,000 genes in the human genome, 231 genes were selected according to its association with the disease outcome. Further bioinformatic analysis using 2-D cluster analysis followed by a leave-one-out cross validation procedure produced 70 critical genes that were shown to correlate best with the likelihood of distant recurrence. These 70 genes affect all steps known to be important for metastasis including cell cycle regulation, angiogenesis, invasion, cell migration and signal transduction (111).The resulting 70-gene signature profile classifies tumors as either high risk or low risk of recurrence. If it is used in conjunction with other risk factors, it helps to identify patients who will benefit from the adjuvant therapy. The 70-

gene signature was constructed as a dichotomy as the discussions between the research team and clinicians, who insisted that the main goal of the test should be to avoid overtreatment of the disease. To accomplish this end, the low-risk group had to be defined inclusively. At the same time, the test developers felt that clinicians expected a clear answer (good/poor signature) from the test, hence the dichotomy (111). This position, once again, contrasts with the Genomic Health's decision to report their Oncotype DX data analysis as a continuous variable that leaves room for clinical judgment (110).

With this 70-gene signature, further validation was needed on a larger, independent patient population. The primary validation was thus carried out via another retrospective study that used samples from 295 patients held in the same NKI bio-bank. The first validation for the 70-gene signature was undertaken in a series of 295 consecutive women with breast cancer. The proportion of patients who remained free from distant metastases at ten years was 87% in the low-risk group and 44% in the high-risk group. The profile was a statistically independent predictor and added to the power of standard clinico-pathologic parameters (125). A research network team called TRANSBIG, an abbreviation for "Translating molecular knowledge into early breast cancer management: building on the BIG network for improved treatment tailoring", used the 70-gene signature as retrospective study in 2006 using 307 pa54tient samples from five European institutions. The results showed that the proportion of patients who remained free from distant metastases at 10 years was 90% in the low-risk group and 71% in the high-risk group. The 70-gene signature was found to provide prognostic information more than what could be determined from patient age, tumor grade, tumor size, and ER status in a population of lymph node negative patients without adjuvant chemotherapy (113). Although they initially favored licensing the technology, the NKI team found no viable taker. So, in 2003 the original researchers, in consultation with the NKI board of directors, established a spin-off company using private venture capital and European Union (EU) funding, and convinced the director of oncology at a leading diagnostic company, Agendia, for Amsterdam Genetic Diagnostics Amersham (110). The Agendia team had a signature but they did not have a test. In other words, it was not immediately obvious how to convert the 70-gene signature into what eventually became MammaPrint, a 'high-throughput diagnostic test' (126). The original signature had been developed using microarrays containing 25,000 oligonucleotides, a highly impractical platform for routine use. The company therefore developed a customized microarray containing a reduced set of probes, whose production was entrusted to Agilent, to whom Rosetta had, in the meantime, sold its technology.

The TRANSBIG Consortium performed another independent validation study of 302 adjuvantly untreated patients with at least ten years of follow-up. For the NKI researchers, the problem was less RNA extraction than the microarray analysis itself. Compared with RT-PCR, microarray analysis was a relatively novel, non-standardized technology and as such, it raised a number of logistic and statistical challenges (127, 128). As a result, in addition to the validation studies of the signature per se, researchers conducted a number of other studies to show that sample collection for the test (as distinct from the centrally performed test itself) was feasible and reproducible in community-based settings (129). Additional studies demonstrated that the MammaPrint classifies greater than 95% of ER-negative cancers as poor prognosis and there was a strong correlation between 70-gene signature-defined poor prognosis and high histological grade (130, 131). Furthermore, the studies demonstrated that the 70-gene signature would outperform the current methods based on clinicopathological parameters for chemotherapy use.

One study revealed that MammaPrint validates in older American breast cancer patients (132). While another study demonstrated that MammaPrint has strong prognostic value in patients with 1-3 positive lymph nodes (133). With more than 14,000 patient results reported to date, the technical robustness and reliability of MammaPrint is well established. MammaPrint is a considerable a step forward in the advancement of personalized cancer treatment. Several other prognostic signatures including the 76-gene signature (134, 135) and genomic grade index (136-139) were also shown to be independent predictors for the cancer outcomes.

i. **MicroarRAy PrognoSTics in Breast CancER (RASTER) study**

To evaluate whether the prognostic signature is suitable for the use in clinical practice, the MammaPrint was used to assess feasibility of implementation of the test as a diagnostic test in community hospitals in the Netherlands. The study aimed to test the effect of the signature on the use of adjuvant systemic treatment; proportion of patients with "poor" versus "good" prognosis in a series of unselected patients with node-negative breast cancer; and finally to examine the concordance between risk predicted by the prognosis signature and risk predicted by commonly used clinicopathological guidelines. The findings of this study show that implementation of the 70-gene prognosis signature as a diagnostic test is feasible in community hospitals in the Netherlands (129).

ii. **MINDACT Trials**

MammaPrint is currently being tested in the MINDACT (Microarray In Node-negative and 1-3 positive lymph-node Disease may Avoid ChemoTherapy) trial (140). This is to determine whether this signature can actually replace clinicopathological parameters for the identification of patients who could be spared from the use of chemotherapy. The more 'confrontational attitude' of the MINDACT leaders toward traditional clinico-pathological tools has resulted in a very different trial design compared to the Oncotype DX TAILORx Trial.In the MINDACT trial, women recruited into the trial are assigned to high- and low-risk categories using both standard clinical-pathological features and the 70-gene MammaPrint test results. An open-access computer program, Adjuvant! Online, developed in the US and widely used by breast cancer clinicians to estimate the outcome in terms of relapse and survival with or without chemotherapy. By confronting the predictions of MammaPrint and Adjuvant! Online, the trial directly compares between these two prognostic tools: women whose Adjuvant! Online and MammaPrint results are discordant (when clinical/pathological features indicate high risk of recurrence and when MammaPrint indicates low risk, or vice versa) are then randomized for chemotherapy.

6.5. Conclusion

Based on the recommendation by the Evaluation of Genomic Applications in Practice and Prevention (EGAPP) Working Group, the general consensus was that retrospective study of samples and data from prospective studies were insufficient, although these studies were superior to studies using 'convenience samples', such as those contained in a general-purpose bio-bank. However, potential for patient selection bias cannot be excluded (141), therefore the working group recommend prospective studies such as TAILORx and MINDACT as the gold standard for testing the value of a multigene molecular test such as Onco*type* or MammaPrint. From their review on these multigene molecular tests, they found insufficient evidence to make a recommendation for or against the use of tumor gene expression profiles to improve outcomes indefined populations of women with breast cancer. The working group found preliminary evidence on the potential benefit of the Oncotype *DX* testing results to some women who face decisions about treatment options (reduced adverse events due to low risk women avoiding chemotherapy) but could not rule out the potential harm for others (breast cancer recurrence that might have been prevented). The evidence is insufficient to assess the balance of benefits and harms of the proposed uses of the tests. The working group therefore encourages further development and evaluation of these technologies. There are still limitations that prevent these multigene molecular test such as the Oncotype *DX*, MammaPrint and other genomic prognostic markers from replacing the microscope for diagnosis, prognosis and treatment of an early breast cancer. However, additional important clinical information from this test has added to traditional histology and IHC determination of ER, PR and HER2 in terms of prognostic and predictive power.

7. Challenges associated with the clinical translation

Advances in laboratory and clinical science has propelled to a transitional period, which requires a redefinition of biology, genomics, and medicine in relation to one another. "Molecular gene signatures" is a new buzz word within the field of personalized medicine in the treatment of breast cancer (111, 118), thyroid cancer (142), endometrial cancer (143), ovarian cancer (144) and other cancers as well. However, the road from the scientific discovery of molecular signatures associated with cancer until it can be translated to clinical application is long and arduous. A recent review on the current status of translational research in cancer genetics has analyzed the extramural grant portfolio of the National Cancer Institute (NCI) from Fiscal Year of 2007. From the study, the funded grants and publications were classified as follows: T_0 as discovery research; T_1 as research to develop a candidate health application (e.g., test or therapy); T_2 as research that evaluates a candidate application and develops evidence-based recommendations; T_3 as research that assesses how to integrate an evidence-based recommendation into cancer care and prevention; and T_4 as research that assesses health outcomes and population impact (145). An "explosion" in gene expression research during the last few years has already led to the development of several genetic classifiers in the genomic discovery (T_0) stage and T_1 stage (which bridges discovery to candidate health application, or "bench to bedside"). However, less genomic research was conducted and published in T_2 and above, with only 1.8% of the grant portfolio and 0.6% of the published literatures in these categories. In addition to discovery research in cancer genetics, a translational research infrastructure is urgently needed to methodically evaluate and translate gene discoveries for cancer care and prevention (146, 147).

	POPULATION ONCOLOGY	TRANSITION	PERSONALIZED ONCOLOGY
Screening	Population-wide risk reduction	Population-wide approaches modified for at-risk subpopulations	Individualized risk estimation and programs adapted to individual risk
Diagnosis	Organ-of-origin-/histology-based	Organ of origin, histology, and some molecular markers	Primarily molecular marker-based
Staging	Anatomic extent of disease	Anatomic extent with some molecular risk profiling	Primarily molecular risk-based
Treatment determination	Typically organ-of-origin- and stage-based	Organ-of-origin- and stage-based with some implementation of molecular markers	Primarily molecular marker-based
Assessment intervals	Based on clinical evaluation/ examination findings	Based on routine interval imaging	Early, frequent serial assessments by imaging, circulating tumor cells, and other marker assessments
Early phase clinical trials	Oriented to maximum tolerated dose	Oriented to "optimum biologic dose"	Determine range of tolerable and active doses
Mid-phase clinical trials	Histology and prior treatment-based eligibility; typically single-arm, noncomparator trials	Histology and prior treatment-based eligibility; some marker-based screening; some randomized controlled trials	Some trials, histology, and prior treatment-based eligibility with rapid, serial assessments; many with eligibility restricted to tumor marker subsets

Table 3. Systemic therapy options for the treatment of invasive breast cancer in the adjuvant and advanced disease settings. Among solid tumors, breast cancer treatment arguably has made some of the greatest advances during the previous 3 decades (148). Advances in laboratories and clinical science have propelled us into the current transitional period and how clinical trials must evolve to lead us into the era of personalized oncology (148)

7.1. Challenges of gene expression profiling studies

In order to understand challenges associated with the clinical translation of molecular gene signature obtained from microarray studies, we must understand the challenges and limitations of gene expression profiling. Although gene expression profiling seems to have value in the discovery of molecular markers for potential use in diagnosis or as a therapeutic target, translating this technology into genomic medicine is still a work in progress. For a better understanding in terms of strengths and limitations of gene expression profiling techniques, we need to understand biological, technological, statistical, and informatics challenges and caveats.

7.2. Biological challenges

A microarray experiment presents a snapshot of the gene expression of the biological system that is dynamic and constantly changing at a given time point, which may not provide the complete picture or accurately depict of what is really happening at cellular level. Thus, the presence of mRNA does not explicitly mean that it was just synthesized. Likewise, the inability to detect an unstable transcript may be due to its high degradation rate (149). The expression of some genes ("housekeeping genes") is thought to be more stable, and these genes are often used as controls for the normalization of expression levels of other genes. However, the expression of traditionally used controls such as ribosomal RNA genes, also changes across different tissues and experimental conditions making it difficult to select "gold standards" (150). Sampling issues such as biopsy method (151), contamination from neighboring tissues may seriously affect in different expression profiles as microarray technology is very sensitive to such variations (152). RNA quality is a critical issue in genome-wide analysis of gene expression. RNA is less stable than DNA and care should be taken and adequate protocols followed to preserve the quality of biological material. This is particularly important in clinical setting. Another limitation in prognostic or predictive markers from gene expression profiling is that microarray covers only part of the whole picture. Most of cellular functions are performed by proteins and physiological changes can be modulated by not only changes in protein levels but also by protein modifications such as glycosalation, methylation, acethylation, and phosphorylation. These modifications could change protein conformation and lead to changes in activity, which is not detectable by gene expression profiling (152).

7.3. Technological challenges

All of the microarray platforms available in the market are proprietary, a general concern for the inter-platform variability in the gene expression profiles has been addressed by the MicroArray Quality Consortium II (MAQC) (153). Despite the high variability in gene expression attributed to differences in microarray platforms, studies have demonstrated that reproducibility across platforms can be dramatically improved when standardized protocols are implemented for RNA labeling, hybridization, data processing, data acquisition, and data normalization. When these technical variables are standardized, different microarray platforms can produce comparable outcomes (154, 155). Nevertheless, the results from comparison across different platforms can be misleading and should be interpreted with great caution (156). Technicalities of the microarray platforms deals with binding efficiency of labeled target to the respective probe as well as technical variation during experiments also may affect the reproducibility of the gene expression profiles (152). With regards to prospective experiments, the uniformity of experimental conduct will help to minimize potential bias and thus improve the validity of a study. The establishment of the Microarray Quality Control (MAQC) project in 2005 to develop procedural guidelines and quality control metrics in the first phase and the second phase aims to evaluate various data analysis method and predictive models (153). One of the serious problems has been a wide diversity of data formats used in microarray experiments. As a result, the Microarray GeneExpression Database Society (MGED) was created in 1999 to develop a common standard for data input and reporting that could be shared among scientists in the microarray field. In 2001, the MGED created the Minimum Information About a Microarray Experiment (MIAME) guidelines, which serve as a template for researchers to report an adequate description of how microarray data were obtained (157).

7.4. Statistical and and bioinformatic challenges

The experimental design of the microarray studies is of paramount importance, as it should have a clear goal and a specific hypothesis to test. In the design of a microarray experiment, all potential sources of variation should be taken into account to avoid any systematic bias. Researchers should adhere to the sound principles of study and match the experimental variables of cases and controls to the fullest extent possible. It is important to select biologically homogenous sample populations, balancing a design with respect to all factors that can confound results among the comparison groups, and handling samples uniformly through the course of the entire experiment when designing a microarray study (158). Randomization of samples will assure baseline equality between the groups being compared. Violation of these principles will lead to biased results and can cause a loss in power. It should be pointed out that statistical analysis of data couldn't solve fundamental problems of study design. Significantly, the validity of gene expression profiles depends on the characteristics of samples and selection bias, eligible criteria of participation and other confounding factors. An adequate sample size is necessary to achieve sufficient power to demonstrate significance of findings, especially in microarray studies where thousands of genes are tested simultaneously (159). Appropriate preprocessing of microarray data, known as "normalization" prior to analysis is critical for identifying differentially expressed genes. Normalization attempts to remove variability among chips and other systematic biases that are unrelated to biological variation so that a meaningful biological comparison can be made. Transformation is used for multiple purposes, including stabilizing variance in data so that underlying assumptions required for the statistical analysis method are met. Although it is expected that the choice of a preprocessing procedure does not affect the core results of microarray data, different normalization and/or transformation methods may result in different outcomes (160).

Application of appropriate analysis methods to the microarray data, for example classification and cluster analysis are typical analytical approaches to categorized microarray data into manageable classes. However, there is no standard 'method' to how to best analyze the genomic data and it's very tempting to present / published the best-looking result, leading to biased evaluation of the statistical prediction rule. Another issue of classification is "overfitting", which occurs when a classifier is made to perfectly fit a set of data that was used in the model development, but has no discriminatory power so that the results cannot be reproduced in a set of completely independent samples (161). This may lead to insufficient evidence of accuracy and reproducibility of multigene signature from gene expression profiles for clinical use, although it showed initial promising and reproducible results in class discovery studies and preclinical analysis (162). An adequate sample size is essential for any cross-validation technique to be effective. Another significant challenge for researchers is to reconstruct network structure from available expression data. Many different methods for network inference have been proposed (163). A common problem of such models is exponential complexity: the number of parameters increases exponentially with the number of variables. Thus, many alternative and equally probable network structures may be constructed from a given dataset. Dupuy and Simon (164) reviewed the cancer literature of studies relating gene expression profiles to patient outcome, either response to treatment, survival or disease-free survival and found that 50% of the publications had at least one flaw so serious as to raise questions about the validity of the conclusions. The three most common serious flaws they found were: misleading use of cluster analysis, lack of adjustment for the multiplicity of analyzing thousands of genes, and erroneous use of partial cross-validation. They pointed out that cluster analysis rarely has a valid role in the development of predictive classifiers. Its wide use in the literature reflects a lack of proper statistical guidance or collaboration in the conduct of expression profiling studies (164).Therefore, cancer research organization need to better appreciate the fundamental changes occurring in the nature of biomedical research and make major commitments to departments for providing professional biostatistical collaboration as an integral part of translational research.

7.5. Challenges in incorporating molecular profiling assays into routine clinical practice

While the first-generation prognostic multigene classifiers, such as the MammaPrint assay and the Oncotype *DX* breast cancer assay, are the closest to clinical practice, the second-generation prognostic multigene assays have not been commercialized. This includes the assessment of breast cancer microenvironment or host immune response. The assay requires further external validation studies to determine their clinical utilities (165). Despite several studies, the translation of predictive multigene classifiers into the clinic is even more challenging than that of prognostic multigene classifiers (166). Most of the predictive assays are derived mainly from cell lines. Microarray as the assay platform is not as quantitative as using a qRT-PCR assay. Therefore, subtle changes in gene expression may not be reflected in microarray-based assays, although these subtle differences may be sufficient to cause resistance to chemotherapeutics. Furthermore, resistance may occur due to low penetrance of the drug being administered and may be unrelated to tumor tissue. To incorporate prognostic and/or predictive multigene classifiers into clinical practice, the following key criteria need to be fulfilled:

First, the platform on which the classifier is based should be suitable for broad clinical application and ensure that the classifier is stable under a variety of operating conditions. If not, the classifier needs to be translated to a clinically applicable platform (167). The assay protocols should be standardized to achieve satisfactory inter-laboratory and intra-laboratory reproducibility, thereby establishing analytic validity. Assay standardization includes pre-analytic parameters, such as sample storage and preparation, and analytic performance parameters, such as the sensitivity and specificity of the system as well as assay reproducibility. The Clinical Laboratory Improvement Amendments of 1988 (CLIA) requires laboratories to independently establish analytic validity and improve assay standardization. To venture from scientific discovery to the beginning of clinical translational research is a challenge as academic scientist are usually funded and rewarded for discovery, rather than to pursue focused translational research as members of a large interdisciplinary team. Funding agencies may not be experience in funding and monitoring focus translational research. In some other developing countries, to fund such large interdisciplinary and multicenter translational research is prohibitively expensive. Because of these limitations in conducting and funding focused translational research, a defined discovery to a product for use in a defined medical context goes untranslated unless they are of interest to the industry (168, 169).

Second, it is critical to classify studies as developmental or validation studies in order to increase the clinical validity of the classifier. For assays that purport to elucidate predictive significance, this strategy needs to be applied to determine the clinical utility of the classifier (167, 170). Developmental studies need to include internal clinical validation; this can be accomplished either by splitting the study population into two populations (the training model and the testing model or by cross-validation based on repeated model development and testing on random data partitions. These approaches will increase the accuracy of the classifier, which in turn makes its further development possible. Independent validation studies are critical to further evaluate the predictive accuracy and usefulness of the classifier in clinical practice. The studies should be prospectively designed, and should verify both clinical validity and clinical utility. Pusztai et al (171) identified out of the 939 publications over twenty years period on prognostic factors for patients with breast cancer, only estrogen receptor, progesterone receptor and HER2 amplification and *Oncotype DX* RS were included alongside the traditional staging variables recommended by the ASCO guidelines. The pitfall for most of these genomics discovery researches is that only a few of the markers studied were properly validated in a cohort. However, most of the studies were performed using convenience sampling of heterogenous collection of patients and difficult to use such results in therapeutic decision making for individual patients. Finally, most of the publications were based on research assays without demonstration of robustness or analytical validity. Without a diagnostic company to develop a robust assay for a test with a clear and important medical application, the publication is unlikely to be part of successful translational research (169).

Third, does the classifier only assess prognosis? Or does it help with selection of a certain type of therapy? What is the therapeutic relevance of the classifier? Prognostic multigene classifiers assess the likelihood of disease recurrence, whereas predictive multigene classifiers evaluate the potential benefit from certain types of chemotherapy or anti-estrogen therapy. However, a prognostic classifier may also exhibit predictive significance. If a classifier is a predictive classifier, the bar for utility is often quite low. For example, approximately half of patients with HER2 positivity respond to trastuzumab. However, if the assay assesses low likelihood for recurrence or metastases (a prognostic assay), patients classified as low risk need to have such a low risk that they can be spared from adjuvant therapy without affecting their long-term prognosis (172).

Fourth, the incorporation of the classifier into the clinic might be more beneficial if it outperforms or adds predictive power to existing prognostic methods; this would help justify the money and time invested in its external validation in a trial of a much larger scale. In other words, it is important to determine cost-effectiveness. The "intrinsic" classification was the first assay to use modern molecular tools to classify breast cancers. MammaPrint

(111) and the *Oncotype DX*(118) have been tested in more than one validation cohort and are being tested for further clinical utility in large prospective trials in Europe (MINDACT; MammaPrint assay) (140) and in the United States (TAILORx; *Oncotype DX* assay)(173). Both assays have completed a cost-benefit analysis on the utility of the assay in clinical practice (174-178). Both assays demonstrate cost effectiveness in guiding adjuvant chemotherapy treatment in patients with early-stage breast cancer. Another assay in an advanced stage of development is a 50-gene assay (PAM50) (179), although the clinically applicable platform of intrinsic subtype classification is still a long away from clinical application.

The Evaluation of Genomic Applications in Practice and Prevention (EGAPP) Working Group (EWG) assessed the value of the *Oncotype DX* and MammaPrint assay. The EWG found insufficient evidence to make a recommendation for or against the use of tumor gene expression profiles to improve outcomes in defined populations of women with breast cancer (180). The EWG encouraged further development and evaluation of these technologies. It is clear that the molecular profiling tests have a great potential to improve clinical decision making, since they address the complexity of breast cancer. It was suggested that the combinatorial use of these assays with the existing traditional clinicopathologic parameters to be more favorable, as clinicians are hesitant to do away with the existing clinicopathologic parameters. Indeed, a recent study used a similar combinatorial approach in which the *Oncotype DX* RS was integrated with clinicopathological parameters to develop a tool, the RS-Pathology-Clinical (RSPC) assessment (181). This model although requires validation, might have the greatest predictive and/or prognostic utility in cases classified as "intermediate risk" by the *Oncotype DX* (182).These studies highlight the difficulties in prognostication in patients with breast cancer and the need to use anatomical, histological, and biological approaches to assist with clinical decision-making. It is indisputable that multigene classifiers cannot replace, but rather strengthen, prognostication and prediction in combination with clinicopathological parameters. They do not have a role in cases in which the patient (or the clinician) has already made the decision to proceed with systemic adjuvant therapy. However, these tests have a role to play in those patients who are undecided or for whom a definite decision cannot be made based on clinicopathological findings. No test should be ordered if its results are not going to influence clinical decisions (168).

i. **Problems related to early detection**

Scientists postulate the basic underlying prognostic microarray studies is that all tumors acquire a metastasis phenotype through the same unique mechanism, and that gene expression data in tumor tissue obtained at resection of the primary tumor can be used to clearly distinguish between tumors that will relapse or will not relapse. The results of the pioneering prognostic microarray study concerning breast cancer (111) are considered proof of concept and have led to general acceptance of the postulate. However, the performances of microarray studies are poorer than initially thought and published gene signature lists are unstable (161). Some of the multi-biomarker scores do show consistent prognostic value such as in breast cancer, but until the recent advent of large validation studies, microarray studies are not significantly better prognostic classification than conventional prognostic models (113, 122). In addition, it has been shown that almost all first-generation gene signatures in breast cancer provide a quantitative read-out of the same biological pathway of proliferation (183, 184). As of today we are still in need of a precise estimation of the incremental value (185-187). Moreover, by assuming a unique mechanism for the metastasis phenotype, the postulation contradicts with the concept of cancer heterogeneity and consequently with personalized treatments. The potential interest of microarrays could not be rejected provided true critical consideration, incorporating, and not opposed to, full clinical evidence is now necessary.

ii. Problems related to prognosis indicator

The validation of "first-generation" prognostic signatures, usually based exclusively on gene expression profiling, has proven particularly challenging (188). It has been even more difficult to identify and validate predictors of response to nontargeted therapies (radiotherapy and chemotherapy), although analysis of large sample sets from clinical trials have already provided preliminary evidence of novel markers (189).

Limitations to the current prognostic multigene signatures

The ability of the *Oncotype Dx* and MammaPrint, to determine prognosis seems to be directly correlated to the assessment of proliferation/cell cycle-related genes (183, 190). The fact that these multigene signatures are mere surrogates of proliferation poses some important problems for their uses. First, given that proliferation has been shown to be prognostic in ER-positive disease and not in ER-negative cancers, first-generation signatures are applicable only for the prognostication of patients with ER-positive and HER2-negative breast cancers (190, 191). As the expression level of proliferation related genes in ER-positive cancers has been demonstrated to follow a continuum rather than a bimodal distribution, the subdivision of ER-positive cancers into good-prognosis (luminal A) and poor-prognosis (luminal B) groups is considered artificial (183, 190). In fact, the continuous nature of the *Oncotype DX* RS is more representative of the ranges of prognosis of patients with ER-positive disease. It should be noted, however, that this approach for clinical decision-making might be problematic. For instance, the prognostication and management of patients with an intermediate RS remain unclear, and up to 40% to 60% of clinically intermediate-risk patients (that is, breast cancers combining ER-positive, HER2-negative, and grade II status) are allocated to the intermediate-risk RS group (175). Therefore, the actual contribution of *Oncotype DX* to the management of this particular group of patients remains to be elucidated, and is currently being examined in the TAILORx trial (173, 175). Lack of prognostic power of first-generation prognostic signatures in ER-negative breast cancer and their associations with proliferation in ER-positive breast cancer have brought to the forefront of cancer research the limitations of histological grading. Classical histological grade is not prognostic in ER-negative disease and is strongly associated with proliferation (190, 192). It should be noted, however, that the levels of intra- and inter-observer agreement of histological grade remain suboptimal, despite the numerous efforts to implement a standardized histological grading system (192). It could be argued, on the basis of the above observations that the major contribution of first-generation prognostic gene signatures is to provide a standardized proliferation assay for breast cancer. A second limitation of the first-generation prognostic signatures stems from the fact that most of them were developed to predict short-term distant recurrence (<5 years) and were shown to have a strong 'time dependence' and a reduced prognostic value after 5 to 10 years of follow-up (113, 193). Hence, these signatures may represent merely early distant recurrence surrogates and are unable to predict late relapses with the same accuracy. Thus, there is still a need to develop signatures that could identify patients who have a higher risk of late relapse and who may benefit from prolonged therapy.

iii. **Problems related to therapeutic response**

There is also increasing evidence that better classifiers and improved prognostication can be derived from combined analysis that profile both tumour DNA and RNA (194-196). Neoadjuvant therapy trials hold great promise as the right framework to identify these predictive biomarkers for chemotherapy (and targeted therapies) response. ER and Her2 are predictors of a lack of benefit from targeted therapies, hormone therapy and anti-Her2-targeted agents, when the cancers do not express the markers. These predictors, however, fail to identify tumours that despite expressing the biomarkers still fail to respond to the targeted therapies (197).

7.6. Gene expression signatures and response to chemotherapy

With the clinical need for predictive markers for specific chemotherapy agents and multidrug regimens, several groups have developed multigene signatures specifically designed to predict response in patients receiving either chemotherapy or endocrine therapy. Using supervised approaches, several studies have attempted to identify multigene signatures of response to chemotherapy by comparing gene expression profiles between high sensitivity and low-responsiveness tumors (198-201). The majority of the studies focused on neoadjuvant chemotherapy and analyzed tumor samples obtained from biopsies taken at diagnosis before initiation of chemotherapy by microarrays or RT-PCR. Chemotherapy sensitivity usually was estimated with rate of pathological complete response to neoadjuvant therapy (pCR) as a surrogate of long-term benefit from the treatment. For example, a 30-gene signature was developed by the MD Anderson Cancer Center group in 82 breast cancer patients receiving T/FAC chemotherapy (paclitaxel, fluorouracil, doxorubicin, cyclophosphamide). This predictor signature was then validated in 51 independent patients and predicted pCR probability with higher sensitivity and negative predictive value than clinical variables based on age, grade, and ER status (198, 200), which were later confirmed in an independent study (202). Despite these interesting preliminary results, the accuracy of the 30-gene predictor was not found in a recent study in which it was not an independent predictor of pCR after multivariate analysis and did not perform better than clinical variables (203). A similar 78-gene signature to MammaPrint that was developed from a dataset of metastatic breast cancerpatients who did and did not respond to tamoxifen treatment was identified as truly predictive of tamoxifen response. They found that their signatures seemed to be more predictive than prognostic compared with the RS in an independent set of tamoxifen-treated ER-positive metastatic breast cancer patients (204). Whilst the metastatic setting may be the most logical way to investigate the true predictive ability of a biomarker, it remains plausible that metastatic breast cancer patients have different disease biology compared with those having early-stage disease. Miller et al (205) used the neoadjuvant or preoperative setting to uncover gene profiles for which baseline expression and relative change with 14 days of treatment differed between breast cancers that were clinically responsive or resistant toletrozole therapy. The advantage of the neoadjuvant settingis that it allows multiple ways of assessment of response to therapy, eg, monitoring of changes in tumor size during the first months of treatment and sequential tumor biopsiesbefore and after neoadjuvant treatment with letrozole. Gene expression profiles were then related to clinical responses as assessed from tumor volume measurements after three months of treatment. This study underscores the potential of the neoadjuvant setting for high-level correlative science, but also supports the need for biologically driven hypotheses and stratification of luminal subtypes, and also highlights the difficulties of serial analyses using high-dimensional data.

An alternative attempt to predict chemosensitivity to specific chemotherapy regimens was developed with the use of *in vitro* models. Using a combination of *in vitro* signatures associated with drug sensitivity in cell lines, a composite signatures that could predict response to multidrug regimens were derived and translated to patients receiving multidrug chemotherapy (206). These 'regimen-specific' signatures tested in patients who, as participants in the European Organization for Research and Treatment of Cancer (EORTC) BIG00-01 clinical trial, received TET (docetaxel, epirubicin-docetaxel) or FEC (fluorouracil, epirubicin, and cyclophosphamide) chemotherapy resulted in a validation study (207). Importantly, problems with the methodology of these studies have been identified (208) and serious concerns about the validity of the published results were raised. Subsequently, after a series of investigations, the findings derived from *in vitro* studies were considered invalid, and this led to the discontinuation of the clinical trials based on these prediction models (166, 209).

Another method to develop multigene classifiers of chemosensitivity is based on the use of metagenes, groups of co-expressed genes associated with a small number of biological processes. A retrospective microarray analysis of prospectively collected ER-negative breast cancer samples demonstrated that increased stromal gene expression predicted resistance to FEC chemotherapy, which was subsequently validated in two independent cohorts (210). Despite the promising initial results, the signatures of chemotherapy sensitivity have so far had limited use in clinical practice. Most of them have been developed in small, convenience cohorts and require further external validation. None of the different predictors of chemosensitivity is commercially available, and additional evidence is still required before they can be implemented in clinical practice. A recent review has discussed the reasons for the limited success of the predictive signatures available to date (166). On the basis of the design employed in most of the studies, the predictive signatures for multidrug regimens are likely to capture the transcriptomic features of sensitivity/resistance to cytotoxic agents in general. These mechanisms may constitute convergent phenotypes, that are multiple genetic/epigenetic aberrations that may lead to resistance to cytoxic agents (211).

8. Conclusion

Cancer is a multi-factorial disease that involves multiple genes and distinct pathways. The ultimate objective in the high throughput gene expression study approach is to fill the gap in the early biomarker detection, prognostication improvement and gene-targetted therapy. Outcomes from these studies can be obtained from the literatures and some are available as open public databases. Scientists have taken steps forward by using the data either as a single gene studies or multiple genes with related molecular pathways to investigate further on an individual cancer. However, there is a great challenge to devise the suitable gene lists from heterogenous data especially for drug discovery studies. With a great amount of genomic data avaiable, nearly all cancers faced the same setbacks of unable to pick the right genes for the right cancer. Among all cancer, breast cancer has the most advance experience in translating the lab findings into the clinical practice with the emergence of multigene signatures. The current array data can provide a platform for future scientists to explain the complexity of cancer in combination with the latest advancement in deep sequencing technology,

Author details

Norfilza M. Mokhtar
Department of Physiology, Faculty of Medicine
UKM Medical Molecular Biology Institute, Universiti Kebangsaan Malaysia, Cheras, Kuala Lumpur, Malaysia

Nor Azian Murad, Then Sue Mian and Rahman Jamal
UKM Medical Molecular Biology Institute, Universiti Kebangsaan Malaysia, Cheras, Kuala Lumpur, Malaysia

Acknowledgement

The authors would like to thank UKM Medical Molecular Biology Institute (UMBI) for providing facilities for some of our previous works.

9. References

[1] Abelev GI, Eraiser TL. On the path to understanding the nature of cancer. Biochemistry (Mosc). 2008 May;73(5):487-97.

[2] Deschoolmeester V, Baay M, Lardon F, Pauwels P, Peeters M. Immune Cells in Colorectal Cancer: Prognostic Relevance and Role of MSI. Cancer Microenviron. 2011 Dec;4(3):377-92.

[3] Allen JI. Molecular biology of colon polyps and colon cancer. Semin Surg Oncol. 1995 Nov-Dec;11(6):399-405.

[4] Al-Sohaily S, Biankin A, Leong R, Kohonen-Corish M, Warusavitarne J. Molecular pathways in colorectal cancer. J Gastroenterol Hepatol. 2012 Jun 13.

[5] Blum HE. [Colon carcinoma: molecular diagnosis and therapy]. Praxis (Bern 1994). 1997 Sep 24;86(39):1504-9.

[6] Bodmer WF. Cancer genetics: colorectal cancer as a model. J Hum Genet. 2006;51(5):391-6.

[7] Cunningham D, Atkin W, Lenz HJ, Lynch HT, Minsky B, Nordlinger B, et al. Colorectal cancer. Lancet. 2010 Mar 20;375(9719):1030-47.

[8] Jin K, Gao W, Lu Y, Lan H, Teng L, Cao F. Mechanisms regulating colorectal cancer cell metastasis into liver (Review). Oncol Lett. 2012 Jan;3(1):11-5.

[9] Salah S, Watanabe K, Welter S, Park JS, Park JW, Zabaleta J, et al. Colorectal cancer pulmonary oligometastases: pooled analysis and construction of a clinical lung metastasectomy prognostic model. Ann Oncol. 2012 Apr 29.

[10] Horton JK, Tepper JE. Staging of colorectal cancer: past, present, and future. Clin Colorectal Cancer. 2005 Jan;4(5):302-12.

[11] Aarts MJ, Lemmens VE, Louwman MW, Kunst AE, Coebergh JW. Socioeconomic status and changing inequalities in colorectal cancer? A review of the associations with risk, treatment and outcome. Eur J Cancer. 2010 Oct;46(15):2681-95.

[12] Fornaro R, Frascio M, Denegri A, Stabilini C, Impenatore M, Mandolfino F, et al. [Chron's disease and cancer]. Ann Ital Chir. 2009 Mar-Apr;80(2):119-25.

[13] Triantafillidis JK, Nasioulas G, Kosmidis PA. Colorectal cancer and inflammatory bowel disease: epidemiology, risk factors, mechanisms of carcinogenesis and prevention strategies. Anticancer Res. 2009 Jul;29(7):2727-37.

[14] Abdul Murad NA, Othman Z, Khalid M, Abdul Razak Z, Hussain R, Nadesan S, et al. Missense Mutations in MLH1, MSH2, KRAS, and APC Genes in Colorectal Cancer Patients in Malaysia. Dig Dis Sci. 2012 Jun 6.

[15] Hewish M, Lord CJ, Martin SA, Cunningham D, Ashworth A. Mismatch repair deficient colorectal cancer in the era of personalized treatment. Nat Rev Clin Oncol. 2010 Apr;7(4):197-208.

[16] Claes K, Dahan K, Tejpar S, De Paepe A, Bonduelle M, Abramowicz M, et al. The genetics of familial adenomatous polyposis (FAP) and MutYH-associated polyposis (MAP). Acta Gastroenterol Belg. 2011 Sep;74(3):421-6.

[17] Hanks H, Veitch C, Harris M. Colorectal cancer management - the role of the GP. Aust Fam Physician. 2008 Apr;37(4):259-61.

[18] Finlay GJ. Genetics, molecular biology and colorectal cancer. Mutat Res. 1993 Nov;290(1):3-12.

[19] Fearon ER. Molecular genetics of colorectal cancer. Annu Rev Pathol. 2011;6:479-507.

[20] Pritchard CC, Grady WM. Colorectal cancer molecular biology moves into clinical practice. Gut. 2011 Jan;60(1):116-29.

[21] Hendry JH. Genomic instability: potential contributions to tumour and normal tissue response, and second tumours, after radiotherapy. Radiother Oncol. 2001 May;59(2):117-26.
[22] Geigl JB, Obenauf AC, Schwarzbraun T, Speicher MR. Defining 'chromosomal instability'. Trends Genet. 2008 Feb;24(2):64-9.
[23] Gagos S, Irminger-Finger I. Chromosome instability in neoplasia: chaotic roots to continuous growth. Int J Biochem Cell Biol. 2005 May;37(5):1014-33.
[24] Guastadisegni C, Colafranceschi M, Ottini L, Dogliotti E. Microsatellite instability as a marker of prognosis and response to therapy: a meta-analysis of colorectal cancer survival data. Eur J Cancer. 2010 Oct;46(15):2788-98.
[25] Iacopetta B, Grieu F, Amanuel B. Microsatellite instability in colorectal cancer. Asia Pac J Clin Oncol. 2010 Dec;6(4):260-9.
[26] Des Guetz G, Uzzan B, Nicolas P, Schischmanoff O, Perret GY, Morere JF. Microsatellite instability does not predict the efficacy of chemotherapy in metastatic colorectal cancer. A systematic review and meta-analysis. Anticancer Res. 2009 May;29(5):1615-20.
[27] Vilar E, Gruber SB. Microsatellite instability in colorectal cancer-the stable evidence. Nat Rev Clin Oncol. 2010 Mar;7(3):153-62.
[28] Barault L, Charon-Barra C, Jooste V, de la Vega MF, Martin L, Roignot P, et al. Hypermethylator phenotype in sporadic colon cancer: study on a population-based series of 582 cases. Cancer Res. 2008 Oct 15;68(20):8541-6.
[29] Hinoue T, Weisenberger DJ, Pan F, Campan M, Kim M, Young J, et al. Analysis of the association between CIMP and BRAF in colorectal cancer by DNA methylation profiling. PLoS One. 2009;4(12):e8357.
[30] Lander ES, Linton LM, Birren B, Nusbaum C, Zody MC, Baldwin J, et al. Initial sequencing and analysis of the human genome. Nature. 2001 Feb 15;409(6822):860-921.
[31] Thean LF, Li HH, Teo YY, Koh WP, Yuan JM, Teoh ML, et al. Association of caucasian-identified variants with colorectal cancer risk in singapore chinese. PLoS One. 2012;7(8):e42407.
[32] Gerber MM, Hampel H, Schulz NP, Fernandez S, Wei L, Zhou XP, et al. Evaluation of allele-specific somatic changes of genome-wide association study susceptibility alleles in human colorectal cancers. PLoS One. 2012;7(5):e37672.
[33] Stadler ZK, Thom P, Robson ME, Weitzel JN, Kauff ND, Hurley KE, et al. Genome-wide association studies of cancer. J Clin Oncol. 2010 Sep 20;28(27):4255-67.
[34] Tenesa A, Farrington SM, Prendergast JG, Porteous ME, Walker M, Haq N, et al. Genome-wide association scan identifies a colorectal cancer susceptibility locus on 11q23 and replicates risk loci at 8q24 and 18q21. Nat Genet. 2008 May;40(5):631-7.
[35] Pomerantz MM, Ahmadiyeh N, Jia L, Herman P, Verzi MP, Doddapaneni H, et al. The 8q24 cancer risk variant rs6983267 shows long-range interaction with MYC in colorectal cancer. Nat Genet. 2009 Aug;41(8):882-4.
[36] Matsuo K, Suzuki T, Ito H, Hosono S, Kawase T, Watanabe M, et al. Association between an 8q24 locus and the risk of colorectal cancer in Japanese. BMC Cancer. 2009;9:379.
[37] Jaeger E, Webb E, Howarth K, Carvajal-Carmona L, Rowan A, Broderick P, et al. Common genetic variants at the CRAC1 (HMPS) locus on chromosome 15q13.3 influence colorectal cancer risk. Nat Genet. 2008 Jan;40(1):26-8.

[38] Roberts AB, Wakefield LM. The two faces of transforming growth factor beta in carcinogenesis. Proc Natl Acad Sci U S A. 2003 Jul 22;100(15):8621-3.

[39] Sillars-Hardebol AH, Carvalho B, de Wit M, Postma C, Delis-van Diemen PM, Mongera S, et al. Identification of key genes for carcinogenic pathways associated with colorectal adenoma-to-carcinoma progression. Tumour Biol. 2010 Apr;31(2):89-96.

[40] Zhou H, Kuang J, Zhong L, Kuo WL, Gray JW, Sahin A, et al. Tumour amplified kinase STK15/BTAK induces centrosome amplification, aneuploidy and transformation. Nat Genet. 1998 Oct;20(2):189-93.

[41] De Luca M, Lavia P, Guarguaglini G. A functional interplay between Aurora-A, Plk1 and TPX2 at spindle poles: Plk1 controls centrosomal localization of Aurora-A and TPX2 spindle association. Cell Cycle. 2006 Feb;5(3):296-303.

[42] Smits VA, Klompmaker R, Arnaud L, Rijksen G, Nigg EA, Medema RH. Polo-like kinase-1 is a target of the DNA damage checkpoint. Nat Cell Biol. 2000 Sep;2(9):672-6.

[43] Wu Y, Wang X, Wu F, Huang R, Xue F, Liang G, et al. Transcriptome profiling of the cancer, adjacent non-tumor and distant normal tissues from a colorectal cancer patient by deep sequencing. PLoS One. 2012;7(8):e41001.

[44] Siegel R, Naishadham D, Jemal A. Cancer statistics, 2012. CA Cancer J Clin. 2012 Jan-Feb;62(1):10-29.

[45] Zainal Ariffin O, Nor Saleha IT. National Cancer Registry Report 2007. Kuala Lumpur: Ministry of Health, Malaysia2011.

[46] Menon U, Jacobs IJ. Ovarian cancer screening in the general population: current status. Int J Gynecol Cancer. 2001;11 Suppl 1:3-6.

[47] Gram IT, Lukanova A, Brill I, Braaten T, Lund E, Lundin E, et al. Cigarette smoking and risk of histological subtypes of epithelial ovarian cancer in the EPIC cohort study. Int J Cancer. 2012 May 1;130(9):2204-10.

[48] Jordan SJ, Siskind V, A CG, Whiteman DC, Webb PM. Breastfeeding and risk of epithelial ovarian cancer. Cancer Causes Control. 2010 Jan;21(1):109-16.

[49] Fekete T, Raso E, Pete I, Tegze B, Liko I, Munkacsy G, et al. Meta-analysis of gene expression profiles associated with histological classification and survival in 829 ovarian cancer samples. Int J Cancer. 2012 Jul 1;131(1):95-105.

[50] Cannistra SA. Cancer of the ovary. N Engl J Med. 2004 Dec 9;351(24):2519-29.

[51] Nakayama N, Nakayama K, Yeasmin S, Ishibashi M, Katagiri A, Iida K, et al. KRAS or BRAF mutation status is a useful predictor of sensitivity to MEK inhibition in ovarian cancer. Br J Cancer. 2008 Dec 16;99(12):2020-8.

[52] Tutt A, Robson M, Garber JE, Domchek SM, Audeh MW, Weitzel JN, et al. Oral poly(ADP-ribose) polymerase inhibitor olaparib in patients with BRCA1 or BRCA2 mutations and advanced breast cancer: a proof-of-concept trial. Lancet. 2010 Jul 24;376(9737):235-44.

[53] Christie M, Oehler MK. Molecular pathology of epithelial ovarian cancer. J Br Menopause Soc. 2006 Jun;12(2):57-63.

[54] Alsop K, Fereday S, Meldrum C, Defazio A, Emmanuel C, George J, et al. BRCA Mutation Frequency and Patterns of Treatment Response in BRCA Mutation-Positive Women With Ovarian Cancer: A Report From the Australian Ovarian Cancer Study Group. J Clin Oncol. 2012 Jul 20;30(21):2654-63.

[55] Aarnio M, Sankila R, Pukkala E, Salovaara R, Aaltonen LA, de la Chapelle A, et al. Cancer risk in mutation carriers of DNA-mismatch-repair genes. Int J Cancer. 1999 Apr 12;81(2):214-8.

[56] Stany MP, Vathipadiekal V, Ozbun L, Stone RL, Mok SC, Xue H, et al. Identification of novel therapeutic targets in microdissected clear cell ovarian cancers. PLoS One. 2011;6(7):e21121.

[57] Yamaguchi K, Mandai M, Oura T, Matsumura N, Hamanishi J, Baba T, et al. Identification of an ovarian clear cell carcinoma gene signature that reflects inherent disease biology and the carcinogenic processes. Oncogene. 2010 Mar 25;29(12):1741-52.

[58] Schwartz DR, Kardia SL, Shedden KA, Kuick R, Michailidis G, Taylor JM, et al. Gene expression in ovarian cancer reflects both morphology and biological behavior, distinguishing clear cell from other poor-prognosis ovarian carcinomas. Cancer Res. 2002 Aug 15;62(16):4722-9.

[59] Schaner ME, Ross DT, Ciaravino G, Sorlie T, Troyanskaya O, Diehn M, et al. Gene expression patterns in ovarian carcinomas. Mol Biol Cell. 2003 Nov;14(11):4376-86.

[60] Tothill RW, Tinker AV, George J, Brown R, Fox SB, Lade S, et al. Novel molecular subtypes of serous and endometrioid ovarian cancer linked to clinical outcome. Clin Cancer Res. 2008 Aug 15;14(16):5198-208.

[61] Shridhar V, Lee J, Pandita A, Iturria S, Avula R, Staub J, et al. Genetic analysis of early- versus late-stage ovarian tumors. Cancer Res. 2001 Aug 1;61(15):5895-904.

[62] Davidson B, Stavnes HT, Holth A, Chen X, Yang Y, Shih Ie M, et al. Gene expression signatures differentiate ovarian/peritoneal serous carcinoma from breast carcinoma in effusions. J Cell Mol Med. 2011 Mar;15(3):535-44.

[63] Vui-Kee K, Mohd Dali AZ, Mohamed Rose I, Ghazali R, Jamal R, Mokhtar NM. Molecular markers associated with nonepithelial ovarian cancer in formalin-fixed, paraffin-embedded specimens by genome wide expression profiling. Kaohsiung J Med Sci. 2012 May;28(5):243-50.

[64] Tomlinson VA, Newbery HJ, Wray NR, Jackson J, Larionov A, Miller WR, et al. Translation elongation factor eEF1A2 is a potential oncoprotein that is overexpressed in two-thirds of breast tumours. BMC Cancer. 2005;5:113.

[65] Sherman ME, Bur ME, Kurman RJ. p53 in endometrial cancer and its putative precursors: evidence for diverse pathways of tumorigenesis. Hum Pathol. 1995 Nov;26(11):1268-74.

[66] Creasman W. Revised FIGO staging for carcinoma of the endometrium. Int J Gynaecol Obstet. 2009 May;105(2):109.

[67] Lax SF. Molecular genetic pathways in various types of endometrial carcinoma: from a phenotypical to a molecular-based classification. Virchows Arch. 2004 Mar;444(3):213-23.

[68] Lax SF, Pizer ES, Ronnett BM, Kurman RJ. Comparison of estrogen and progesterone receptor, Ki-67, and p53 immunoreactivity in uterine endometrioid carcinoma and endometrioid carcinoma with squamous, mucinous, secretory, and ciliated cell differentiation. Hum Pathol. 1998 Sep;29(9):924-31.

[69] Moreno-Bueno G, Sanchez-Estevez C, Cassia R, Rodriguez-Perales S, Diaz-Uriarte R, Dominguez O, et al. Differential gene expression profile in endometrioid and

nonendometrioid endometrial carcinoma: STK15 is frequently overexpressed and amplified in nonendometrioid carcinomas. Cancer Res. 2003 Sep 15;63(18):5697-702.
[70] Kok Ying N, Ganesalingam M, Sabaratnam S. Cancer Incidence in Peninsular Malaysia. Kuala Lumpur2008.
[71] Doll A, Abal M, Rigau M, Monge M, Gonzalez M, Demajo S, et al. Novel molecular profiles of endometrial cancer-new light through old windows. J Steroid Biochem Mol Biol. 2008 Feb;108(3-5):221-9.
[72] Llaurado M, Ruiz A, Majem B, Ertekin T, Colas E, Pedrola N, et al. Molecular bases of endometrial cancer: new roles for new actors in the diagnosis and the therapy of the disease. Mol Cell Endocrinol. 2012 Jul 25;358(2):244-55.
[73] Felix AS, Weissfeld JL, Stone RA, Bowser R, Chivukula M, Edwards RP, et al. Factors associated with Type I and Type II endometrial cancer. Cancer Causes Control. 2010 Nov;21(11):1851-6.
[74] Deligeoroglou E, Michailidis E, Creatsas G. Oral contraceptives and reproductive system cancer. Ann N Y Acad Sci. 2003 Nov;997:199-208.
[75] Aoki Y, Watanabe M, Amikura T, Obata H, Sekine M, Yahata T, et al. Adjuvant chemotherapy as treatment of high-risk stage I and II endometrial cancer. Gynecol Oncol. 2004 Aug;94(2):333-9.
[76] Burbos N, Musonda P, Crocker SG, Morris EP, Duncan TJ, Nieto JJ. Outcome of investigations for postmenopausal vaginal bleeding in women under the age of 50 years. Gynecol Oncol. 2012 Apr;125(1):120-3.
[77] Lacey JV, Jr., Yang H, Gaudet MM, Dunning A, Lissowska J, Sherman ME, et al. Endometrial cancer and genetic variation in PTEN, PIK3CA, AKT1, MLH1, and MSH2 within a population-based case-control study. Gynecol Oncol. 2011 Feb;120(2):167-73.
[78] Seeger A, Kolbl H, Petry IB, Gebhard S, Battista MJ, Bohm D, et al. p53 is correlated with low BMI negative progesterone receptor status and recurring disease in patients with endometrial cancer. Gynecol Oncol. 2012 Apr;125(1):200-7.
[79] Singh M, Darcy KM, Brady WE, Clubwala R, Weber Z, Rittenbach JV, et al. Cadherins, catenins and cell cycle regulators: impact on survival in a Gynecologic Oncology Group phase II endometrial cancer trial. Gynecol Oncol. 2011 Nov;123(2):320-8.
[80] Gurin CC, Federici MG, Kang L, Boyd J. Causes and consequences of microsatellite instability in endometrial carcinoma. Cancer Res. 1999 Jan 15;59(2):462-6.
[81] Maxwell GL, Chandramouli GV, Dainty L, Litzi TJ, Berchuck A, Barrett JC, et al. Microarray analysis of endometrial carcinomas and mixed mullerian tumors reveals distinct gene expression profiles associated with different histologic types of uterine cancer. Clin Cancer Res. 2005 Jun 1;11(11):4056-66.
[82] Mokhtar NM, Ramzi NH, Yin-Ling W, Rose IM, Hatta Mohd Dali AZ, Jamal R. Laser capture microdissection with genome-wide expression profiling displayed gene expression signatures in endometrioid endometrial cancer. Cancer Invest. 2012 Feb;30(2):156-64.
[83] Pavelic J, Radakovic B, Pavelic K. Insulin-like growth factor 2 and its receptors (IGF 1R and IGF 2R/mannose 6-phosphate) in endometrial adenocarcinoma. Gynecol Oncol. 2007 Jun;105(3):727-35.

[84] Sugiyama Y, Sugiyama K, Hirai Y, Akiyama F, Hasumi K. Microdissection is essential for gene expression profiling of clinically resected cancer tissues. 2002 [updated Jan; cited 117 1]; 2002/01/16:[109-16]. Available from: http://www.ncbi.nlm.nih.gov/entrez/query.fcgi?cmd=Retrieve&db=PubMed&dopt=Citation&list_uids=11789716.

[85] Mannelqvist M, Stefansson IM, Bredholt G, Hellem Bo T, Oyan AM, Jonassen I, et al. Gene expression patterns related to vascular invasion and aggressive features in endometrial cancer. Am J Pathol. 2011 Feb;178(2):861-71.

[86] Ferguson SE, Olshen AB, Levine DA, Viale A, Barakat RR, Boyd J. Molecular profiling of endometrial cancers from African-American and Caucasian women. Gynecol Oncol. 2006 May;101(2):209-13.

[87] Metcalfe K, Lubinski J, Lynch HT, Ghadirian P, Foulkes WD, Kim-Sing C, et al. Family history of cancer and cancer risks in women with BRCA1 or BRCA2 mutations. J Natl Cancer Inst. 2010 Dec 15;102(24):1874-8.

[88] Sariego J. Breast cancer in the young patient. Am Surg. 2010 Dec;76(12):1397-400.

[89] Ross JS. Multigene classifiers, prognostic factors, and predictors of breast cancer clinical outcome. Adv Anat Pathol. 2009 Jul;16(4):204-15.

[90] Ross JS, Fletcher JA, Linette GP, Stec J, Clark E, Ayers M, et al. The Her-2/neu gene and protein in breast cancer 2003: biomarker and target of therapy. Oncologist. 2003;8(4):307-25.

[91] Eroles P, Bosch A, Alejandro Perez-Fidalgo J, Lluch A. Molecular biology in breast cancer: Intrinsic subtypes and signaling pathways. Cancer Treat Rev. 2012 Oct;38(6):698-707.

[92] This P, de la Rochefordiere A, Savignoni A, Falcou MC, Tardivon A, Thibault F, et al. Breast and ovarian cancer risk management in a French cohort of 158 women carrying a BRCA1 or BRCA2 germline mutation: patient choices and outcome. Fam Cancer. 2012 Jun 19.

[93] de Bruin MA, Kwong A, Goldstein BA, Lipson JA, Ikeda DM, McPherson L, et al. Breast cancer risk factors differ between Asian and white women with BRCA1/2 mutations. Fam Cancer. 2012 May 26.

[94] Keogh RH, Park JY, White IR, Lentjes MA, McTaggart A, Bhaniani A, et al. Estimating the alcohol-breast cancer association: a comparison of diet diaries, FFQs and combined measurements. Eur J Epidemiol. 2012 May 29.

[95] Saslow D, Hannan J, Osuch J, Alciati MH, Baines C, Barton M, et al. Clinical breast examination: practical recommendations for optimizing performance and reporting. CA Cancer J Clin. 2004 Nov-Dec;54(6):327-44.

[96] McDonald S, Saslow D, Alciati MH. Performance and reporting of clinical breast examination: a review of the literature. CA Cancer J Clin. 2004 Nov-Dec;54(6):345-61.

[97] Murphy CG, Morris PG. Recent advances in novel targeted therapies for HER2-positive breast cancer. Anticancer Drugs. 2012 Sep;23(8):765-76.

[98] Cai Q, Wen W, Qu S, Li G, Egan KM, Chen K, et al. Replication and functional genomic analyses of the breast cancer susceptibility locus at 6q25.1 generalize its importance in women of chinese, Japanese, and European ancestry. Cancer Res. 2011 Feb 15;71(4):1344-55.

[99] Stacey SN, Sulem P, Zanon C, Gudjonsson SA, Thorleifsson G, Helgason A, et al. Ancestry-shift refinement mapping of the C6orf97-ESR1 breast cancer susceptibility locus. PLoS Genet. 2010 Jul;6(7):e1001029.

[100] Turnbull C, Ahmed S, Morrison J, Pernet D, Renwick A, Maranian M, et al. Genome-wide association study identifies five new breast cancer susceptibility loci. Nat Genet. 2010 Jun;42(6):504-7.

[101] Gold B, Kirchhoff T, Stefanov S, Lautenberger J, Viale A, Garber J, et al. Genome-wide association study provides evidence for a breast cancer risk locus at 6q22.33. Proc Natl Acad Sci U S A. 2008 Mar 18;105(11):4340-5.

[102] Bessarabova M, Kirillov E, Shi W, Bugrim A, Nikolsky Y, Nikolskaya T. Bimodal gene expression patterns in breast cancer. BMC Genomics. 2010;11 Suppl 1:S8.

[103] Sun Z, Asmann YW, Kalari KR, Bot B, Eckel-Passow JE, Baker TR, et al. Integrated analysis of gene expression, CpG island methylation, and gene copy number in breast cancer cells by deep sequencing. PLoS One. 2011;6(2):e17490.

[104] Ma XJ, Dahiya S, Richardson E, Erlander M, Sgroi DC. Gene expression profiling of the tumor microenvironment during breast cancer progression. Breast Cancer Res. 2009;11(1):R7.

[105] Kao J, Salari K, Bocanegra M, Choi YL, Girard L, Gandhi J, et al. Molecular profiling of breast cancer cell lines defines relevant tumor models and provides a resource for cancer gene discovery. PLoS One. 2009;4(7):e6146.

[106] Aaroe J, Lindahl T, Dumeaux V, Saebo S, Tobin D, Hagen N, et al. Gene expression profiling of peripheral blood cells for early detection of breast cancer. Breast Cancer Res. 2010;12(1):R7.

[107] Iwamoto T, Bianchini G, Booser D, Qi Y, Coutant C, Ya-Hui Shiang C, et al. Gene pathways associated with prognosis and chemotherapy sensitivity in molecular subtypes of breast cancer. J Natl Cancer Inst. 2011;103:264-72.

[108] Goldhirsch A, Wood WC, Gelber RD, Coates AS, Thürlimann B, Senn HJ, 10th St. Gallen conference. Meeting highlights: updated international expert consensus on the primary therapy of early breast cancer. J Clin Oncol. 2003;21:3357-65.

[109] NCCN Guidelines for Breast Cancer, NCCN Task Force Report: adjuvant therapy for breast cancer. . J Natl Compr Canc Netw.; 2006. p. S1-26.

[110] Kohli-Laven N, Bourret P, Keating P, Cambrosio A. Cancer clinical trials in the era of genomic signatures: Biomedical innovation, clinical utility, and regulatory scientific hybrids. Soc Stud Sci. 2011;41(4):487-513.

[111] van 't Veer LJ, Dai H, van de Vijver MJ, He YD, Hart AA, Mao M, et al. Gene expression profiling predicts clinical outcome of breast cancer. Nature. 2002;415(6871):530-6.

[112] Simon RM, Paik S, Hayes DF. Use of Archived Specimens in Evaluation of Prognostic and Predictive Biomarkers. J Natl Cancer Inst. 2009;101:1446-52.

[113] Buyse M, Loi S, van't Veer L, Viale G, Delorenzi M, Glas AM, et al. Validation and clinical utility of a 70-gene prognostic signature for women with node-negative breast cancer. J Natl Cancer Inst. 2006;98:1183-92.

[114] Bourreta P, Keating P, Cambrosio A. Regulating diagnosis in post-genomic medicine: Re-aligning clinical judgment? Soc Stud Sci. 2011;73(6):816-24.

[115] Glück S, Yip AYS, Ng ELY. Can we replace the microscope with microarrays for diagnosis, prognosis and treatment of early breast cancer? Expert Opin Ther Targets. 2012;16((Suppl.1)):S17-S22.

[116] Cronin M, Ghosh K, Sistare F, Quackenbush J, Vilker V, O'Connell C. Universal RNA reference materials for gene expression. Clinical Chemistry 2004;50:1464–71.

[117] Cronin MT, Dutta D, Pho M, Nguyen A, Jeong J, Liu ML. Tumor marker discovery by expression profiling RNA from formalin fixed paraffin embedded tissues. . Methods in Molecular Biology. 2009;520:177–93.

[118] Paik S, Shak S, Tang G, Kim C, Baker J, Cronin M, et al. A multigene assay to predict recurrence of tamoxifen-treated, node-negative breast cancer. N Engl J Med 2004;351:2817-26.

[119] Paik S, Tang G, Shak S, Kim C, Baker J, Kim W, et al. Gene Expression and Benefit of Chemotherapy in Women with Node-Negative, Estrogen Receptor-Positive Breast Cancer. J Clin Oncol 2006;24(23):3726-34

[120] Ross JS, Hatzis C, Symmans WF, Pusztai L, Hortobágyi GN. Commercialized multigene predictors of clinical outcome for breast cancer. The Oncologist. 2008;13:477-93.

[121] Habel LA, Shak S, Jacobs M, Capra A, Alexander C, Pho M, et al. A Population-Based Study of Tumor Gene Expression and Risk of Breast Cancer Death Among Lymph Node-Negative Patients. Breast Cancer Res 2006;8(3):R25.

[122] Albain KS, Barlow W, Shak S, Hortobagyi G, Livingston R, Yeh I-T, et al. Prognostic and predictive value of the 21-gene recurrence score assay in post-menopausal women with node-positive, oestrogen-receptor-positive breast cancer on chemotherapy: a retrospective analysis of a randomised trial. Lancet Oncol. 2010;11(1):55-65.

[123] Jessup JM, Lively TG, Taube SE. Program for the assessment of cancer clinical tests (PACCT): Implementing promising assays into clinical practice. Expert Review of Molecular Diagnostics. 2005;5:271–3.

[124] Harris L, Fritsche H, Mennel R, Norton L, Ravdin P, Taube S, et al. American Society of Clinical Oncology: Update of recommendations for the use of tumor markers in breast cancer. J Clin Oncol. 2007;25:5287-312.

[125] van de Vijver MJ, He YD, van't Veer LJ, Dai H, Hart AA, Voskuil DW, et al. A gene-expression signature as a predictor of survival in breast cancer. N Engl J Med. 2002;347:1999-2009.

[126] Glas AM, Floore A, Delahaye LJ, Witteveen AT, Pover RC, Bakx N, et al. Converting a breast cancer microarray signature into a high-throughput diagnostic test. BMC Genomics. 2006;7:278.

[127] Keating P, Cambrosio A. Too many numbers: Microarrays in clinical cancer research. Stud Hist Philos Biol Biomed Sci. 2012;43:37-51.

[128] Rogers S, Cambrosio A. Making a new technology work: The standardization and regulation of microarrays. Yale Journal of Biology and Medicine. 2007;80:165–78.

[129] Bueno-de-Mesquita JM, van Harten WH, Retel VP, van't Veer LJ, van Dam FS, Karsenberg K, et al. Use of 70-gene signature to predict prognosis of patients with node-negative breast cancer: a prospective community-based feasibility study (RASTER). Lancet Oncol. 2007;8:1079-87.

[130] Beuno-de-Mesquita JM, Linn SC, Keijzer R, Wesseling J, Nuyten DS, van Krimpen C, et al. Validation of 70-gene prognosis signature in node-negative breast cancer. Breast Cancer Res Treat. 2009;117(3).

[131] Wittner BS, Sgroi DC, Ryan PD, Bruinsma TJ, Glas AM, Male A, et al. Analysis of the MammaPrint breast cancer assay in a predominantly postmenopausal cohort. Clin Cancer Res. 2008 May 15;14(10):2988-93.

[132] Wittner BS, Sgroi DC, Ryan PD, Bruinsma TJ, Glas AM, Male A, et al. Analysis of the MammaPrint breast cancer assay in a predominantly postmenopausal cohort. Clin Cancer Res. 2008;14(10):2988-93.

[133] Mook S, Schmidt MK, Viale G, Pruneri G, Eekhout I, Floore A, et al. The 70-gene prognosis-signature predicts disease outcome in breast cancer patients with 1-3 positive lymph nodes in an independent validation study. Breast Cancer Res Treat. 2009;116(2):295-302.

[134] Wang Y, Klijn JG, Zhang Y, Sieuwerts AM, Look MP, Yang F, et al. Gene-expression profi les to predict distant metastasis of h-node-negative primary breast cancer. Lancet Oncol. 2005;365:671-9.

[135] Foekens JA, Atkins D, Zhang Y, Sweep FC, Harbeck N, Paradiso A, et al. Multicenter validation of a gene expression-based prognostic signature in h node-negative primary breast cancer. J Clin Oncol. 2006;24:1665-71.

[136] Sotiriou C, Wirapati P, Loi S, Harris A, Fox S, Smeds J, et al. Gene expression profiling in breast cancer: understanding the molecular basis of histologic grade to improve prognosis. J Natl Cancer Inst 2006;98:262-72.

[137] Loi S, Haibe-Kains B, Desmedt C, Lallemand F, Tutt AM, Gillet C, et al. Definition of clinically distinct molecular subtypes in estrogen receptor-positive breast carcinomas through genomic grade. J Clin Oncol. 2007;25:1239-46.

[138] Liedtke C, Hatzis C, Symmans WF, Desmedt C, Haibe-Kains B, Valero V, et al. Genomic grade index is associated with response to chemotherapy in patients with breast cancer. . J Clin Oncol 2009;27:3185-91.

[139] Desmedt C, Giobbie-Hurder A, Neven P, Paridaens R, Christiaens MR, Smeets A, et al. The Gene expression Grade Index: a potential predictor of relapse for endocrine-treated breast cancer patients in the BIG 1-98 trial. . BMC Med Genomics 2009;2:40.

[140] Cardoso F, Van't Veer L, Rutgers E, Loi S, Mook S, Piccart-Gebhart MJ. Clinical application of the 70-gene profile: the MINDACT trial. J Clin Oncol. 2008;26:729-35.

[141] Cardoso F. Show me the genes - I will tell you who/how to treat! Breast Cancer Research. 2005;7:77-9.

[142] Handkiewicz-Junak D, Czarniecka A, Jarzab B. Molecular prognostic markers in papillary and follicular thyroid cancer: Current status and future directions. . Mol Cell Endocrinol. 2010;322:8-28.

[143] Risinger JI, Maxwell GL, Chandramouli GVR, Jazaeri A, Aprelikova O, Patterson T, et al. Microarray Analysis Reveals Distinct Gene Expression Profiles among Different Histologic Types of Endometrial Cancer. Cancer Res. 2003;63:6-11.

[144] Schwartz DR, Kardia SLR, Shedden KA, Kuick R, Michailidis G, Taylor JMG, et al. Gene Expression in Ovarian Cancer Reflects Both Morphology and Biological Behavior, Distinguishing Clear Cell from Other Poor-Prognosis Ovarian Carcinomas. Cancer Res. 2002;62:4722-9.

[145] Khoury MJ, Gwinn M, Yoon PW, Dowling N, Moore CA, Bradley L. The continuum of translation research in genomic medicine how can we accelerate the appropriate integration of human genome discoveries into health care and disease prevention? . Genet Med. 2007;9:665-74.

[146] Khoury MJ, Coates RJ, Fennell ML, Glasgow RE, Scheuner MT, Schully SD, et al. Multilevel research and the challenges of implementing genomic medicine. J Natl Cancer Inst Monogr. 2012;44:112-20.

[147] Schully SD, Benedicto CB, Gillanders EM, Wang SS, Khoury MJ. Translational Research in Cancer Genetics: The Road Less Traveled. Public Health Genomics 2010;14:1-8.

[148] Maitland ML, Schilsky RL. Clinical trials in the era of personalized oncology. CA Cancer J Clin. 2011;61:365-81.

[149] Cheadle C, Fan J, Cho-Chung YS, Werner T, Ray J, Do L, et al. Stability regulation of mRNA and the control of gene expression. Ann N Y Acad Sci. 2005;1058:196–204.

[150] Thorrez L, Van Deun K, Tranchevent LC, Van Lommel L, Engelen K, Marchal K, et al. Using ribosomal protein genes as reference: a tale of caution. . PLoS ONE. 2008;3:e1854.

[151] Mutch DM, Tordjman J, Pelloux V, Hanczar B, Henegar C, Poitou C, et al. Needle and surgical biopsy techniques differentially affect adipose tissue gene expression profiles. Am J Clin Nutr. 2009;89:51-7.

[152] Kim K, Zakharkin SO, Allison DB. Expectations, validity and reality in gene expression profiling J Clin Epidemiol. 2010;63:950–9.

[153] Shi L, Reid LH, Jones WD, Shippy R, Warrington JA, Baker SC, et al. The MicroArra Quality Control (MAQC) projects shoes inter- and intraplatform reproducibility of gene expression measureament. Nat Biotechnol. 2006;24:1151-61.

[154] Larkin JE, Frank BC, Gavras H, Sultana R, Quackenbush J. Independence and reproducibility across microarray platforms. Nat Methods. 2005;2:337–44.

[155] Irizarry RA, Warren D, Spencer F, Kim IF, Biswal S, Frank BC, et al. Multiple-laboratory comparison of microarray platforms. Nat Methods. 2005;2:345–50.

[156] Standardizing global gene expression analysis between laboratories and across platforms, (2005).

[157] Brazma A, Hingamp P, Quackenbush J, Sherlock G, Spellman P, Stoeckert C, et al. Minimum information about a microarray experiment (MIAME)-toward standards for microarray data. Nat Genet. 2001 Dec;29(4):365-71.

[158] Ransohoff DF. How to improve reliability and efficiency of research about molecular markers: role of phases, guidelines and study design. J Clin Epidemiol. 2007;60:1205-19.

[159] Zakharkin SO, Kim K, Mehta T, Chen L, Barnes S, Scheirer KE, et al. Sources of variation in Affymetrix microarray experiments. BMC Bioinformatics. 2005;6:214.

[160] Bolstad BM, Irizarry RA, Astrand M, Speed TP. A comparison of normalization methods for high density oligonucleotide array data based on variance and bias. Bioinformatics. 2003;19:185–93.

[161] Michiels S, Kramar A, Koscielny S. Multidimentionality of microarrays: Statiscal challenges and (im)possible solutions. Mol Onco. 2011;5:190-6.

[162] Kim K, Zakharkin SO, Allison DB. Expectations, validity, and reality in gene expression profiling. J Clin Epidemiol. 2010 Sep;63(9):950-9.

[163] Lee WP, Tzou WS. Computational methods for discovering gene networks from expression data. Brief Bioinform. 2009;10:408-23.

[164] Dupuy A, Simon RM. Critical review of published microarray studies for cancer outcome and guidelines on statistical analysis and reporting. J Natl Cancer Inst. 2007;99:147-57.

[165] Reis-Filho JS, Weigelt B, Fumagalli D, Sotiriou C. Molecular profiling: moving away from tumor philately. Sci Transl Med. 2010;2:47ps3.

[166] Borst P, Wessels L. Do predictive signatures really predict response to cancer chemotherapy? . Cell Cycle. 2010;9:4836-40.

[167] Simon R. Roadmap for developing and validating therapeutically relevant genomic classifiers. J Clin Oncol. 2005;23:7332-41.

[168] Gökmen-Polar YBS. Molecular profiling assays in breast cancer: are we ready for prime time? Oncology (Willston Park). 2012;26(4):350-7.

[169] Simon R. Lost in translation problems and pitfalss in translating laboratory observation to clinical utility. Eur J Cancer. 2008;44:27072-2713.

[170] Simon R. Development and validation of therapeutically relevant multi-gene biomarker classifiers. J Natl Cancer Inst. 2005;97:866-7.

[171] Pusztai L, Ayers M, Stec J, Hortobagyi GN. Clinical application of cDNA microarrays in oncology. The Oncologist. 2003;8:252-8.

[172] Sparano JA, Solin LJ. Defining the clinical utility of gene expression assays in breast cancer: the intersection of science and art in clinical decision making. J Clin Oncol. 2010;28:1625-7.

[173] Sparano JA, Paik S. Development of the 21-gene assay and its application in clinical practice and clinical trials. J Clin Oncol. 2008;26:721-8.

[174] Lyman GH, Cosler LE, Kuderer NM, Hornberger J. Impact of a 21-Gene RT-PCR Assay on Treatment Decisions in Early-Stage Breast Cancer: An Economic Analysis Based on Prognostic and Predictive Validation Studies. Cancer. 2007;109(6):1011-8.

[175] Kelly CM, Krishnamurthy S, Bianchini G, Litton JK, Gonzalez-Angulo AM, Hortobagyi GN, et al. Utility of oncotype DX risk estimates in clinically intermediate risk hormone receptor-positive, HER2-normal, grade II, lymph node-negative breast cancers. Cancer. 2010;116:5161-7.

[176] Retèl VP, Joore MA, Knauer M, Linn SC, Hauptmann M, Harten WH. Cost-effectiveness of the 70-gene signature versus St. Gallen guidelines and Adjuvant Online for early breast cancer. Eur J Cancer. 2010;46:1382-91.

[177] Chen E, Tong KB, Malin JL. Cost-effectiveness of 70-gene MammaPrint signature in node-negative breast cancer. Am J Manag Care. 2010;16:e333-42.

[178] Hornberger J, Cosler LE, Lyman GH. Economic Analysis of Targeting Chemotherapy Using a 21-Gene RT-PCR Assay in Lymph-Node–Negative, Estrogen-Receptor–Positive, Early-Stage Breast Cancer. Am J Manag Care. 2005;11:313-24.

[179] Parker JS, Mullins M, Cheang MC, Leung S, Voduc D, Vickery T, et al. Supervised risk predictor of breast cancer based on intrinsic subtypes. J Clin Oncol. 2009;27:1160-7.

[180] Recommendations from the EGAPP Working Group: can tumor gene expression profiling improve outcomes in patients with breast cancer?, 11 (2009).

[181] Tang G, Cuzick J, Costantino JP, al. e. Risk of recurrence and chemotherapy benefit for patients with node-negative, estrogen receptor-positive breast cancer: recurrence score alone and integrated with pathologic and clinical factors. J Clin Oncol. 2011;29:4365-72.

[182] Pusztai L. Anatomy and biology: two complementary sides of breast cancer prognostication. J Clin Oncol. 2011;29:4347-8.
[183] Wirapati P, Sotiriou C, Kunkel S, Farmer P, Pradervand S, Haibe-Kains B, et al. Meta-analysis of gene expression profiles in breast cancer: toward a unified understanding of breast cancer subtyping and prognosis signatures. Breast Cancer Res Treat. 2008;10:R65.
[184] Haibe-Kains B, Desmedt C, Sotiriou C, Bontempi G. A comparative study of survival models for breast cancer prognostication based on microarray data: does a single gene beat them all? Bioinformatics [serial on the Internet]. 2008; 24.
[185] Recommendations from the EGAPP Working Group: can tumor gene expression profiling improve outcomes in patients with breast cancer?, 11 (2009).
[186] Koscielny S, Michiels S. Clinical usefulness of microarrays for cancer prognosis in 2010--letter. n Cancer Res. 2010;16:6180-1.
[187] Marchionni L, Wilson RF, Marinopoulos SS, Wolff AC, Parmigiani G, Bass EB, et al. Impact of gene expression profiling tests on breast cancer outcomes. Evid Rep Technol Assess (Full Rep). 2007;160:1-105.
[188] Pharoah PD, Caldas C. How to validate a breast cancer prognosticature. Nat Rev Clin Oncol. 2010;7:615–6.
[189] Bartlett JM, Munro AF, Dunn JA, McConkey C, Jordan S, Twelves CJ, et al. Predictive markers of anthracycline benefit: a prospectively planned analysis of the UK National Epirubicin Adjuvant Trial (NEAT/BR9601). . Lancet Oncol. 2010;11:266–74.
[190] Desmedt C, Haibe-Kains B, Wirapati P, Buyse M, Larsimont D, Bontempi G, et al. Biological processes associated with breast cancer clinical outcome depend on the molecular subtypes. Clin Cancer Res. 2008;14:5158-65.
[191] Wang Y, Klijn JG, Zhang Y, Sieuwerts AM, Look MP, Yang F, et al. Gene-expression profiles to predict distant metastasis of lymph-node-negative primary breast cancer. Lancet Oncol. 2005;365:671-9.
[192] Rakha EA, Reis-Filho JS, Baehner F, Dabbs DJ, Decker T, Eusebi V, et al. Breast cancer prognostic classification in the molecular era: the role of histological grade. Breast Cancer Res. 2010;12:207.
[193] Desmedt C, Piette F, Loi S, Wang Y, Lallemand F, Haibe-Kains B, et al. Strong time dependence of the 76-gene prognostic signature for node-negative breast cancer patients in the TRANSBIG multicenter independent validation series. Clin Cancer Res. 2007;13:3207-14.
[194] Chin S-F, Teschendorff AE, Marioni JC, Wang Y, Barbosa-Morais NL, Thorne NP, et al. High-resolution array-CGH and expression profiling identifies a novel genomic subtype of ER negative breast cancer. Genome Biol. 2007;8:R215.
[195] Blenkiron C, Goldstein LD, Thorne NP, Spiteri I, Chin SF, Dunning MJ, et al. MicroRNA expression profiling of human breast cancer identifies new markers of tumour subtype. . Genome Biol. 2007;8:R214.
[196] Russnes HG, Vollan HK, Lingjaerde OC, Krasnitz A, Lundin P, Naume B, et al. Genomic architecture characterizes tumor progression paths and fate in breast cancer patients. . Sci Transl Med. 2010;2:38ra47.
[197] Berns K, Horlings HM, Hennessy BT, Madiredjo M, Hijmans EM, Beelen K, et al. A functional genetic approach identifies the PI3K pathway as a major determinant of trastuzumab resistance in breast cancer. . Cancer Cell. 2007;12:395-402.

[198] Ayers M, Symmans WF, Stec J, Damokosh AI, Clark E, Hess K, et al. Gene expression profiles predict complete pathologic response to neoadjuvant paclitaxel and fluorouracil, doxorubicin, and cyclophosphamide chemotherapy in breast cancer. J Clin Oncol. 2004;22:2284-93.

[199] Iwao-Koizumi K, Matoba R, Ueno N, Kim SJ, Ando A, Miyoshi Y, et al. Prediction of docetaxel response in human breast cancer by gene expression profiling. J Clin Oncol. 2005;23:422-31.

[200] Hess KR, Anderson K, Symmans WF, Valero V, Ibrahim N, Mejia JA, et al. Pharmacogenomic predictor of sensitivity to preoperative chemotherapy with paclitaxel and fluorouracil, doxorubicin, and cyclophosphamide in breast cancer. J Clin Oncol. 2006;24:4236-44.

[201] Thuerigen O, Schneeweiss A, Toedt G, Warnat P, Hahn M, Kramer H, et al. Gene expression signature predicting pathologic complete response with gemcitabine, epirubicin, and docetaxel in primary breast cancer. J Clin Oncol 2006;24:1839-45.

[202] Peintinger F, Anderson K, Mazouni C, Kuerer HM, Hatzis C, Lin F, et al. Thirty-gene pharmacogenomic test correlates with residual cancer burden after preoperative chemotherapy for breast cancer. . Clin Cancer Res. 2007;13:4078-82.

[203] Tabchy A, Valero V, Vidaurre T, Lluch A, Gomez H, Martin M, et al. Evaluation of a 30-gene paclitaxel, fluorouracil, doxorubicin, and cyclophosphamide chemotherapy response predictor in a multicenter randomized trial in breast cancer. Clin Cancer Res. 2010;16:5351-61.

[204] Kok M, Linn S, Laar R. Comparison of gene expression profiles predicting progression in breast cancer patients treated with tamoxifen. Breast Cancer Res Treat. 2009;113:275–83.

[205] Miller WR, Larionov A, Renshaw L, Anderson TJ, Walker JR, Krause A, et al. Gene expression profiles differentiating between breast cancer clinically responsive or resistant to letrozole. J Clin Oncol. 2009;27:1382–7.

[206] Potti A, Dressman HK, Bild A, Riedel RF, Chan G, Sayer R, et al. Genomic signatures to guide the use of chemotherapeutics. Nat Med. 2006;12:1294-300.

[207] Bonnefoi H, Potti A, Delorenzi M, Mauriac L, Campone M, Tubiana-Hulin M, et al. Validation of gene signatures that predict the response of breast cancer to neoadjuvant chemotherapy: a substudy of the EORTC 10994/BIG 00-01 clinical trial. Lancet Oncol. 2007;8:1071-8.

[208] Liedtke C, Wang J, Tordai A, Symmans WF, Hortobagyi GN, Kiesel L, et al. Clinical evaluation of chemotherapy response predictors developed from breast cancer cell lines. Breast Cancer Res Treat. 2010;121:301-9.

[209] Collingridge D. Expression of concern--validation of gene signatures that predict the response of breast cancer to neoadjuvant chemotherapy: a substudy of the EORTC 10994/BIG 00-01 clinical trial. Lancet Oncol. 2010;11:813-4.

[210] Farmer P, Bonnefoi H, Anderle P, Cameron D, Wirapati P, Becette V, et al. A stroma-related gene signature predicts resistance to neoadjuvant chemotherapy in breast cancer. Nat Med. 2009;15:68-74.

[211] Ashworth A, Lord CJ, Reis-Filho JS. Genetic interactions in cancer progression and treatment. Cell. 2011;145:30-8.

Chapter 2

Biomarkers in Lung Cancer: Integration with Radiogenomics Data

Elena Aréchaga-Ocampo, Nicolas Villegas-Sepulveda, Eduardo Lopez-Urrutia, Mayra Ramos-Suzarte, César López-Camarillo, Carlos Perez-Plasencia, Claudia H. Gonzalez-de la Rosa, Cesar Cortes-Gonzalez and Luis A. Herrera

Additional information is available at the end of the chapter

http://dx.doi.org/10.5772/53426

1. Introduction

Lung cancer remains as one of the most aggressive cancer types with nearly 1.6 million new cases worldwide each year. There are an estimated 222,520 new cases and 157,300 deaths from lung cancer in the United States in 2010 [1]. Non-small cell lung cancer (NSCLC) is the most common subtype of lung cancer, comprising three major histological subtypes: adenocarcinoma, squamous cell carcinoma, and large cell carcinoma. Chronic exposure to carcinogens drives genetic and epigenetic damage that can result in lung epithelial cells progressively acquiring growth and/or survival advantages, giving as a result the generation of tumor cells. Studies have shown that some specific molecules contribute to sporadic tumors of lung cancer; even now, they are useful as predictive biomarkers. Mutations in at least one of the established lung cancer driver genes including *egfr, kras, braf, her2, akt1, nras, pik3ca, mek1, eml4-alk* and *met* amplification are found in approximately 60% of tumor specimens, and greater than 90% were "exclusive": only one mutation was found in a particular tumor [2]. Epidermal growth factor receptor (EGFR) exhibits overexpression or aberrant activation by mutations in 50 to 90% of NSCLC. Much effort has been focused on the development of targeted molecular inhibitors for this molecule, but it has become clear that molecular-targeted cancer therapies can only reach their full potential through appropriate patient selection. Conventional therapies as chemo- and radiotherapy continue being the first option of treatment for lung cancer patients, even their mutation status of NSCLC driver genes. Radiotherapy, alone or in combination with surgery, chemotherapy or biological therapies, play a critical role in the management of lung cancer. Currently, there are several clinical studies in radiation response of NSCLC tumors, which exhibit a wide spectrum of response to this modality treatment. Thus, a successful radiation sensitivity assay to calculate individual tumor radioresponse is central for the development of personalized strategies in radio-oncology. Some research groups have done effort in radiogenomics and proteomics in lung cancer with the purpose of finding specific molecules to predict resistance or sensibility to radiotherapy. NSCLC tumors with mutations in well-known molecular markers as EGFR and KRAS represent two molecularly distinct tumor entities, with different clinical behaviors. In this chapter we focus on the biomarkers used as biological therapy targets in lung cancer and their impact on resistance to therapeutic interventions. Moreover, we highlight genomic and proteomic data in radiation response to lung cancer.

2. Lung cancer

Lung cancer remains as one of the most aggressive cancer types with nearly 1.6 million new cases worldwide each year. In 2010, in the United States were estimated 222,520 new cases and 157,300 deaths from lung cancer [1]. Non-small cell lung cancer (NSCLC) subtype represents 85% of all cases of lung cancer, while small cell lung cancer (SCLC) subtype comprises 15%. Histologically, NSCLC is classified as adenocarcinoma, squamous cell carcinoma, and large cell carcinoma. This classification has important implications for the clinical management and prognosis of the disease [3]. Yet early detection methods are not extensively used in the wider population, malignancy is most commonly diagnosed at a late stage resulting in poor patient survival. Overall 5-year survival rates for lung cancer vary globally but are consistently low (7.5-16%) [1]. Approximately 40% of patients with advanced unresectable disease at the time of diagnosis have a poor prognosis. At present, no single chemo-radiation therapy regimen can be considered standard; despite the treatment choice for unresectable stage III NSCLC, a platinum-based chemotherapy regimen and thoracic radiation are concurrently administered. Chemotherapy concurrently with chest radiation therapy significantly improves the survival of patients with unresectable stage IIIA and IIIB disease. Decades of research have increased understanding the lung cancer as a multistep process involving genetic and epigenetic alterations, through which, resulting DNA damage transforms normal epithelial cells that progressively acquire growth and/or survival advantages until cancer arises [2,4-7]. Malignant transformation of lung epithelial cells is characterized by genetic instability, which can exist at the chromosomal level (with large-scale loss or gain of genomic material, translocations, and microsatellite instability) or at the nucleotide level (with single or several nucleotide base changes). Moreover, lung cancer is also related to genomic and epigenomic changes at the transcriptome (with altered gene and microRNA expression) and proteome [8-11] level. As many kinds of tumors, molecular abnormalities in lung cancer cells are typically targeted to proto-oncogenes, tumor suppressor genes, DNA repair genes, and other genes that can promote outgrowth and immortality of affected cells [12,13]. It is accepted that the successful discovery, validation and implementation of specific molecular markers for early diagnosis, clinical surveillance and determination of tumor response to therapeutic intervention could improve survival rates for patients, but only few biomarkers turned out to be useful in the clinic. *egfr* and *kras* gene mutations are prognosis markers in NSCLC [2,12,14]. Because of the importance of EGFR as a prognostic factor in NSCLC, mutated EGFR has been the target for development of biological therapies; at present, these therapies are being used in treatment of a certain group of patients [15]. In this context, current research focuses on identifying other potential molecular targets for the development of new agents and the assessment of better combinations of established therapies. Intensive research has originated numerous potential lung carcinoma molecular biomarkers related to therapy response in order to establish an appropriate molecular selection of patients, with focus on personalized medicine.

3. Genome biomarkers: The opening to personalized medicine in lung cancer

Nowadays, molecular and genetic studies have shown that some specific molecules contribute to sporadic tumors of lung cancer; they are useful as therapeutic targets and predictive biomarkers [16]. Recently, the National Cancer Institute's lung cancer mutation consortium (NCI's LCMC) performed such a study on more than 800 lung adenocarcinoma tumor specimens, examining mutations in established lung cancer driver genes (*egfr, kras, braf, her2, akt1, pik3ca, mek1, eml4-alk, met* amplification) [2]. Mutations in at least one of these genes were found in approximately 60% of tumor specimens, and greater than 90% were "exclusive", namely, only one mutation was found in a particular tumor. EGFR regulates important tumorigenic processes, including proliferation, apoptosis, angiogenesis, and invasion. EGFR, along with its ligands, is frequently overexpressed during the development and progression of NSCLC. *egfr* gene are amplified and over-expressed in 6% of NSCLC. However, activating mutations in exons 18 to 21 comprised in the kinase domain of EGFR (Figure 1) occur early in the development of adenocarcinomas with clinic characteristics like never-smoking, female sex and Asian ethnicity [7,15].

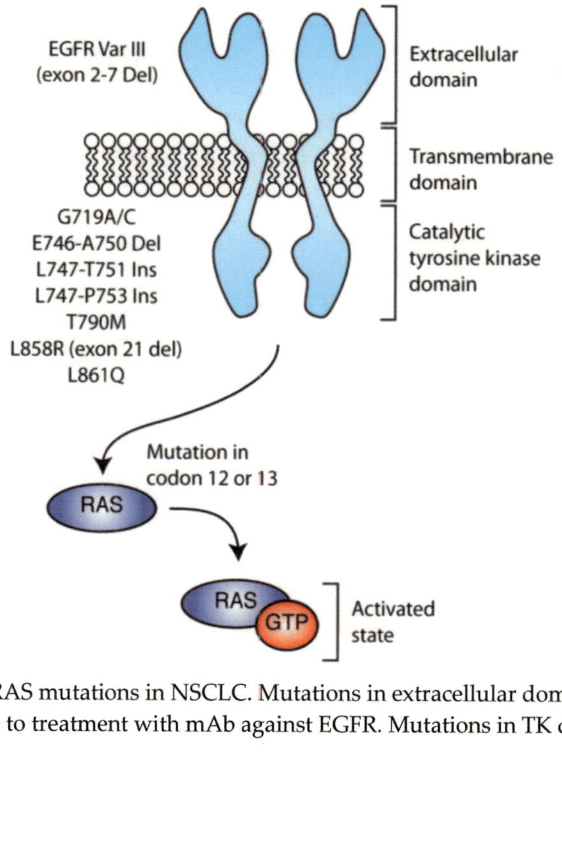

Figure 1. EGFR and KRAS mutations in NSCLC. Mutations in extracellular domain of EGFR have been implicated in resistance to treatment with mAb against EGFR. Mutations in TK domain are most

common in NSCLC, including L858R and E746-A750 deletion in exon 19. These mutations are target for small molecules inhibitors of tyrosine kinases domain (TKI). T790M is a mutation related to resistance to TKI treatment. Mutations in codon 12 or 13 of *kras* gene can lead to constantly union of GTP to KRAS protein, this represent the activate state of KRAS. GTP/KRAS induces activation of signaling depending to KRAS, permitting uncontrolled cell proliferation.

Mutated EGFR are present in 10-15% of NSCLC tumors [2,17]. Mutant EGFRs (either by exon 19 deletion or punctual mutation in exon 21 known as L858R) show an increased amount and duration of EGFR activation compared with wild-type receptors [18]. Mutated EGFR can activate RAS/RAF/MEK/MAPK and phosphoinositide 3-kinase (PI3K)/AKT and STAT3/STAT5 pathways [19-21]. Beside the importance of EGFR on lung carcinogenesis, some other molecules have been described as molecular markers for prognosis and therapeutic targets. Gene amplification and mutations in the kinase domain of C-erbB2 (HER-2/neu), a member of EGFR family, have been identified in patients with lung adenocarcinomas with a frequency of less than 5% and 5 to 10% respectively, and its overexpression are involved in ~25% of NSCLC cases [22]. EGFR and HER-2 kinase domain mutations have similar associations with female sex, non-smoking status and Asian background in patients with adenocarcinoma [15,22]. RAS/RAF/MEK/MAPK pathway is involved in signaling downstream from EGFR leading the growth and tumor progression in NSCLC. Activating *kras* gene mutation occurs in ~30% of cases of NSCLC, mostly adenocarcinomas. KRAS mutations are localized in exon 12 (in 90% of patients) or exon 13, and they are smoking-related G→T transversion and nonsmoking-related G→A transition [23]. KRAS mutations appear to be an early event in smoking-related lung adenocarcinoma, representing a poor prognosis in these patients. Another promising predictive markers in NSCLC are BRAF [24] and the oncogenic fusion gene of EML4-ALK [25]. BRAF, an effector molecule of RAS pathway, is mutated in about 2% of adenocarcinomas that does not show *kras* gene mutations. While *eml4-alk* is present in 2% to 7% of NSCLC cases; essentially, this fusion gene is present in young patients with adenocarcinoma and no exposure to smoking [26] (Figure 2).

Some other molecules have been identified based on expression and genomic data such as MYC and Cyclin D1 which are amplified and over-expressed in 2.5–10% and 5% of NSCLC respectively, while BCL-2 over-expression is involved in ~25% of cases of NSCLC [8,16]. Recent data have shown that methylation of the promoter regions of genes is a common event in NSCLC, which contributes to oncogenes over-expression or tumor genes suppressors silenced. These epigenetic changes may be an early event in NSCLC, since that promoter region of p16 gene is frequently methylated in smokers and premalignant lesion of lung cancer [27]. PI3K-AKT-mTOR pathway is altered in NSCLC. AKT overexpression has been described in a subgroup of NSCLC tumors jointly with mutations or amplification of PIK3CA gene. These genomic modifications are related with enhanced activity of PI3-K pathway mainly in squamous cell carcinoma tumors [28]. On the other hand, tissues of smoker patients show higher levels of angiogenic factors such as VEGF. VEGF expression increases in relationship with tumoral grade, which in turn, correlates with increased microvessel density, development and poor prognosis of lung cancer. Tumoral angiogenesis and angiogenic factors are regulated by hypoxic inductor factor (HIF) 1α and 2α or through oncogenes as *egfr, kras* and *p53* [29]. Genomics and proteomics tools have permitted the identification of molecules associated with a specific phenotype in cancer. Gene, microRNA and protein-expression signatures in lung cancer have allowed for the identification of molecules that show promise as biomarkers or therapeutic target for diagnosis, prognosis and therapeutic treatments [review 11,30]. The research focused on improving anti-tumor treatments in lung cancer has focused on genomic and proteomic study of tumors with specific genetic background, such as tumors with mutations in EGFR and KRAS. This molecular classification has had an influence on the response to biological therapies based on monoclonal antibodies (mAb) and tyrosine kinase inhibitors (TKIs) in lung cancer patients [15, 31-32], but now, we also know that the genetic background of lung tumors has an impact on the response to chemotherapy [33] and radiotherapy [34,35].

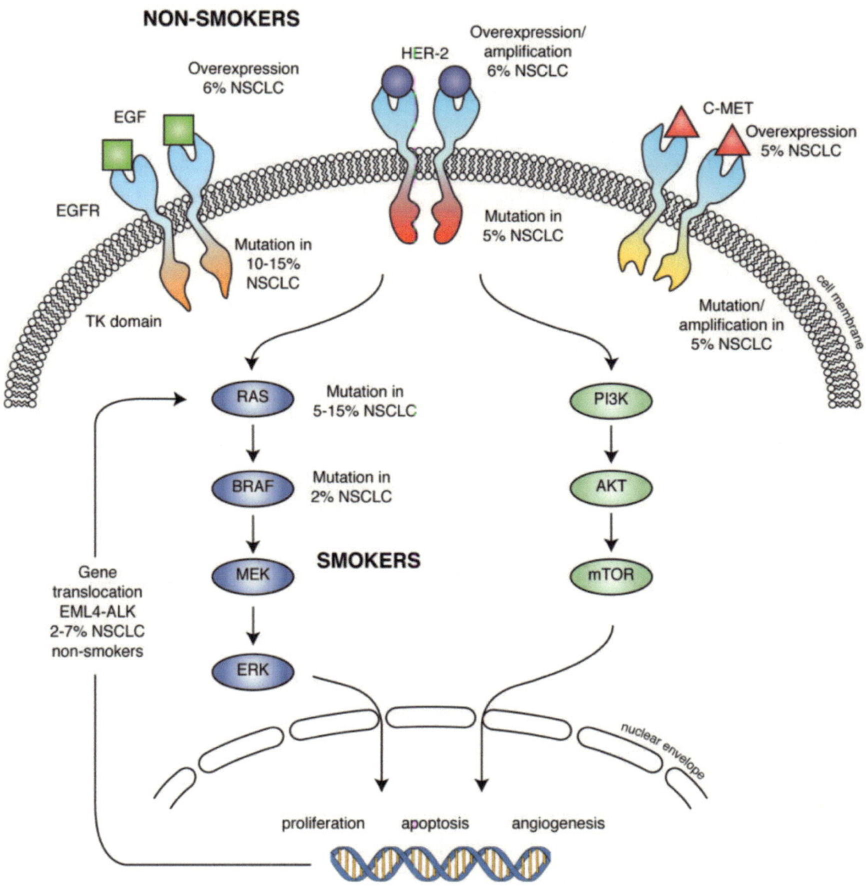

Figure 2. EGFR pathway in NSCLC. Mutations, amplification or overexpression of growth factors receptors such as EGFR, HER-2 and C-MET are most frequent in NSCLC tumors from non-smokers patients. All these genetic alterations have been observed commonly in adenocarcinomas, women and Asiatic ethnicity. EML4/ALK fusion gene is associated to NSCLC from young and non-smokers patients. KRAS mutations and signaling pathway depending to KRAS are most frequent in smoker patients. PI3K signaling pathway modifications are most frequently observed in squamous cell carcinomas.

4. Molecular and radiology therapies in lung cancer

4.1. Molecular therapy: Response and biological resistance

EGFR exhibits overexpression or aberrant activation in 50 to 90% of NSCLC. Mutations in EGFR allow sustained activation of EGF signaling for tumor cell survival, therefore, has been development targeted inhibitors for this molecule [16]. mAbs target the extracellular domain of EGFR and small molecules that inhibit intracellular EGFR tyrosine kinase domain function. In 2004, a significant advancement in the treatment of NSCLC was made following the observation that somatic mutations in the kinase domain of EGFR strongly correlated with sensitivity to EGFR TKIs [31, 32]. EGFR mutations are particularly prevalent in a patient subgroups with specific characteristics as adenocarcinoma histology, women, never smokers, and East Asian ethnicity [36]. This subgroup shows an exquisite sensitivity and marked tumor response to TKIs treatment. Despites the results obtained with biological therapies, there is a group of patients who do not respond to molecular therapy. Moreover, there is another group of patients with EGFR mutant lung cancer who initially respond to TKI treatment, but subsequently develop disease progression after a median of 10 to 14 months on treatment with biological therapy [37,38]. Hence, no optimal therapy thereafter has yet been established. Presumably, tumors do not respond because their molecular lesions are downstream of the therapeutic target [39]. Resistance to biologic therapy in NSCLC has been associated with EGFR exon-20 insertions [40] or a secondary T790M mutation [41], KRAS mutation [42], or amplification of the MET proto-oncogene [43,44], where MET is a transmembrane receptor with a tyrosine kinase domain, which activates signaling survival depending to PI3K and MAPK pathways. Of importance, Some reports showed that inhibition of MET signaling can restore sensitivity to TKIs [45]. HER-2 kinase domain mutations are associated with resistance to EGFR TKIs, but also with sensitivity to HER-2-targeted therapy [46].

Genomics data have provided information for developing targeted therapies in lung cancer patients based upon identification of cancer-specific vulnerabilities and set the stage for molecular biomarkers that provide information on clinical outcome and response to treatment. It has become clear that molecular-targeted cancer therapies can only reach their full potential through appropriate patient selection. In addition, there are now large clinical studies of lung cancer showing distinct chemotherapy and radiation responses. The majority of patients with lung cancer display advanced disease, these patients have obtained modest improvements in overall survival and quality of life through the use of systemic chemotherapy; however, the survival is still low, getting a median survival of 8 to 10 months [1]. Once recurred or metastasized, the disease is essentially incurable with survival rates at 5 years of less than 5%, and this has improved only marginally during the past 25 years [1]. The substantial genetic heterogeneity inherent to human cancers as an indicator of distinct phenotypes makes the identification of patients most likely to benefit from a given anticancer agent challenging. The description of molecules associated with resistance or sensitivity to cytotoxic treatments will improve personalized therapy for lung cancer. Radiotherapy, alone or in combination with surgery or chemotherapy, plays a critical role in the management of lung cancer. More than 60% of lung cancer patients receive radiotherapy at least once during the course of their disease [47].

4.2. Role of EGFR pathways in resistance and sensibility to radiotherapy

NSCLC tumors exhibit a wide response spectrum to radiation therapy but the molecular basis for this responsiveness is unknown. Some patients with NSCLC have a good response to radiation therapy with long-term local control while others relapse even with high dose treatment [48]. Many factors are involved in biological process of lung damage induced by radiation. At the molecular level, it is established that ionizing radiation causes various types of cellular damage; the creation of DNA breaks represents the principal damage induced by direct action of ionizing radiation or indirect action provoked by reactive species oxygen (ROS). Inadequately repaired DNA breaks leads to loss of cell clonogenicity via the generation of lethal chromosomal aberrations or the direct induction of apoptosis [49]. In addition to DNA breaks, ROS rapidly triggers the production of cytokines, growth factors, and more ROS, ultimately leading to chronic oxidative stress, hypoxia and the nonhealing tissue response in the lung [50,51]. Tumor radioresistance, including intrinsic resistance before treatments and acquired resistance during radiotherapy, is one of the main obstacles for radiotherapy efficiency for NSCLC. Some of the most important mechanisms associated with radioresistance in cancer including checkpoint pathway, mismatch repair process, and DNA damage repair [52-54]. Accumulating evidence suggests that radioresistance is often correlated with some genes, such as p53 [55] and EGFR [56]. In this regard, targeting EGFR pathway activation radiosensitizes human cancer cells [57-59], suggesting that the presence of overexpressed or activated oncogenes such as EGFR or RAS may be a mechanism for increased cellular resistance to radiation. In some models, it has been demonstrated that EGFR/Ras/Raf/MEK/ERK signaling may be activated in response to radiation, promoting cancer cell survival and proliferation [52-54,60] (Figure 3).

Variations in NSCLC responses to radiotherapy alone or in combination with chemotherapy or biological therapy are most likely due in the majority of cases to the genetic and epigenetic constitution of tumors [61,62]. In NSCLC, EGFR and KRAS oncogenes play an important role as prognostic factors; therefore, their role in radioresistance has been documented [63]. NSCLC cell lines harboring EGFR with mutations in tyrosine kinase domain were many folds more sensitive to radiation compared to cell lines with wild type EGFR. Radiosensitivity of NSCLC cell lines with mutant EGFR and human bronchial epithelial cells stably expressing mutant forms of EGFR was attributed to delayed DNA repair kinetics, defective radiation-induced arrest during DNA synthesis or mitosis, and pronounced increases in apoptosis or the occurrence of micronuclei [63]. Apparently, mutant EGFR is unable to translocate into the nucleus, which hinders its interaction with DNA-dependent protein kinase (DNA-PK), which is a fundamental enzyme for repair radiation-induced double strand breaks [63]. Besides of the promising role of mutant EGFR in radiosensitivity, the effort by blocking EGFR pathway to induce better response to radiotherapy has been limited. Inhibition of the EGFR by TKI or mAb, has been shown to

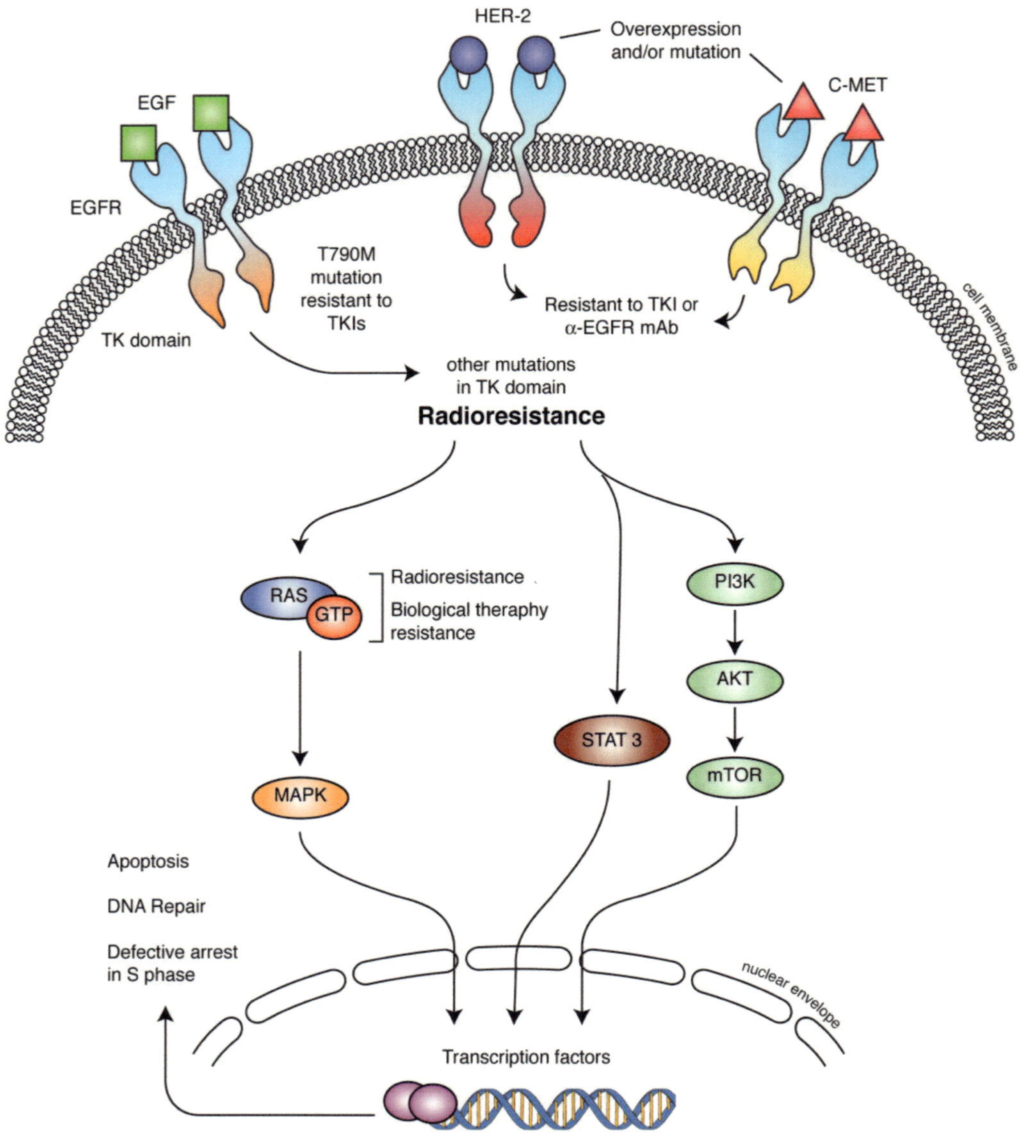

Figure 3. Role of EGFR pathway in radioresistance and radiosensibility in NSCLC. Aberrantly activation of EGFR pathways, including receptor mutations, KRAS activation, PI3K/AKT/mTOR pathway activation allows expression of specific genes for to regulate apoptosis, DNA repair, cell cycle and cell proliferation in order to get resistance to radiation.

radiosensitize a limited number of NSCLC cell lines *in vitro* and *in vivo* [34,35,63-65]. In NSCLC cell lines with wild-type or mutant p53, cell proliferation and clonogenic survival could be disturbed by senescence induced by EGFR inhibition and double strand breaks (DSB) produced by radiation. Apparently, radiosensitization by EGFR inhibitors is due to an increase in the levels of non-repairable DSB and disturbance of the MEK-ERK pathway [66]. Although a variety of signaling pathways downstream of EGFR have been implicated in radioresistance, including PI3K-AKT, MEK-ERK, and PLC-PKC [67-69], no evidence of a common molecular pathway of radiosensitization, and cellular mechanisms by which EGFR TKI and mAb may cause radiosensitization remained largely elusive. Activating KRAS mutations is a marker for worse prognosis in NSCLC [23, 26]. Sun *et al.* evaluated whether the presence of mutation could be a potential factor for radioresistance. The results showed a reduced level of apoptosis in response to radiation in lung cancer cell line HCC2429 transfected with mutant KRAS 12V (mutation in codon 12). The authors suggested that phosphorylation of ERK could contribute to the low levels of apoptosis induced by radiotherapy in mutated KRAS lung cancer cells. This work suggests that KRAS mutation status is one potential factor associated with increased resistance to radiation-induced apoptosis in lung cancer cells [70]. The same group has recently shown that the specific inhibition of JAK2 by the novel molecule TG101209, induces radiosensibility through inhibition of phosphorylation of STAT3 and reduced expression of survivin in HCC2429 lung cancer cells. Moreover, the inhibition of survivin by treatment with TG101209 in experiments *in vivo*, was related to increased apoptosis, reducing tumor proliferation and vascular density [70]. Lu *et al.* demonstrated that overexpression of survivin leads to radioresistance in H460 lung cancer cells by inhibiting apoptosis and promoting cell survival, however, when survivin is inhibited by antisense oligonucleotides the cytotoxic effect of radiation is enhanced [71]. These results suggested that survivin might be a molecular marker for prognostic response to radiotherapy in NSCLC. While inhibition of survivin expression in HCC2429 and H460 cells were related to radiosensibility, both cell lines showed different apoptosis levels which were related to radioresistance depending on KRAS mutation status.

5. Lung cancer radiogenomics

Radiotherapy has played a key role in the control of tumor growth in many cancer patients, including lung cancer. Studies that originated more than 40 years ago [72,73] have indicated that tumors respond to radiotherapy by initiating a process called accelerated repopulation. In this process, the few surviving cells that escaped death after exposure to radiotherapy or chemotherapy can rapidly repopulate the badly damaged tumor by proliferating at a markedly faster pace. This phenomenon suggested that tumoral heterogeneity permits a cell population in the tumor to have advantages to avoid cell death induced by radiation. Cellular senescence, DNA repair and cell cycle checkpoint are cellular mechanisms that influence the resistance to radiotherapy. However, the molecular mechanisms that regulate the radioresistance phenotype have not been clear in cancer. For this reason, some research groups have focused in the study of biological models to obtain genomic and proteomic signatures in order to find genes and proteins that could predict radiosensitivity or radioresistance in lung tumors (Table 1). Although such researches have contributed to a partial understanding of the mechanisms underlying cellular radioresistance, the comprehensive functional mechanisms remain largely elusive. This may be quite reasonable since the mechanisms of radioresistance are a complex multigene interaction. In this sense, Torres-Roca *et al.* [74] in 2005, hypothesized that a radiation sensitivity classifier or predictor could be developed based on gene expression profiles derived from DNA microarrays. This hypothesis was based in the fact of three main biological mechanisms partially correlated with clinical failure to radiotherapy, which are: hypoxia, intrinsic radiosensitivity and proliferation. These mechanisms, in turn, are handled by changes in gene expression.

Radiosensibility	
c-Jun*	[75]
HDAC-1	
RELA (p65 subunit NFkB	
PKC-beta	
Sumo1	
c-Ab1	
STAT1	
AR	
CDK1	
IRF1	
Innate Radioresistance	
Up-regulated in basal condition	[76]
XRCC5	
ERCC5	
ERCC1	
RAD9A	
ERCC4	
Up-regulated after radiation	[76]
MDM2*	
BCL-2	
PKC-2	
PIM2	
Acquired Radioresistance	
Up-regulated	[77]
DDB2	
LOX	
CDH2	
CR4AB	
Livin α*	[79]
Down-regulated	[77]
GBP-1	
CD83	
TNNC1	
TP53I3*	[78]

* Validated genes

Table 1. Genes associated to radiation response in NSCLC from genomics data

The authors developed a radiation classifier to calculate the radiosensitivity of tumor cell lines based on basal gene expression profiles obtained from the literature. They predicted the survival fraction to 2 Gy (SF2) value in 22 of 35 cell lines from the National Cancer Institute, a result significantly different from chance ($P = 0.0002$). In their approach, radiation sensitivity as a continuous variable, significance analysis of microarrays is used for gene selection, and a multivariate linear regression model is used for radiosensitivity prediction. In gene selection, they identified three novel genes: RbAp48, RGS19, and R5PIA, whose expression values correlated with radiation sensitivity. Exogenous overexpression of RbAp48 into three cancer cell lines (HS-578T, MALME-3M, and MDA-MB-231) induced radiosensitization (1.5- to 2-fold), moreover, higher proportion of transfected cells with RbAp48 were in G2-M phase of the cell cycle (27% versus 5%). Finally, RbAp48 overexpression is correlated with dephosphorylation of Akt, suggesting that RbAp48 might be exerting its effect radiosensitized by antagonizing the Ras pathway, but it could also do so through PI3K. The authors establish that radiation sensitivity can be predicted based on gene expression profiles and they introduce a genomic approach to the identification of novel molecular markers of radiation sensitivity. Despite of results in different tumor cell lines, this work included only four NSCLC cell lines and they were able to predict correct SF2 values for only two of them [74]. So, the study should be performed on a broader panel of NSCLC cell lines. In lung cancer, multiple studies have identified a wide array of genetic and epigenetic alterations, including mutations in DNA sequence, DNA copy number changes, aberrant DNA promoter methylation, changes in mRNA, microRNAs and protein expression [8], revealing many potential determinants and signaling pathways governing lung tumorigenesis and progression. Gene expression profiling analysis allows for an increase in the understanding of the molecular mechanisms and pathways that involve radioresistance. Thus, the strategy followed by Torres-Roca and collaborators can be applied to gene expression data reported in lung cancer, in order to identify new molecular targets for radiotherapy response. In this sense, we know that the response of tumor cells to radiation is accompanied by complex changes in the gene expression pattern. Based on mRNA expression profiles and systems-biology approach, Eschrich *et al.* [75] applied a linear regression algorithm that integrates gene expression with biological variables, including RAS and p53 status (mut/wt), and tissue of origin, with the aim of understanding radiosensitivity and identifying radiation specific markers. The modeling of radiosensitivity represented for the survival fraction at 2 Gy of 48 human cancer cell lines reported a direct correlation between gene expression and radiosensitivity of the lung cancer cell lines. The authors developed a model that classified four different clusters of genes that were markers for radiosensitivity. They identified 10 gene networks comprised by c-Jun, HDAC1, RELA (p65 subunit of NFKB), PKC-beta, SUMO-1, c-Abl, STAT1, AR, CDK1 and IRF1. Interestingly, RAS was a dominant variable in the analysis, as was the tissue of origin (lung), and their interaction with gene expression but not with p53. Moreover, when they knocked-down c-Jun in eight different cancer cell lines (lung, colon and breast cancer) there was an overall trend toward radioresistance, predominantly in lung cancers, but not in breast or colon cancers, implying that the origin of the tissue was important [75].

A problem in radiogenomics research is the difficulty to determine what fraction of the tumor cell population is radioresistant after a course of radiotherapy. For understand the radiation-mediated changes in gene expression that might result in different responses to radiation, Guo W *et al.* in 2005 [76] designed an oligonucleotide microarray to analyze the expression of 143 genes in lung cancer cell lines that differed in radiosensitivity. In the radioresistant A549 cells, 8 genes were significantly up-regulated and 10 genes were down-regulated compared to radiosensitivity NCI-H446 cells. When the lung cancer cell lines were irradiated with 5Gy of γ rays, they identified genes showing altered expression and potential candidate genes that might confer radioresistance. In A549 cells, 19 up-regulated and 3 down-regulated genes, and 8 up-regulated and 18 down-regulated genes were found 6 and 24 h after irradiation, respectively. In NCI-H446 cells, the expression of 9 up-regulated and 8 down-regulated genes, and 8 up-regulated and 12 down-regulated genes was altered 6 and 24 h after irradiation, respectively. They found that MDM2, BCL2, PKCZ and PIM2 expression levels were increased in A549 cells and decreased in NCI-H446 cells after irradiation. Whereas, XRCC5, ERCC5, ERCC1, RAD9A, ERCC4 and the gene encoding DNA-PK were found to be increased to a higher level in A549 cells than in NCI-H446 cells. Inhibition of MDM2 by an antisense oligonucleotide in A549 cells resulted in increased radiosensitivity. The authors demonstrate the possibility that a group of genes involved in DNA repair, regulation of the cell cycle, cell proliferation and apoptosis are responsible for the different endogenous radioresistance between these two lung cancer cell lines [76]. To continue searching for new molecular evidences for radioresistance, Qing-Yong *et al.* in 2008 identified gene expression profiles in lung adenocarcinoma cell line Anip973 and obtained radioresistant phenotype cells (Anip973R). Expression profiles were obtained by oligonucleotide microarrays consisting of 21,522 human genes, while radioresistant cells Anip973R were obtained by fractionated ionizing radiation treatment of 4 Gy until a total dose of 60 Gy. In Anip973R cells, the authors reported 59 up-regulated genes associated with DNA damage repair (DDB2), extracellular matrix (LOX), cell adhesion (CDH2), and apoptosis (CRYAB); and 43 down-regulated genes associated with angiogenesis (GBP-1), immune response (CD83), and calcium signaling pathway (TNNC1). Validation of the selected eleven genes, including CD24, DDB2, IGFBP3, LOX, CDH2, CRYAB, PROCR, ANXA1 DCN, GBP-1 and CD83 by Q-RT-PCR was consistent with microarray analysis [77]. In 2010, Lee *et al.*. analyzed expression profiles of H460 NSCLC radiosensitive cell lines and their radioresistant counterpart (H460R) cells established by fractionated irradiation. By utilizing a cDNA microarray, they identified 1,463 genes altered more than 1.5-fold in H460R compared with parental H460. Tumor protein p53-inducible protein 3 (TP53I3) gene was significantly down-regulated in radioresistant H460R cells predicting a link to p53-dependent cell death signaling. Interestingly, mRNA expression of TP53I3 differed in X-ray–irradiated H460 and H460R cells, and overexpression of TP53I3 significantly affected the cellular radiosensitivity of H460R cells [78]. These works showed that fractionated ionizing radiation can lead to the development of acquired radiation resistance across altered gene profiles. Genomic profile using *in vivo* models of radioresistance may provide new insights into mechanisms underlying the promotion of clinical resistance for NSCLC. Some other researches have been focused in describing specific molecules that revert the radioresistant phenotype. It is well known that there is a large amount of cell death during cytotoxic cancer therapy such as radiotherapy; therefore, radioresistance is associated with deregulation of apoptosis proteins. Sun *et al.* in 2011 reported the role of livin in radioresistance of lung adenocarcinomas cell lines A549 and SPC-A1. Livin is a IAPs family member whose expression is related with apoptosis inhibition, in some studies, it has been suggested that livin may be of clinical significance [79]. This work showed that A549 lung adenocarcinoma cells do not express livin in basal condition, but it is expressed after cells were irradiated. Moreover, gene silencing of livin by siRNA in SPC-A1 lung cell line induced a remarkable sensibility to radiation. Additionally, the authors showed that the isoform livin α had more impact on radioresistance that livin β had. These results suggested that livin expression in lung adenocarcinoma cells could be a radioresistance mechanism through down-regulation of apoptosis. The cytotoxicity of oncological therapies is highly dependent on the cell cycle phase. G2/M phase is the one most sensitive to ionizing radiation. A work published in 2010 determined that arresting time on G2/M cell cycle phase is different between NSCLC cell lines sensitive and resistance to ionizing radiation. Radiosensitive H460 NSCLC cell line showed a significant G2/M arrest after 12 h of irradiation with 5 Gy of γ rays, while radioresistant A549 cell lines showed a significant G2/M arrest after 12 h of radiation. Interestingly, the arrest in A549 completely disappeared after 24 h of radiation. The arrest on G2/M correlated with higher methylated CpG sites of PTEN gene and consequently, reducing expression of the protein. PTEN negatively regulate pAKT which regulate negatively to p53. Therefore, radioresistance of A549 may depend to over activation of p53 signaling pathways. Epigenetic gene modification may be a way for regulating genes that participate in radiation response [80]. Signal transduction pathways depending to STAT have been explored. In A549 and SK-MES-1 cells, the exogenous over-expression of STAT3 was evaluated for its role in radioresponse. STAT3 over-expression enhanced the sensitivity to ionizing radiation *in vitro* and *in vivo*. Apparently, the radiosensibility may induce through STAT3-dependent inhibition of growth and induction of apoptosis [81]. These works showed that the regulation of signaling molecules that control apoptosis, cell growth and cell cycle has an important role in positive or negative radiation response.

6. Proteomics of radiation response in lung cancer

Despite proteomics being useful to find molecular markers associated to lung cancer cells [82], in radiation resistance research there are very few studies focused on applying proteomics to find new markers associated to radiotherapy response in lung cancer. Recently, Wei R *et al.* [83] in 2012 evaluated the multidrug resistance (MDR) effect on the radioresistance (RDR) in human lung adenocarcinoma cell lines and tissues. In this work, the authors screen MDR- and RDR-related proteins after irradiation of A549 and A549/DDP (resistant to cisplatin) human lung adenocarcinoma cells. The cell lines were analyzed by colony-forming assay and flow cytometry. Two-dimensional electrophoresis (2-DE) and matrix-assisted laser desorption/ionization time-of-flight mass spectrometry (MALDI-

TOF–MS) were utilized to identify differentially expressed proteins between irradiated A549 and A549/DDP. The SF2 value increased and the mean percentage of G2 phase and apoptosis rate decreased significantly in A549/DDP cells compared with A549 cells. Forty spots were found, and among them, 27 were identified through proteomics. Four up-regulated proteins (HSPB1, Vimentin, Cofilin-1, and Annexin A4) were confirmed by Western blot in MDR cells as compared with non-MDR cells. Immunohistochemistry showed that they were also over-expressed in MDR tissues compared with non-MDR counterparts of human lung adenocarcinomas. These results proved that the MDR in lung adenocarcinoma cells and tissues increased the radioresistance. HSPB1, Vimentin, Cofilin-1, and Annexin A4 are potential biomarkers for predicting lung adenocarcinomas response to chemo- and radiotherapy, as well as novel targets for treatment of lung adenocarcinomas [83].

7. Conclusion

One of the most important problems in lung oncology is lack of suitable biomarkers as therapeutic targets or the absence of predictors of therapy response. The genetic heterogeneity of the lung tumors influences the initial molecular resistance to therapies, but also in the development of resistance during treatment. The molecular mechanisms that influence the resistance to biological or radiological treatments, referring to the resistance mechanisms occurring naturally because of the carcinogenic process, or those developing as a result of evolutionary pressure that tumor cells undergoing during the treatment administration, is a barrier that has not been fully elucidated. With current genomics and proteomics studies in lung cancer focused on solving the mystery of therapeutic resistance, it has been possible to identify molecules that may serve as prognostic markers of response to radiological and molecular therapy resistance. Genes and proteins that regulate cell proliferation and survival, including signaling molecules and transcription factors such as KRAS, BRAF, PI3K, MAPK, mTOR, JAK2, STAT, survivin and others have demonstrated to be part of the molecular machinery that regulates therapeutic resistance. Moreover, gene and protein expression profiling of lung cancer has focused specifically on searching predictive markers to radiotherapy. Some studies have generated data on molecules involved in radioresistance or radiosensitivity either natural or acquired. Using therapeutic doses of radiation in *in vitro* models, it have described proteins implicated in DNA repair, cell cycle checkpoint and cell death. Mutations in EGFR pathway have played an important role as therapeutic targets for development of new therapies, moreover, mutations in this pathway represent a mechanism of radioresistance, suggesting that aberrant activation of EGFR pathway, including activated mutations in EGFR and KRAS might be an innate radioresistance mechanism in NSCLC. Despite advances in proteomics and radiogenomics in lung cancer, an enormous need to implement *in vivo* and clinical models for identification of effective biomarkers predictive in radio-oncology has also became evident. This is currently a promising field of cancer research in which genomics, tumor molecular biology and clinical experience interact to achieve more effective combination therapies adjusted to the patient profile. Understanding the mechanisms of radioresistance of cells from solid tumors is of prime importance for further improvement of radiotherapy.

Author details

Elena Aréchaga-Ocampo*
Oncogenomics Lab, National Institute of Cancerology, Mexico

Nicolas Villegas-Sepulveda
Department of Molecular Biomedicine. Center for Research and Advanced Studies of the National Polytechnic Institute, Mexico

Eduardo Lopez-Urrutia
Molecular Biochemistry Lab, UBIPRO, FES-I, National Autonomous University of Mexico, Mexico

Mayra Ramos-Suzarte
Center of Molecular Immunology, Atabey, Havana, Cuba

César López-Camarillo
Genomics Science Program, Oncogenomics and Cancer Proteomics Lab, Autonomous University of Mexico City, Mexico

Carlos Perez-Plasencia
Oncogenomics Lab, National Institute of Cancerology, Mexico
Massive Sequencing Unite, National Institute of Cancerology-Genomics Lab, FES-I, UBIMED, National Autonomous University of Mexico, Mexico

Claudia H. Gonzalez-de la Rosa
Department of Natural Science, Metropolitan Autonomous University-C, Mexico

Cesar Cortes-Gonzalez and Luis A. Herrera
Cancer Biomedical Research Unit, National Institute of Cancerology-Biomedical Research Institute National Autonomous University of Mexico, Mexico

Acknowledgement

Authors gratefully acknowledge the financial support from the National Council of Science and Technology (CONACyT), Mexico (grants 115552 and 115591), and The Institute of Science and Technology (ICyT-DF), Mexico (grant PIUTE147).

8. References

[1] Jemal A, Bray F, Center MM, Ferlay J, Ward E, Forman D. Global cancer statistics. CA Cancer Journal for Clinician 2011; 61(2) 69-90.

---

* Corresponding Author

[2] Kris MG, Johnson BE, Kwiatkowski DJ, Iafrate AJ, Wistuba II, Aronson SL, Engelman JA, Shyr Y, Khuri FR, Rudin CM, Garon EB, Pao W, Schiller JH, Haura EB, Shirai K, Giaccone G, Berry LD, Kugler K, Minna JD, Bunn PA. Identification of driver mutations in tumor specimens from 1000 patients with lung adenocarcinoma: the NCI's lung cancer mutation consortium (LCMC) [abstract CRA7506]. Journal of Clinical Oncology 2011; 29(Suppl).

[3] Wistuba II, Gazdar AF. Lung cancer preneoplasia. Annual Review of Pathology 2006; 1 331-348.

[4] Sekido Y, Fong KM, Minna JD. Progress in understanding the molecular pathogenesis of human lung cancer. Biochemical and Biophysical Acta 1998; 1378(1) F21-59.

[5] Silvestri GA, Alberg AJ, Ravenel J. The changing epidemiology of lung cancer with a focus on screening. British Medical Journal 2009; 339 451-454.

[6] Mao L, Lee JS, Kurie JM, Fan YH, Lippman SM, Lee JJ, Ro JY, Broxson A, Yu R, Morice RC, Kemp BL, Khuri FR, Walsh GL, Hittelman WN, Hong WK. Clonal genetic alterations in the lungs of current and former smokers. Journal of National Cancer Institute 1997; 89(12) 857-862.

[7] Sun S, Schiller JH, Gazdar AF. Lung cancer in never smokers-a different disease. Nature Reviews Cancer 2007; 7(10) 778-790.

[8] Nikliński J, Niklińska W, Laudanski J, Chyczewska E, Chyczewski L. Prognostic molecular markers in non-small cell lung cancer. Lung Cancer 2001; 4-Suppl 2 S53-58.

[9] Enfield KS, Pikor LA, Martinez VD, Lam WL. Mechanistic roles of noncoding RNAs in lung cancer biology and their clinical implications. Genetic Research International 2012; 2012 ID:737416.

[10] Belinsky SA. Gene-Promoter Hypermethylation as a biomarker in lung cancer. Nature Reviews Cancer 2004; 4(9) 707-717.

[11] Cho JY, Sung HJ. Proteomic approaches in lung cancer biomarker development. Expert Review of Proteomics 2009; 6(1) 27-42.

[12] Sato M, Shames DS, Gazdar AF, Minna JD. A translational view of the molecular pathogenesis of lung cancer. Journal of Thoracic Oncology 2007; 2(4) 327-343.

[13] Lee W, Jiang Z, Liu J, Haverty PM, Guan Y, Stinson J, Yue P, Zhang Y, Pant KP, Bhatt D, Ha C, Johnson S, Kennemer MI, Mohan S, Nazarenko I, Watanabe C, Sparks AB, Shames DS, Gentleman R, de Sauvage FJ, Stern H, Pandita A, Ballinger DG, Drmanac R, Modrusan Z, Seshagiri S, Zhang Z. The mutation spectrum revealed by paired genome sequences from a lung cancer patient. Nature 2010; 465(7297) 473-477.

[14] Aviel-Ronen S, Blackhall FH, Shepherd FA, Tsao MS. K-ras mutations in non-small-cell lung carcinoma: a review. Clinical Lung Cancer 2006; 8(1) 30-38.

[15] Pao W, Miller V, Zakowski M, Doherty J, Politi K, Sarkaria I, Singh B, Heelan R, Rusch V, Fulton L, Mardis E, Kupfer D, Wilson R, Kris M, Varmus H. EGF receptor gene mutations are common in lung cancers from "never smokers" and are associated with sensitivity of tumors to gefitinib and erlotinib. Proceedings of the National Academy of Science USA 2004; 101(36) 13306-13311.

[16] Choong NW, Salgia R, Vokes EE. Key signaling pathways and targets in lung cancer therapy. Clinical Lung Cancer 2007; 8 Suppl 2 S52-S60.

[17] Tang X, Shigematsu H, Bekele BN, Roth JA, Minna JD, Hong WK, Gazdar AF, Wistuba II. EGFR tyrosine kinase domain mutations are detected in histologically normal respiratory epithelium in lung cancer patients. Cancer Research 2005; 65(17) 7568-7572.
[18] Lynch TJ, Bell DW, Sordella R, Gurubhagavatula S, Okimoto RA, Brannigan BW, Harris PL, Haserlat SM, Supko JG, Haluska FG, Louis DN, Christiani DC, Settleman J, Haber DA. Activating mutations in the epidermal growth factor receptor underlying responsiveness of non-small-cell lung cancer to gefitinib. New England Journal of Medicine 2004; 350(21) 2129-2139.
[19] Sordella R, Bell DW, Haber DA, Settleman J. Gefitinib sensitizing EGFR mutations in lung cancer activate anti-apoptotic pathways. Science 2004; 305(5687) 1163-1167.
[20] de Mello RA, Marques DS, Medeiros R, Araujo AM. Epidermal growth factor receptor and K-Ras in non-small cell lung cancer-molecular pathways involved and targeted therapies. World Journal of Clinical Oncology 2011; 2(11) 367-376.
[21] Li H, Schmid-Bindert G, Wang D, Zhao Y, Yang X, Su B, Zhou C. Blocking the PI3K/AKT and MEK/ERK signaling pathways can overcome gefitinib-resistance in non-small cell lung cancer cell lines. Advances in Medical Science 2011; 56(2) 275-284.
[22] Shigematsu H, Takahashi T, Nomura M, Majmudar K, Suzuki M, Lee H, Wistuba II, Fong KM, Toyooka S, Shimizu N, Fujisawa T, Minna JD, Gazdar AF. Somatic mutations of the HER2 kinase domain in lung adenocarcinomas. Cancer Research 2005; 65(5) 1642-1646.
[23] Riely GJ, Kris MG, Rosenbaum D, Marks J, Li A, Chitale DA, Nafa K, Riedel ER, Hsu M, Pao W, Miller VA, Ladanyi M. Frequency and distinctive spectrum of KRAS mutations in never smokers with lung adenocarcinoma. Clinical Cancer Research 2008; 14(18) 5731-5734.
[24] Kobayashi M, Sonobe M, Takahashi T, Yoshizawa A, Ishikawa M, Kikuchi R, Okubo K, Huang CL, Date H. Clinical significance of BRAF gene mutations in patients with non-small cell lung cancer. Anticancer Research 2011; 31(12) 4619-4623.
[25] Soda M, Choi YL, Enomoto M, Takada S, Yamashita Y, Ishikawa S, Fujiwara S, Watanabe H, Kurashina K, Hatanaka H, Bando M, Ohno S, Ishikawa Y, Aburatani H, Niki T, Sohara Y, Sugiyama Y, Mano H. Identification of the transforming EML4-ALK fusion gene in non-small cell lung cancer. Nature 2007; 448(7153) 561-566.
[26] Brose MS, Volpe P, Feldman M, Kumar M, Rishi I, Gerrero R, Einhorn E, Herlyn M, Minna J, Nicholson A, Roth JA, Albelda SM, Davies H, Cox C, Brignell G, Stephens P, Futreal PA, Wooster R, Stratton MR, Weber BL. BRAF and RAS mutations in human lung cancer and melanoma. Cancer Research 2002; 62(23) 6997-7000.
[27] Belinsky SA, Liechty KC, Gentry FD, Wolf HJ, Rogers J, Vu K, Haney J, Kennedy TC, Hirsch FR, Miller Y, Franklin WA, Herman JG, Baylin SB, Bunn PA, Byers T. Promoter hypermethylation of multiple genes in sputum precedes lung cancer incidence in a high-risk cohort. Cancer Research 2006; 66(6) 3338-3344.
[28] Rekhtman N, Paik PK, Arcila ME, Tafe LJ, Oxnard GR, Moreira AL, Travis WD, Zakowski MF, Kris MG, Ladanyi M. Clarifying the spectrum of driver oncogene mutations in biomarker-verified squamous carcinoma of lung: lack of EGFR/KRAS and presence of PIK3CA/AKT1 mutations. Clinical Cancer Research 2012; 18(4) 1167-1176.

[29] Giatromanolaki A. Prognostic role of angiogenesis in non-small cell lung cancer. Anticancer Research 2001; 6B 4373-4382.

[30] Vrabec-Branica B, Gajovic S. Molecular biomarkers of lung carcinoma. Front Bioscience. (Elite Ed). 2012; 4 865-875.

[31] Lynch TJ, Bell DW, Sordella R, Gurubhagavatula S, Okimoto RA, Brannigan BW, Harris PL, Haserlat SM, Supko JG, Haluska FG, Louis DN, Christiani DC, Settleman J, Haber DA. Activating mutations in the epidermal growth factor receptor underlying responsiveness of non-small-cell lung cancer to gefitinib. New England of Journal Medicine 2004; 350(21) 2129-2139.

[32] Paez JG, Jänne PA, Lee JC, Tracy S, Greulich H, Gabriel S, Herman P, Kaye FJ, Lindeman N, Boggon TJ, Naoki K, Sasaki H, Fujii Y, Eck MJ, Sellers WR, Johnson BE, Meyerson M. EGFR mutations in lung cancer: correlation with clinical response to gefitinib therapy. Science 2004; 304(5676) 1497-500.

[33] Eberhard DA, Johnson BE, Amler LC, Goddard AD, Heldens SL, Herbst RS, Ince WL, Jänne PA, Januario T, Johnson DH, Klein P, Miller VA, Ostland MA, Ramies DA, Sebisanovic D, Stinson JA, Zhang YR, Seshagiri S, Hillan KJ. Mutations in the epidermal growth factor receptor and in KRAS are predictive and prognostic indicators in patients with non-small-cell lung cancer treated with chemotherapy alone and in combination with erlotinib. Journal of Clinical Oncology 2005; 23(25) 5900-5909.

[34] Das AK, Sato M, Story MD. Non-small-cell lung cancers with kinase domain mutations in the epidermal growth factor receptor are sensitive to ionizing radiation. Cancer Research 2006; 66(19) 9601-9608.

[35] Raben D, Helfrich B, Bunn PA Jr. Targeted therapies for non-small-cell lung cancer: biology, rationale, and preclinical results from a radiation oncology perspective. International Journal of Radiation Oncology Biology Physic 2004; 59(2 Suppl) 27-38.

[36] Fujino S, Enokibori T, Tezuka N, Asada Y, Inoue S, Kato H, Mori A. A comparison of epidermal growth factor receptor levels and other prognostic parameters in non-small cell lung cancer. European Journal of Cancer 1996; 32A(12) 2070-2074.

[37] Rosell R, Moran T, Queralt C, Porta R, Cardenal F, Camps C, Majem M, Lopez-Vivanco G, Isla D, Provencio M, Insa A, Massuti B, Gonzalez-Larriba JL, Paz-Ares L, Bover I, Garcia Campelo R, Moreno MA, Catot S, Rolfo C, Reguart N, Palmero R, Sánchez JM, Bastus R, Mayo C, Bertran-Alamillo J, Molina MA, Sanchez JJ, Taron M; Spanish Lung Cancer Group. Screening for epidermal growth factor receptor mutations in lung cancer. New England of Journal Medicine 2009; 361(10) 958-967.

[38] Mok TS, Wu YL, Thongprasert S, Yang CH, Chu DT, Saijo N, Sunpaweravong P, Han B, Margono B, Ichinose Y, Nishiwaki Y, Ohe Y, Yang JJ, Chewaskulyong B, Jiang H, Duffield EL, Watkins CL, Armour AA, Fukuoka M. Gefitinib or carboplatin-paclitaxel in pulmonary adenocarcinoma. New England Journal of Medicine 2009; 361(10) 947-957.

[39] Gazdar AF. Activating and resistance mutations of EGFR in non-small-cell lung cancer: role in clinical response to EGFR tyrosine kinase inhibitors. Oncogene 2009; 28(Suppl 1) S24-31.

[40] Yasuda H, Kobayashi S, Costa DB. EGFR exon 20 insertion mutations in non-small-cell lung cancer: preclinical data and clinical implications. Lancet Oncology 2012; 13(1) e23-31.

[41] Pao W, Miller VA, Politi KA, Riely GJ, Somwar R, Zakowski MF, Kris MG, Varmus H. Acquired resistance of lung adenocarcinomas to gefitinib or erlotinib is associated with a second mutation in the EGFR kinase domain. PLoS Medicine 2005; 2(3) e73.

[42] Pao W, Wang TY, Riely GJ, Miller VA, Pan Q, Ladanyi M, Zakowski MF, Heelan RT, Kris MG, Varmus HE. KRAS mutations and primary resistance of lung adenocarcinomas to gefitinib or erlotinib. PLoS Medicine 2005; 2(1) e17.

[43] Bean J, Brennan C, Shih JY, Riely G, Viale A, Wang L, Chitale D, Motoi N, Szoke J, Broderick S, Balak M, Chang WC, Yu CJ, Gazdar A, Pass H, Rusch V, Gerald W, Huang SF, Yang PC, Miller V, Ladanyi M, Yang CH, Pao W. MET amplification occurs with or without T790M mutations in EGFR mutant lung tumors with acquired resistance to gefitinib or erlotinib. Proceedings of the National Academy of Science USA 2007; 104(52) 20932-20937.

[44] Engelman JA, Zejnullahu K, Mitsudomi T, Song Y, Hyland C, Park JO, Lindeman N, Gale CM, Zhao X, Christensen J, Kosaka T, Holmes AJ, Rogers AM, Cappuzzo F, Mok T, Lee C, Johnson BE, Cantley LC, Jänne PA. MET amplification leads to gefitinib resistance in lung cancer by activating ERBB3 signaling. Science 2007; 316(5827) 1039-1043.

[45] Xu L, Kikuchi E, Xu C, Ebi H, Ercan D, Cheng KA, Padera R, Engelman JA, Jänne PA, Shapiro GI, Shimamura T, Wong KK. Combined EGFR/MET or EGFR/HSP90 inhibition is effective in the treatment of lung cancers codriven by mutant EGFR containing T790M and MET. Cancer Research 2012; 72(13) 3302-3311.

[46] Wang SE, Narasanna A, Perez-Torres M, Xiang B, Wu FY, Yang S, Carpenter G, Gazdar AF, Muthuswamy SK, Arteaga CL. HER2 kinase domain mutation results in constitutive phosphorylation and activation of HER2 and EGFR and resistance to EGFR tyrosine kinase inhibitors. Cancer Cell 2006; 10 25-38.

[47] Kong FM, Ten Haken RK, Schipper MJ, Sullivan MA, Chen M, Lopez C, Kalemkerian GP, Hayman JA. High-dose radiation improved local tumor control and overall survival in patients with inoperable/unresectable non-small-cell lung cancer: long-term results of a radiation dose escalation study. International Journal of Radiation Oncology Biology Physics 2005; 63(2) 324-333.

[48] Bradley JD, Paulus R, Graham MV, Ettinger DS, Johnstone DW, Pilepich MV, Machtay M, Komaki R, Atkins J, Curran WJ; Radiation Therapy Oncology Group. Phase II trial of postoperative adjuvant paclitaxel/carboplatin and thoracic radiotherapy in resected stage II and IIIA non-small-cell lung cancer: promising long-term results of the Radiation Therapy Oncology Group-RTOG 9705. Journal of Clinical Oncology 2005; 23(15) 3480-3487.

[49] Willers H, Dahm-Daphi J, Powell SN. Repair of radiation damage to DNA. British Journal of Cancer 2004; 90 1297-1301.

[50] Marks LB, Yu X, Vujaskovic Z, Small W Jr, Folz R, Anscher MS. Radiation-induced lung injury. Seminars in Radiation Oncology 2003; 13(3) 333-345.

[51] Fleckenstein K, Gauter-Fleckenstein B, Jackson IL, Rabbani Z, Anscher M, Vujaskovic Z. Using biological markers to predict risk of radiation injury. Seminars Radiation Oncology 2007; 17(2) 89-98.

[52] Contessa JN, Hampton J, Lammering G, Mikkelsen RB, Dent P, Valerie K, Schmidt-Ullrich RK. Ionizing radiation activates Erb-B receptor dependent Akt and p70 S6 kinase signaling in carcinoma cells. Oncogene 2002; 21(25) 4032-4041.

[53] Bernhard EJ, Stanbridge EJ, Gupta S, Gupta AK, Soto D, Bakanauskas VJ, Cerniglia GJ, Muschel RJ, McKenna WG. Direct evidence for the contribution of activated N-ras and K-ras oncogenes to increased intrinsic radiation resistance in human tumor cell lines. Cancer Research 2000; 60(23) 6597-6600.

[54] Rodemann HP, Dittmann K, Toulany M. Radiation-induced EGFR signaling and control of DNA-damage repair. International Journal of Radiation Biology 2007; 83 781-791.

[55] Biard DS, Martin M, Rhun YL, Duthu A, Lefaix JL, May E, May P. Concomitant p53 gene mutation and increased radiosensitivity in rat lung embryo epithelial cells during neoplastic development. Cancer Research 1994; 54(13) 3361-3364.

[56] Wang H, Yu JM, Yang GR, Song XR, Sun XR, Zhao SQ, Wang XW, Zhao W. Further characterization of the epidermal growth factor receptor ligand 11C-PD153035. Chinese Medical Journal (Engl) 2007; 120(11) 960-964.

[57] Camp ER, Summy J, Bauer TW, Liu W, Gallick GE, Ellis LM. Molecular mechanisms of resistance to therapies targeting the epidermal growth factor receptor. Clinical Cancer Research 2005; 11 397-405.

[58] Chinnaiyan P, Huang S, Vallabhaneni G, Armstrong E, Varambally S, Tomlins SA, Chinnaiyan AM, Harari PM. Mechanisms of enhanced radiation response following epidermal growth factor receptor signaling inhibition by erlotinib (Tarceva). Cancer Research. 2005; 65(8) 3328-3335.

[59] Schmidt-Ullrich RK, Mikkelsen RB, Dent P, Todd DG, Valerie K, Kavanagh BD, Contessa JN, Rorrer WK, Chen PB. Radiation-induced proliferation of the human A431 squamous carcinoma cells is dependent on EGFR tyrosine phosphorylation. Oncogene 1997; 15(10) 1191-1197.

[60] Yacoub A, McKinstry R, Hinman D, Chung T, Dent P, Hagan MP. Epidermal growth factor and ionizing radiation up-regulate the DNA repair genes XRCC1 and ERCC1 in DU145 and LNCaP prostate carcinoma through MAPK signaling. Radiation Research 2003;159 439-452.

[61] Pao W, Kris MG, Iafrate AJ. Integration of molecular profiling into the lung cancer clinic. Clinical Cancer Research 2009; 15(17) 5317-5322.

[62] Minna JD, Girard L, Xie Y. Tumor mRNA expression profiles predict responses to chemotherapy. Journal of Clinical Oncology 2007; 25(28) 4329-4336.

[63] Das AK, Chen BP, Story MD. Somatic mutations in the tyrosine kinase domain of epidermal growth factor receptor (EGFR) abrogate EGFR-mediated radioprotection in non-small cell lung carcinoma. Cancer Research 2007; 67(11) 5267-5274.

[64] Chinnaiyan P, Huang S, Vallabhaneni G. Mechanisms of enhanced radiation response following epidermal growth factor receptor signaling inhibition by erlotinib (Tarceva). Cancer Research 2005; 65(8) 3328-3335.

[65] Shibuya K, Komaki R, Shintani T. Targeted therapy against VEGFR and EGFR with ZD6474 enhances the therapeutic efficacy of irradiation in an orthotopic model of human non-small-cell lung cancer. International Journal of Radiation Oncology Biology Physics 2007; 69(5) 1534-1543.

[66] Wang M, Morsbach F, Sander D, Gheorghiu L, Nanda A, Benes C, Kriegs M, Krause M, Dikomey E, Baumann M, Dahm-Daphi J, Settleman J, Willers H. EGF receptor inhibition radiosensitizes NSCLC cells by inducing senescence in cells sustaining DNA double-strand breaks. Cancer Research 2011; 71(19) 6261-6269.

[67] Kriegs M, Kasten-Pisula U, Rieckmann T, Holst K, Saker J, Dahm-Daphi J, Dikomey E. The epidermal growth factor receptor modulates DNA double-strand break repair by regulating non-homologous end-joining. DNA Repair (Amst). 2010; 9(8) 889-897.

[68] Sturla LM, Amorino G, Alexander MS, Mikkelsen RB, Valerie K, Schmidt-Ullrichr RK. Requirement of Tyr-992 and Tyr-1173 in phosphorylation of the epidermal growth factor receptor by ionizing radiation and modulation by SHP2. Journal of Biological Chemistry 2005; 280 14597-14604.

[69] Toulany M, Dittmann K, Kruger M, Baumann M, Rodemann HP. Radioresistance of K-Ras mutated human tumor cells is mediated through EGFR-dependent activation of PI3K-AKT pathway. Radiotherapy Oncology 2005; 76 143-150.

[70] Sun Y, Moretti L, Giacalone NJ, Schleicher S, Speirs CK, Carbone DP, Lu B. Inhibition of JAK2 signaling by TG101209 enhances radiotherapy in lung cancer models. Journal of Thoracic Oncology 2011; 6(4) 699-706.

[71] Lu B, Mu Y, Cao C, Zeng F, Schneider S, Tan J, Price J, Chen J, Freeman M, Hallahan DE. Survivin as a therapeutic target for radiation sensitization in lung cancer. Cancer Research. 2004; 64 2840-2845.

[72] Hermens AF, Barendsen GW. Changes of cell proliferation characteristics in a rat rhabdomyosarcoma before and after x-irradiation. European Journal of Cancer 1969; 5 173-189.

[73] Stephens TC, Currie GA, Peacock JH. Repopulation of gamma-irradiated Lewis lung carcinoma by malignant cells and host macrophage progenitors. British Journal of Cancer 1978; 38(5) 573-582.

[74] Torres-Roca JF, Eschrich S, Zhao H, Bloom G, Sung J, McCarthy S, Cantor AB, Scuto A, Li C, Zhang S, Jove R, Yeatman T. Prediction of radiation sensitivity using a gene expression classifier. Cancer Research 2005; 65(16) 7169-7176.

[75] Eschrich S, Zhang H, Zhao H. Systems biology modeling of the radiation sensitivity network: a biomarker discovery platform. International Journal of Radiation Oncology Biology Physics 2009; 75(2) 497-505.

[76] Guo WF, Lin RX, Huang J, Zhou Z, Yang J, Guo GZ, Wang SQ. Identification of differentially expressed genes contributing to radioresistance in lung cancer cells using microarray analysis. Radiation Research 2005; 164 27-35.

[77] Qing-yong X, Yuan G, Yan L, Wei-zhi Y, Xiang-ying X. Identification of differential gene expression profiles of radioresistant lung cancer cell line established by fractionated ionizing radiation *in vitro*. Chinese Medicine Journal 2008; 121(18) 1830-1837.

[78] Lee YS, Oh JH, Yoon S, Kwon MS, Song CW, Kim KH, Cho MJ, Mollah ML, Je YJ, Kim YD, Kim CD, Lee JH. Differential gene expression profiles of radioresistant non-small-cell lung cancer cell lines established by fractionated irradiation: tumor protein p53-inducible protein 3 confers sensitivity to ionizing radiation. International Journal of Radiation Oncology Biology Physics 2010; 77(3) 858-866.

[79] Sun JG, Liao RX, Zhang SX, Duan YZ, Zhuo WL, Wang XX, Wang ZX, Li DZ, Chen ZT. Role of inhibitor of apoptosis protein Livin in radiation resistance in non small cell lung cancer. Cancer Biotherapy and Radiopharmacy 2011; 26(5) 585-592.

[80] Jung IL, Kang HJ, Kim KC, Kim IG. PTEN/pAkt/p53 signaling pathway correlates with the radioresponse of non-small cell lung cancer. International Journal of Molecular Medicine 2010; 25(4) 517-523.

[81] Yin ZJ, Jin FG, Liu TG, Fu EQ, Xie YH, Sun RL. Overexpression of STAT3 potentiates growth, survival, and radioresistance of non-small-cell lung cancer (NSCLC) cells. Journal of Surgical Research 2011; 171(2) 675-683.

[82] Indovina P, Marcelli E, Pentimalli F, Tanganelli P, Tarro G, Giordano A. Mass spectrometry-based proteomics: The road to lung cancer biomarker discovery. Mass Spectrometry Reviews. 2012; DOI: 10.1002/mas.21355.

[83] Wei R, Zhang Y, Shen L, Jiang W, Li C, Zhong M, Xie Y, Yang D, He L, Zhou Q. Comparative proteomic and radiobiological analyses in human lung adenocarcinoma cells. Molecular and Cellular Biochemistry 2012; 359(1-2) 151-159.

Chapter 3

Functional Roles of microRNAs in Cancer: microRNomes and oncomiRs Connection

César López-Camarillo, Laurence A. Marchat, Elena Aréchaga-Ocampo, Elisa Azuara-Liceaga, Carlos Pérez-Plasencia, Lizeth Fuentes-Mera, Miguel A. Fonseca-Sánchez and Ali Flores-Pérez

Additional information is available at the end of the chapter

http://dx.doi.org/10.5772/53981

1. Introduction

Cancer is a complex group of diseases characterized by the presence of cells with uncontrolled growth, and high proliferation capacity. The complexity of cancer properties was outlined as the "hallmarks of cancer" a decade ago by Hanahan and Weinberg [1], and it comprises six alterations in cell physiology that dictate malignant growth including: (i) self-sufficiency in growth signals and uncontrolled growth of cells; (ii) insensitivity to anti-growth signals; (iii) evasion of apoptosis; 4 (iv) limitless replicative potential; (v) sustained angiogenesis; and (vi) acquisition of invasive properties to adjacent tissues and organs [1, 2]. These processes are regulated by protein-encoding genes whose expression switches-on or -off during development and in response to cellular environment. Altered versions of the genes (tumor-suppressor genes and proto-oncogenes) which control the normal cellular processes arise from mutations, or expression deregulation in a multistep process resulting in cancer [3]. At the end of the transformation process, the malignant cells acquire growth independence, invasiveness and resistance to senescence and apoptosis. The acquired capabilities of cells to metastasize to other tissues and organs represent the most deadly hallmark of cancer [4-6].

Recently it has been noted that the level of complexity in the mechanisms leading to tumorigenesis has increased as new molecular players in cancer have been identified. Particularly, it has been reported that an abundant class of small non-coding single-stranded RNAs of ~22 nucleotides including microRNAs, and long non-coding RNAs may have relevant roles in cancer. It has been well documented that the expression of microRNAs is strongly deregulated in almost all human malignancies. Functional characterization of these aberrantly expressed microRNAs indicates that they might also function as oncogenes and tumor suppressors, thus they have been collectively named as "oncomiRs" [5]. Deregulation of microRNAs expression strongly alters key events leading to cancer, including differentiation, proliferation, apoptosis, migration, invasion and metastasis, and chemotherapy resistance. In consequence, the identification of deregulated microRNAs in cancer and their respective targets may provide potential diagnostic and prognostic tumor biomarkers and represent new therapeutic targets for cancer therapy.

2. MicroRNAs biogenesis

MicroRNAs are a class of small non-coding single-stranded RNAs around 21-23 nucleotides length which inhibit gene expression through transcriptional repression and degradation of protein-coding messenger RNAs, in animals, plants and unicellular eukaryotes [7, 8]. The process of microRNAs biosynthesis involves a transcription of hairpin-shaped long transcripts generated by RNA polymerase II (RNA pol II), followed by the endonucleolytic cleavage, mediated by two type III ribonucleases enzymes (RNAse III) known as Drosha (in nuclei) and Dicer (in cytoplasm). The first microRNA (lin-4) was discovered in 1993 in the nematode *Caenorhabditis elegans*. Since it has been estimated the existence of around 17,341 mature microRNAs in 142 species and it has been estimated 1,223 human microRNAs by computational predictions [9, 10]. Analysis of complete genomes sequences from diverse species indicates that most microRNAs genes are located in intergenic non-coding regions, but they are also found within exonic or intronic regions in either sense or antisense orientation and are independently transcribed from their own promoters. The microRNAs localized within introns of protein-encoding or -non-encoding genes (pseudo-genes) have been denominated "mirtrons" [11]. These mirtrons are co-transcribed with their host genes. MicroRNAs genes can be grouped into families by their sequence similarity and function, and they can be localized as single units or grouped in clusters in the genome. It has been estimated that a single microRNA can negatively regulate hundreds or even thousands of target genes indicating that about 30% of human genes could be regulated by microRNAs [12]. However, the functions and cellular targets of most of microRNAs remain to be determined.

The first step in canonical microRNAs biogenesis pathway in animals begins with the transcription of the microRNA gene by the RNA pol II producing a long primary transcript denominated as primary miRNA (pri-miRNA). Clustered microRNAs might be transcribed from a single transcription unit as a polycistronic pri-miRNA. Primary microRNAs contain both 5′-cap structure (7MGpppG) as well as 3′-end polyadenylated tails [13]. After the synthesis of pri-miRNA, the molecule is folded itself into a specific secondary structure of stem-loop that is recognized and cleaved by the microprocessor complex comprised of the RNAse III enzyme Drosha and the DiGeorge syndrome critical region protein 8 (DGCR8). The DGCR8 protein interacts with the pri-miRNA and function as a molecular driver to determine the precise cleavage site. After cleavage of primary microRNA a molecule of 70-100 nucleotides length with a stem-loop structure called precursor microRNA (pre-microRNA) is produced [14, 15]. This post-transcriptional maturation of microRNAs precursors is regulated in response to diverse cellular stimuli. In non-canonical microRNAs biogenesis pathway, mirtrons are produced without the intervention of the microprocessor complex. Like canonical microRNAs, these "mirtrons" are encoded within short stem–loop structures. However, these stem–loops are located within short introns of protein-coding genes, which are released upon pre-mRNA splicing mechanism [16]. The pre-miRNA excised by splicing exhibits a lariat intron form which is subsequently linearized by the debranching enzyme DBR1. Today, it has been described in humans about 13 different mirtrons [17]. These pre-microRNAs are transported to cytoplasm by exportin 5 and Ran-GTP. Pre-miRNAs present a short stem plus a ~2-nt 3′ overhang, which is recognized by the nuclear export factor exportin 5 (Figure 1).

Once in the cytoplasm the pre-miRNAs are processed by DICER enzyme (dicing process), another RNAse III enzyme, which together with the dsRNA-binding protein TRBP2 cuts out of the loop and generates an imperfect double stranded RNA formed by the guide (miRNA) and transient strand (miRNA*) which is degraded by AGO2. However, it has been recently established that miRNA* strand is also functional. Subsequently, TRBP2 recruits the protein Argonaut 2 (AGO2) to the complex microRNA/DICER forming the silencing complex induced by RNA (RISC), which preferentially includes the mature single-stranded miRNA molecule and AGO proteins (AGO2-4), acting as guiding molecules to deliver the complex to target mRNA[18]. The mature microRNA then hybridizes to nearly complementary sites in the 3′ untranslated region (3′-UTR) of mRNA targets. Negative gene expression regulation mediated by microRNAs depends on the degree of complementarity between the microRNA and its target mRNA. Translational repression of transcripts is driven when microRNA binds to target with imperfect complementarity. This imperfect miRNA:miRNA interaction means that a single microRNA can potentially target tens to hundreds of mRNAs. When microRNAs binds to its mRNA targets with a high complementarity, the degradation of the messenger is induced [19]. Notably, the microRNAs mediated-decay of mRNA targets is initiated by shortening of poly(A^+) transcripts by the canonical deadenylation machinery that includes the CAF1 deadenylase.

Importantly, translation repression and/or degradation of mRNA targets by microRNAs occurs in cytoplasmic foci denoted as mRNA processing bodies (P-bodies) which are enriched in mRNA decay factors and pools of stored messenger ribonucleoproteins [20]. P-bodies are mRNA processing centers within which non-translating transcripts are sorted and either silenced or degraded. Although the protein inventory of P-bodies has not been defined in detail, around 25 different factors have been detected within these cytoplasmic foci. The P-bodies observed in yeast, insect, nematode and mammalian cells have critical roles in mRNA degradation, mRNA storage, mRNA surveillance and RNA-based gene silencing mechanisms [21]. Moreover, it has been demonstrated that P-bodies have high concentration of target transcripts and the AGO2, DICER, and GW182 proteins involved in RNA interference by microRNAs and small interfering RNAs [22, 23].

Although the main function of microRNAs is the gene regulation at the post-transcriptional level, it has been observed that microRNAs can also activate or repress gene expression at transcriptional level. Recently, it has been evidenced that mature microRNAs may also be localized in nucleus, through a specific hexanucleotide (AGUGUU) sequence which acts as a transferable nuclear localization element [24]. An example of this is the positive regulatory effect on transcriptional level of mir-122 in liver cells [25]. Moreover, it has been shown that vesicles of endocytic origin known as exosomes may contain both mRNA and microRNAs, which can be delivered to adjacent cells, and can be functional therein. These novel RNA molecules are known as exosomal shuttle RNAs as they mediate exchange of microRNAs with other cells which represents a exciting mechanism of genetic exchange [26].

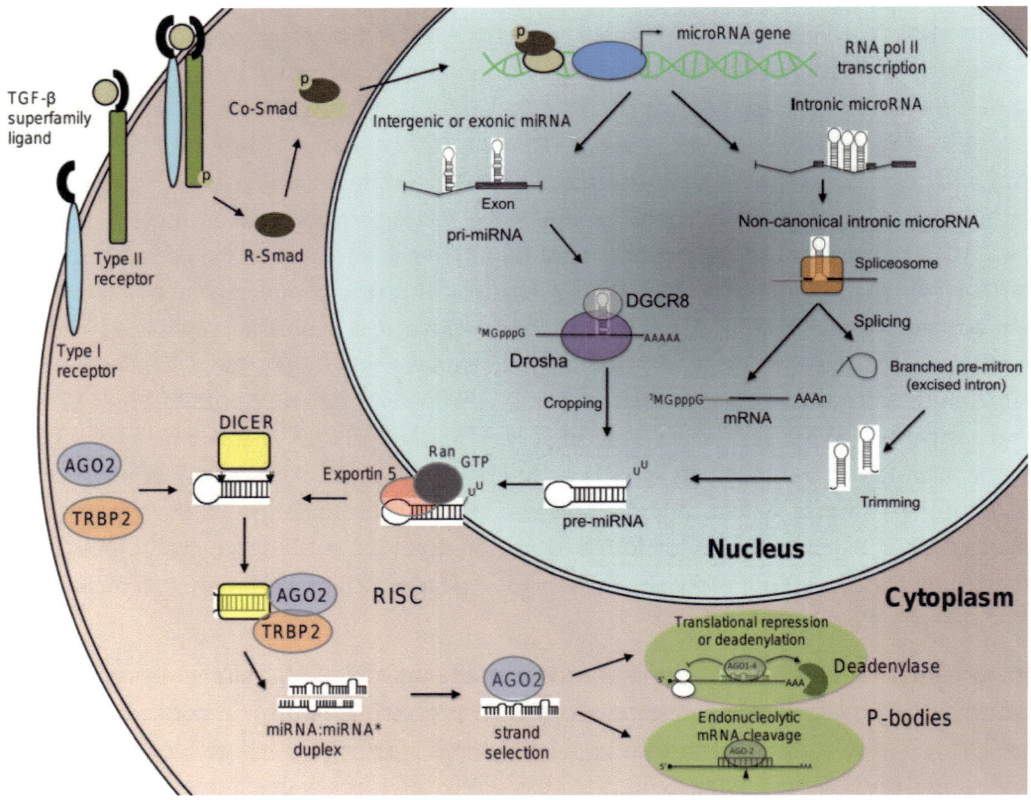

Figure 1. MicroRNAs biogenesis in mammals. The activation of microRNAs transcription by transforming growth factor beta (TGF-β) ligands and sequential phosphorylation of type II receptors activating type I receptors, which in turn activate R-Smads receptors and Smad signaling is depicted. MicroRNAs are transcribed by RNA Pol II in nuclei to generate the primary microRNA (pri-miRNA). These large non-coding RNAs are processed by the endoribonuclease Drosha and DGCR8 proteins (microprocessor complex) to produce the precursor microRNA (pre-miRNA). Mirtrons are alternatively produced during splicing of introns of messenger RNAs. Then, pre-miRNA is exported to cytoplasm by exportin 5/Ran-GTP system. In cytosol, pre-miRNA is processed by Dicer and TRBP2 complex to generate the mature microRNA which then binds to Argonaute family of proteins (AGO1-4) forming the RNA induced silencing complex (RISC). Finally, microRNAs may either inhibit the translation of mRNA or promote mRNA degradation. These events occur in discrete cytoplasmic structures denoted as P-bodies.

2.1. Regulation of microRNAs biogenesis

The biosynthesis of the microRNAs can be regulated at different levels. It has been defined that microRNAs are transcribed by RNA pol II. Primary transcripts present the same characteristics of the mRNAs, including 7-methylguanylate cap structure at the 5′-end, and poly (A) tail at the 3′-end. The majority of DNA-binding elements and transcription factors binding sites in microRNAs promoters largely overlap with those that control protein-coding genes, such as *c-myc* or *p53*. On the other hand, transcription of primary miRNA transcripts can be dynamically regulated in response to growth factor stimulation, including platelet-derived growth factor (PDGF), transforming growth factor beta (TGF-β) and Smad [27]. Epigenetic control of microRNAs expression is another regulation level which includes DNA methylation and histones modifications. For example, the expression of miRNA-127 is reduced due to promoter hypermethylation in bladder cancer [28]. Another example is the regulation of miRNA-1 by inhibition of histone deacetylase (HDAC) enzyme in breast and lung cancers [29]. In addition, it has been reported that mutations in genes coding for Drosha and Dicer occurs in a variety of cancers.

3. MicroRNAs and cancer: OncomiRs

Deregulation of microRNAs expression is common in all types of human cancer. Early studies showed a differential microRNAs expression profiles between tumors and normal tissues [30-32]. Moreover, alterations in microRNAs expression correlate with severity of disease, as they regulate key transcripts involved in initiation and progression of tumors. However, these observations does not imply that deregulated microRNAs are directly involved in tumor development and progression, as they could be indirectly altered by the genetic and epigenomic changes that arise during carcinogenesis. MicroRNAs can act as truly oncogenes or tumor suppressors to inhibit or exacerbate the expression of cancer-related target genes, and to promote or suppress tumorigenesis, thus they have been denominated as oncomiRs [33]. Those microRNAs whose expression is increased in tumors may be considered as oncogenes, as they usually promote tumor development by inhibiting tumor suppressor genes and/or genes that control cell cycle, cell differentiation and apoptosis [34]. Contrarily, when the expression of microRNAs is diminished in cancer cells, they are considered as tumor suppressor genes. Tumor suppressor microRNAs usually prevent tumor development by inhibiting oncogenes and/or genes that control cell differentiation or apoptosis [33]. Deregulation of microRNAs expression frequently arises from genetic or epigenetic alterations, represented by deletions, amplifications, point mutations and aberrant DNA methylation events. Remarkably, about half of the human microRNAs are located within fragile regions of chromosomes, which are domains of the genome that are frequently lost in various human cancers [35].

Of clinical interest, the large high-throughput studies in patients revealed that microRNAs profiling has the potential to classify tumors and predict patient outcome with high accuracy [31, 32, 36]. For example, it was shown that high levels of miR-155 and low let-7a-2 expression correlate with poor survival in patients with lung adenocarcinoma [37]. In addition, microRNA profiling in lung cancer identified five microRNAs important for prognosis. Results showed that high levels of miR-221 and let-7a appeared to be protective, while high levels of miR-137, miR-372, and miR-182 were correlated with worse clinical outcome [38]. Another study in colorectal cancer showed that high miR-21 expression was associated with poor survival and poor therapeutic outcome [39]. Moreover, components of the microRNA-based gene silencing machinery have also been implicated in tumorigenesis. Reduced expression of Dicer has been shown to be down-regulated in lung cancer and associated with poor prognosis [40]. These findings are in agreement with previous reports of Dicer loss in some tumors. In addition, other reports showed that low expression levels of Drosha were significantly associated with advanced tumor stage in ovarian cancer [41]. Other components of the microRNA machinery that have been implicated in cancer include Argonaute family members Ago1, Ago3, and Ago4 which cluster on the 1p34-35 chromosomal region, that is often lost in in human cancers such as Wilms tumors, neuroblastoma and breast, liver and colon carcinomas [42]. In summary, emerging evidence suggests that oncomiRs play important roles in human cancers. Several microRNAs may be directly involved in cancer development by controlling cell differentiation and apoptosis, while others may be involved in cancer by targeting cancer oncogenes and/or tumor suppressors. Next, we will discuss the roles of microRNAs in metastasis, the more deadly hallmark in cancer.

4. MetastamiRs: microRNAs driving invasion and metastasis

4.1. Mechanisms of invasion and metastasis

The ability of cancer cells to metastasize is a hallmark of malignant tumors. Metastatic development from primary tumor to a secondary organ or tissue should be successfully complete in multiple sequential steps that include spreading of tumoral cells from primary tumor, enhanced motility, intravasation, extravasation and colonization in a secondary site to form a distant tumor [43, 44]. Each step in this complex cellular process represents a physiological barrier that must be overcome by the tumor cells for successful metastasis [45]. These events are regulated by genetic and epigenetic programs that are acquired during tumor progression [46]. However, it remains unclear if oncogenic transformation is sufficient for metastatic competence. The long latency period of certain tumor types suggests a further evolution of malignant cells in the microenvironments of particular organs [47]. Metastasis initiation genes allow cancer cells to invade the surrounding tissues, attract a supportive stroma and facilitate cellular dispersion and infiltration in distant tissues [6]. These genes participate in the regulation of motility, epithelial-mesenchymal transition (EMT), adhesion and proteolysis. They determine tumor cells interactions with other cells and with the extracellular matrix, and activate migration, angiogenesis and survival [48]. These genes codified for transcription factors, growth factors receptors, protein kinases and importantly microRNAs [49, 50]. Tumor cells interactions with the extracellular matrix are mediated by integrins which trigger invasion and spread. These proteins promote invasion and proliferation and they determine whether cells migrate and proliferate in response to cytokines and growth factors [51]. Metastatic cells loss their adherent junctions, which, in epithelial cells, are constituted primarily by E-cadherin. E-cadherin is replaced by N-cadherin, which plays an important role in invasion by regulating fibroblast growth factor receptor (FGFR) function [52]. This process, known as the cadherin switch, is associated with EMT, allowing the conversion of epithelial cells to motile fibroblast-like cells that express mesenchymal rather than epithelial cell markers [53]. The communication of epitheliai cell with their microenvironment is regulated by E-cadherin-mediated cell-cell interaction and β1-integrin-mediated adhesion to the basement membrane (BM), which is the first barrier to invasion by carcinoma cells. Other proteins involved in the metastatic process include the matrix metalloproteinases (MMP), COX2 and cytokines. MMP can degrade the components of the BM such as collagen IV. Importantly, MMP promotes angiogenesis, one of the prerequisites for metastatic tumor growth by degradation of the fibrin matrix that surrounds newly formed blood vessels, facilitating endothelial cell penetration of tumor tissues [54].

In the "omics" era, the genomic profiling, second-generation sequencing, proteomics and other global level analytical techniques have dramatically accelerated the efforts to comprehensively characterize metastatic tumour cells and to understand their natural history of evolution from primary tumors [55]. Discovered gene signatures in metastatic tumors have been applied to identify functional drivers of metastasis. Comparing the expression profiles of highly metastatic cells with their weakly metastatic counterparts from an isogenic background allowed for the identification of metastasis-promoting [56-58] and metastasis-suppressing genes [59-61]. In addition, gain-of-function or loss-of-function genomic screens, cross-species integrated genomic analyses and computational reanalysis of genomic profiling data have also led to the identification of functional mediators of metastasis with direct clinical relevance [61]. However, despite great advancements in the knowledge of metastasis biology, the molecular mechanisms are still not completely understood. Remarkably, a regulatory role for microRNAs in metastasis has been established, thus they have been denominated metastamiRs, as they have pro- and anti-metastatic effects [62]. The term metastamiRs was recently introduced by Welch and colleagues to refer to those regulatory microRNAs which promote or suppress various steps in migration and metastasis of cancer cells [63]. It seems that these metastamiRs regulate key steps in the metastatic program and processes, such as EMT and angiogenesis. Most commonly, metastamiRs promoting cell migration and invasion have been described [62]. Next, we will review some of the identified microRNAs with a relevant role in metastasis in human cancers.

4.2. MetastamiRs in prostate cancer

Prostate cancer is the second more lethal cancer type in men in America [64]. Once it has progressed to metastasis (manly to bone) the disease is currently incurable, since metastatic cells are highly resistant to conventional therapies. The involvement of microRNAs in human prostate cancer has been well documented and some aberrantly expressed microRNAs with critical roles in the progression and metastasis of prostate cancer have been discovered [65]. For example, miR-21 expression levels significantly correlate with advanced clinical stage, metastasis and poor prognosis in prostate cancer. In these studies it has been evidenced that miR-21 targets myristoylated alanine rich protein kinase c substrate (MARCKS), which is involved in cellular processes, such as cell adhesion and cell motility through regulation of the actin cytoskeleton [66]. In another study, Watahiki and coworkers discovered differentially expressed known and novel microRNAs from a transplantable metastatic compared with non-metastatic prostate cancer xenograft line, both derived via subrenal capsule grafting, and from one patient's primary cancer tissue [67]. These microRNAs seem to have specific roles in the metastasis of prostate cancer. In another report, Gandellini and coworkers showed that miR-205 is overexpressed in normal prostate tissue and RWPE-1 cells, whereas it was almost undetectable in both androgen-dependent and androgen-independent prostate cancer cells [68]. Authors showed that overexpression of miR-205 in prostate cancer cells promotes up-regulation of E-cadherin and reduction of cell locomotion and invasion, suggesting a relation with EMT. Peng and colleagues reported that the expression of five microRNAs (miRs-508-5p, -145, -143, -33a and -100) was significantly decreased in bone metastasis when compared with primary tumor prostate [69]. Notably, miRs-143 and -145, were up-regulated, and they were able to repress migration and invasion *in vitro*, tumor development and bone invasion *in vivo,* as well as EMT of PC-3 derived from metastatic cells. Since the principal problem arising from prostate cancer is its propensity to metastasize to bone, these findings could be important for the understanding of organ specific metastasis in this neoplasia [69].

4.3. MetastamiRs in colorectal cancer

Colorectal cancer is the third most common malignant disease and the fourth leading cause of cancer-related deaths worldwide. Metastases have occurred in about 25% of patients at the time of diagnosis, and an additional 40% to 50% develop secondary metastases during the course of their disease after diagnosis. Currently about 100 miRNAs have been implicated in colorectal cancer [70]. The most up-regulated miRNAs are miR-21, miR 17-92 cluster, miR-135a/b, miR-471 and miR-675, whereas miR-143, miR-14, let-7 and miR-101 showed a decreased expression in colorectal cancer. The main targets of these miRNAs include transcription factors like c-MYC, STAT, OCT4, SOX, E2F1, ZEB1, ZEB2, NFIB and some kinases, such as ERK and YES1, and proteins involved in matrix metalloproteinases regulation like RECK and TIMP3 that functions as metastasis suppressors [71]. It has been reported that up-regulation of miR-21 in colorectal cancer cells increases their migratory and invasive abilities, through regulation of RECK and TIMP3 genes., Dews and coworkers used a mouse model of colon cancer to demonstrate that the angiogenic activity of c-MYC is due at least in part to downstream activation of the miR-17-92 cluster. Authors showed that vascularization of tumors can be induced by expression of either c-MYC or the miR-17-92 cluster [72].

4.4. MetastamiRs in breast cancer

Because of the availability of robust metastasis models, the vast majority of these metastamirs have been identified in breast and/or mammary tumor cell lines [62]. Ma and coworkers from Robert Weinberg's group evidenced that up-regulation of miR-10b suppressed homeobox D10 (HOXD10) expression, allowing the activation of the pro-metastatic gene RHOC and initiation of breast cancer invasion and metastasis [73]. They showed that miR-10b was overexpressed in metastatic MDA-MB-231 cell line, in comparison with tumorigenic non-metastatic MCF7 cells. Interestingly, the ectopic expression of miR-10b results in increased migration and invasion properties in two different human breast cell lines. In contrast, silencing of miR-10b using antisense inhibitor oligonucleotides led to a 10-fold reduction of the invasive properties from transfected cells. Importantly, overexpression of miR-10b in non-metastatic tumorigenic cell lines promoted robust invasion, and lung distant micro-metastases *in vivo*. Moreover, Ma and coworkers evidenced that TWIST1 [74], a metastasis promoting transcription factor specifically binds to the putative promoter of *mir-10b* gene activating its expression. This induces the inhibition of homeobox HOXD10 transcription [75], leading to an increased expression of the pro-metastatic gene RHOC, a signaling GTPase-protein involved in metastasis. Importantly, it has been described that HOXD10 expression is lost in breast tumors [76]. Finally, Ma and coworkers showed that silencing of RHOC by small interfering RNAs caused repression of miR-10b induced cell migration and invasion. In another outstanding study it was reported that systemic therapeutic silencing of miR-10b in tumor-bearing mice significantly suppressed breast cancer metastasis and increased the levels of its target HOXD10 [77]. In another study it was established that miR-373 and miR-520c promote tumor invasion and metastasis by regulating the cell-surface glycoprotein encoding gene CD44 (cell surface receptor for hyaluronan) [78]. Huang and coworkers from Agami's group set up a genetic screen using the non-metastatic MCF7 cell line, and found that miR-373 and miR-520c stimulated cell migration and invasion both *in vitro* and *in vivo*. Interestingly, authors evidenced that miR-373 and miR-520c "seed" sequences were similar and both CD44 target mRNA. Moreover, enhanced expression of a CD44 gene that was unresponsive to miR-373/miR-520c, inhibited the migratory activity of MCF7 cells overexpressing miR-373 and miR-520c.

The team led by Joan Massague performed an array-based miRNA profiling in MDA-MB-231 breast cancer cell derivatives highly metastatic to bone and lung, and found a signature of six genes (miR-335, miR-126, miR-206, miR-122a, miR-199a*, and miR-489) whose expression was highly decreased in metastatic cells [79]. Restoring the expression of miR-335, miR-126 or miR-206 in LM2 cells decreased the lung colonizing activity of these cells by more than fivefold. Interestingly, miR-126 restoration reduced overall tumor growth and proliferation, whereas miR-335 inhibited metastatic cell invasion. In addition, low expression of miR-335 or miR-126 in primary tumors from patients was associated with poor distal metastasis-free survival. In addition they profiled LM2 cells overexpressing miR-335 and identified 756 genes whose expression was decreased including genes previously implicated in extracellular matrix and cytoskeleton control (type 1 collagen COL1A1) and signal transduction (receptor-type tyrosine protein phosphatase PTPRN2, c-Mer tyrosine kinase (MERTK) 21 and phospholipase PLCB1), as well as in cell migration, such as the tenascin C (TNC), an extracellular matrix glycoprotein of stem cells niches [80] and the SRY-box containing transcription factor SOX4. Knockdown of SOX4 and TNC using RNA interference diminished *in vitro* invasive ability and *in vivo* metastatic potential, evidencing that both genes are key effectors of metastasis.

It has been reported that miR-146a and b inhibited invasion and migration of breast cancer cells by down-regulating NFκB through IRAK1 and TRAF6 targeting [81]. Both miR-146a and b suppressed metastasis through targeting of EGF receptor and ROCK1 which are involved in promoting invasion and metastasis. In another study, Hurst and coworkers showed that breast cancer metastasis suppressor 1 (BRMS1), a protein that regulates expression of multiple genes leading to suppression of metastasis, significantly up-regulates miR-146a and miR-146b in metastatic breast cancer cells. Moreover, transduction of miR-146a or miR-146b into MDA-MB-231 down-regulated expression of epidermal growth factor receptor, inhibited invasion and migration *in vitro,* and suppressed experimental lung metastasis [82].

In a seminal paper, it was reported that miR-31 inhibited multiple steps of metastasis including invasion, anoikis, and colonization leading to almost a complete reduction in lung metastasis [83]. Clinically, miR-31 levels were lower in breast cancer patients with metastasis. In another study, it was reported that suppression of miR-21 in metastatic MDA-MB-231 breast cancer cells significantly reduced invasion and lung metastasis, by targeting programmed cell death 4 (PDCD4) and maspin, which have been involved in invasion and metastasis. Li and coworkers reported that down-regulation of miR-193b contributes to enhance urokinase-type plasminogen activator expression and tumor progression and invasion in human breast cancer [84]. In other study, it was evidenced that overexpression of miR-200, which promotes a mesenchymal to epithelial cell transition by inhibiting Zeb2 expression, unexpectedly enhances macroscopic metastases in mouse breast cancer cell lines [85]. Vetter and coworkers showed that miR-661 expression in MCF7 breast cancer cells conditionally overexpressing the EMT master regulator SNAI1, contributes to breast cancer cell invasion by targeting cell-cell adhesion Nectin-1 and the lipid transferase StarD10 messengers [86].

5. MicroRNAs and angiogenesis

5.1. Regulation of angiogenesis

The term angiogenesis refers to the growth of new blood vessels from pre-existing vessels. It normally occurs during embryonic development, wound healing, and the menstruation cycle. During angiogenesis, quiescent endothelial cells are activated by angiogenic factors and start to migrate, proliferate and organize themselves in tubular structures [87]. Angiogenesis is a physiological process during development, and plays essential roles in the recovery of blood flow in ischemic tissues. Unregulated angiogenesis is seen in pathological conditions, such as cancer and is a fundamental step in tumor growth. During tumor growth, angiogenesis is required for proper nourishment and removal of metabolic wastes from tumor sites. Inhibition of tumor angiogenesis leads to repression of tumor growth and has been identified as a potential therapeutic strategy.

Angiogenesis is induced by hypoxia as a result of the expression of pro-angiogenic factors through hypoxia-inducible factor-H1 (HIF-1). HIF-1 is the major oxygen homeostasis regulator. It has a key role as transcriptional regulator, orchestrating the expression of a wide variety of genes thought to be critical for adaptation to low oxygen. Under normoxic conditions, HIF-1 is rapidly degraded by the proteasome. However, under hypoxic conditions, HIF-1 is stabilized and activates a highly complex transcription program, comprising hundreds of genes that regulate processes such as angiogenesis (vascular endothelial growth factor (VEGF), endothelial growth factor receptor 1, plasminogen inhibitor 1), glucose metabolism (lactate dehydrogenase A, aldolase A and C, and phosphofructo-kinase L), survival and death (BNIP3, p21, Nip-3 like protein) [88-90]. When pro-angiogenic factors are in excess in comparison with of anti-angiogenic factors, the switch to an angiogenic phenotype can occurs.

6. MicroRNAs and hypoxia

Hypoxia has recently been shown to induce the expression of a number of microRNAs, which have been termed "hypoxamirs" [89, 94]. Members of this group seem to affect apoptotic signaling in a hypoxic environment and are also predicted to target genes of critical importance for tumor biology. Interestingly, most hypoxia-induced microRNAs are also overexpressed in human cancers, suggesting their role in tumorigenesis [92, 94]. Using miRNA expression arrays different hypoxia-regulated microRNAs (HRMs) were determined to be induced in response to hypoxia in breast and colon cancer cells. These HRM were miR-21, miR-23a, miR-23b, miR-24, miR-26a, miR-26b, miR-27a, miR-30b, miR-93, miR-103, miR-106a, miR-107, miR-125b, miR-181a, miR-181b, miR-181c, miR-192, miR-195, miR-210 and miR-213. *In silico* analysis revealed a highly complex spectrum of candidate targets, including genes involved in proliferation, apoptosis, DNA repair, chromatin remodeling, metabolism, and migration. For example, component of the apoptotic machinery were found to be potentially targeted by HRMs: BID (miR-23), BIM (miR-24); CASP3 (miR-30), CASP 7 (miR-23), APAF1 (miR-27), BAK1 (miR-26), Bnip3L (miR-23) [91]. Recently experimentally data confirmed an important regulatory role in HIF-1 for miR-210, 26 and 181 hypoxia-induced microRNAs [91, 92]

In addition to the microRNAs that respond to hypoxia by up-regulation of their expression, the following microRNAs were identified as downregulated in hypoxic cells: miR-122a, miR-565, miR-195, miR-30e-5p, miR-374, 19a, miR-101, miR-424, miR-29b, miR-186, miR-141, miR-320, miR-422b, and miR-197 in SCC cells; miR-15b, miR-16, miR-20a, miR-20b, 30b and miR-224 in CNE cells, and miR-424 in trophoblasts [93]. In addition it has been reported that several microRNAs, including miR-16, miR-20a, miR-20b and miR-320, control expression of VEGF[92, 93].

6.1. Relationships among HIFs and hypoxamirs

The response to hypoxia generates hypoxamirs that can be grouped into three clusters (Table 1):

a. **Hypoxamirs induced by HIF**: Among the HIF-dependent hypoxamirs are miR-210 and miR-373. The most robustly induced hypoxamir, miR-210, is induced by HIF-1α and suppresses expression of the cell-cycle regulator E2F transcription factor 3 (E2F3), the receptor tyrosine kinase ligand ephrin A3, and the DNA repair protein RAD52. In addition, recently it was shown that miR-210 has an important role in suppression of mitochondrial metabolism in hypoxic states by decreasing expression of the iron-sulfur cluster assembly proteins ISCU1/2, thereby limiting cytochrome assembly and ROS generation from inefficient mitochondrial electron transport under low oxygen tensions [94].
b. **Hypoxamirs that affect HIF:** These hypoxamirs are induced by hypoxia and have an effect on HIF expression [94]. Three hypoxamirs have been shown to affect HIF expression: miR20b, miR-199a, and, most recently, miR-424. The miR-20b targets HIF-1α and suppresses its expression in MCF-7 breast cancer cells, and downregulation of miR-199a derepresses HIF-1α in cardiomyocytes. miR-424 regulates HIF-α isoforms in endothelial cells by targeting cullin 2 (CUL2), the scaffolding protein on which the ubiquitin ligase system assembles, thereby stabilizing HIF-α isoforms by impairing their prolyl hydroxylation [94].
c. **MicroRNAs that affect HIF independently of hypoxia.** At least four microRNAs have been shown to influence HIF expression independently of hypoxia. Induced by p53, miR-107 decreases the expression of HIF-β. Induced by c-MYC, the miR17-92 cluster suppresses the expression of HIF-1α. Suppressed by hepatocyte growth factor, miR-519c suppresses the expression of HIF-1α. In contrast, miR-31, by decreasing expression of the HIF regulatory factor factor-inhibiting HIF (FIH), increases the expression of HIF-1α [94].

Hypoxamirs induced by HIF	Hypoxamirs that affect HIF	MicroRNAs that affect HIF independent of hypoxia
miR-210	miR-20b	miR-107
miR-373	miR-199a	miR-17-92 cluster
	miR-424	miR-31
		miR-519c

Based on [94].

Table 1. MicroRNAs regulated by hypoxia

6.2. Transcriptional regulation of hypoxamirs

The expression of microRNAs requires the basic transcription machinery used for protein-encoding genes transcription. Most of the microRNAs transcription depends on RNA polymerase II. Such resemblances hinted to the possibility that microRNA induction/repression could also be controlled by transcription factors. Delineating the promoter regions of microRNAs is a necessary step for an expanded understanding of microRNA expression control. The main challenge comes from the fact that only few microRNA promoters have been identified experimentally [95]. Kulshereshtha and coworkers analyzed a set of promoters for all the predicted microRNAs in human genome; they predicted HIF-binding sites by position weight matrix approach. The results showed that approximately 6% of the human microRNAs exhibit significantly conserved HIF sites, which could reflect their functional importance. Additional candidate sites for Oct-C, AP2, PPAR γ and E2F transcription factors were also identified in the miR-210 promoter.[96]. These sequences could potentially regulate its expression as part of the hypoxia response. Finally, several studies have shown that microRNA biogenesis machinery is not altered in response to hypoxia. Expression of microRNA processing proteins like Ago2, Drosha, Exp5, Dicer and DP103 does not suffer any expression changes during hypoxia. Additionally Dicer impairs angiogenesis *in vitro* and *in vivo* [97].

6.3. Hypoxamirs expression and cellular context

In the case of hypoxia-regulated microRNAs, *in silico* searches reveal a highly complex spectrum of candidate targets, including genes involved in proliferation, apoptosis, DNA repair, chromatin remodeling, metabolism and migration. One set of targets are cell death regulators, given the importance of this process in a stressful environment, such as hypoxia. Using PicTar, Target-Scan and MirBase prediction programs, a number of core component genes of the apoptotic machinery were found to be potentially targeted by hypoxamirs:: BID (miR-23), BIM (miR-24); CASP3 (miR-30), CASP 7 (miR-23), APAF1 (miR-27), BAK1 (miR-26), Bnip3L (miR-23). Additionally, Bcl2 is also an experimentally confirmed target of miR15 and 16, which were found to respond to hypoxia by down-regulation, at least in CNE cells.

Another process known to be affected by hypoxia is proliferation, since many cell types undergo cell cycle slowdown or arrest during oxygen deprivation. A plethora of cell cycle genes are identified as putative HRMs targets, such as: cdc25A (miR-21, miR-103/107), cyclin D2 (miR-26, miR-103/107), cyclin E1 (miR-26), cyclin H (miR-23), cdk6 (miR-26, miR-103/107) [92]. An additional gene of relevance for this subject is VEGF for which a group of regulatory microRNAs have been identified, including miR-16, miR-20a, miR-20b, let-7b, miR-17-5p, miR-27a, miR-106a, miR-106b, miR-107, miR-193a, miR-210, and miR-320. Interestingly, most of these microRNAs have been identified by at least one of the recent studies as responsive to hypoxia, either by induction or by repression, which could lead to an extra layer of complexity in the angiogenic response. Targeting microRNAs involved in hypoxia control could be applied in clinical oncology, as the majority microRNA identified are overexpressed in some tumor subtypes, suggesting that hypoxia represents a contributing element for microRNA alterations in cancer. Moreover, manipulation of select microRNAs could synergize with conventional therapies.

7. Conclusions

The recent discovery of the role of microRNAs as tumor-suppressor genes or oncogenes has added an additional level of complexity to the mechanisms leading to tumorigenesis. In particular, the review presented here evidences that metastamiRs have emerged as new molecular players that regulate growth, angiogenesis, invasion, and metastasis events in cancer. Understanding how metastamiRs are involved in regulating tumor invasion and metastasis process will provide a promising strategy for the identification of molecular markers of progression and prognosis, for response to chemotherapy, early biomarkers of aggressive tumors, and the development of new metastamiRs-based treatments. In addition, we highlight the prominent roles of hypoxamirs in cancer. Targeting microRNAs involved in hypoxia control could be applied in clinical oncology. However, further investigations about the role of microRNAs in cancer are required in order to use them as targets for therapy, prognosis and diagnosis in the near future.

Author details

César López-Camarillo*, Miguel A. Fonseca-Sánchez and Ali Flores-Pérez
Genomics Sciences Program, Oncogenomics and Cancer Proteomics Lab, Autonomous University of México City, México

Laurence A. Marchat
Biotechnology Program and Institutional Program of Molecular Biomedicine, National School of Medicine and Homeopathy-IPN, México

Elena Aréchaga-Ocampo
Oncogenomics Lab, National Institute of Cancerology, México

Elisa Azuara-Liceaga
Genomics Sciences Program, Autonomous University of México City, México

Carlos Pérez-Plasencia
Oncogenomics Lab, and Massive Sequencing Unit, National Institute of Cancerology, México
Genomics Lab, FES-I, UBIMED, National Autonomous University of México, México

Lizeth Fuentes-Mera
Molecular Biology and Histocompatibility Laboratory, Research Direction, General Hospital "Dr. Manuel Gea González", México

Acknowledgement

Authors gratefully acknowledge the financial support from the National Council of Science and Technology (CONACyT) Mexico, grants 115552 and 115306, and The Institute of Science and Technology (ICyT-DF) Mexico, grants PIFUTP09-269 and PIUTE147.

8. References

[1] Hanahan D, Weinberg RA. The hallmarks of cancer. Cell 2000; 100, 57–70.

* Corresponding Author

[2] Lazebnik, Y. What are the hallmarks of cancer? Nature Reviews Cancer 2010; 10, 232–233.
[3] Vogelstein B, Kinzler KW. The multistep nature of cancer. Trends Genetics 1993; 9, 138–141.
[4] Schmidt-Kittler, O, Ragg T, Daskalakis A, Granzow M, Ahr A, Blankenstein TJ, Kaufmann M, Diebold J, Arnholdt H, Muller P, Bischoff J, Harich D, Schlimok G, Riethmuller G, Eils R, Klein CA. From latent disseminated cells to overt metastasis: Genetic analysis of systemic breast cancer progression. Proceedings of the National Academy of Sciences of the United States of America 2003; 100, 7737–7742.
[5] Esquela-Kerscher A, Slack FJ. Oncomirs-microRNAs with a role in cancer. Nature Reviews Cancer 2006; 6, 259–269.
[6] Nguyen DX, Bos PD, Massague J. Metastasis: From dissemination to organ-specific colonization. Nature Reviews Cancer 2009; 9, 274–284.
[7] Davis-Dusenbery BN, Hata A. Mechanisms of control of microRNA biogenesis. Journal of Biochemistry 2010; 148, 381–392
[8] Bartel DP. MicroRNAs: Genomics, biogenesis, mechanism, and function. Cell 2004; 116, 281–297
[9] Berezikov E, Guryev V, van de Belt J, Wienholds E, Plasterk RH, Cuppen E. Phylogenetic shadowing and computational identification of human microRNA genes. Cell 2005; 120, 21–24.
[10] Dai R, Ahmed SA. microRNA, a new paradigm for understanding immunoregulation, inflammation, and autoimmune diseases. Translation Research 2011; 157(4), 163–179.
[11] Ruby JG, Jan CH, Bartel DP. Intronic microRNA precursors that bypass Drosha processing. Nature 2007; 448, 83–86.
[12] Miranda KC, Huynh T, Tay Y, Ang YS, Tam WL, Thomson AM, Lim B, Rigoutsos I. A pattern-based method for the identification of MicroRNA binding sites and their corresponding heteroduplexes. Cell 2006; 126, 1203–1217.
[13] Cai X, Hagedorn CH, Cullen BR. Human microRNAs are processed from capped, polyadenylated transcripts that can also function as mRNAs. RNA 2004; 10, 1957–1966.
[14] Han J, Lee Y, Yeom KH, Kim YK, Jin H, Kim VN. The Drosha-DGCR8 complex in primary microRNA processing. Genes and Development 2004; 18, 3016–3027.
[15] Denli AM, Tops BB, Plasterk RH, Ketting RF, Hannon GJ. Processing of primary microRNAs by the microprocessor complex. Nature 2004; 432, 231–235.
[16] Chong MM, Zhang G, Cheloufi S, Neubert TA, Hannon GJ, Littman DR. Canonical and alternate functions of the microRNA biogenesis machinery. Genes and development 2010; 24, 1951–1960
[17] Berezikov E, Chung WJ, Willis J, Cuppen E, Lai EC. Mammalian mirtron genes. Molecular Cell 2007; 28, 328–336.
[18] Chendrimada TP, Gregory RI, Kumaraswamy E, Norman J, Cooch N, Nishikura K, Shiekhattar R. TRBP recruits the Dicer complex to Ago2 for microRNA processing and gene silencing. Nature 2005; 436, 740-744.
[19] Vasudevan S, Tong Y, Steitz JA. Switching from repression to activation: microRNAs can up-regulate translation. Science 2007; 318, 1931–1934.
[20] Eulalio A, Behm-Ansmant I, Izaurralde E. P-bodies: at the crossroads of post-transcriptional pathways. Nature Reviews Molecular and Cellular Biology 2007; 8, 9-22.

[21] Sen GL, Blau HM. Argonaute 2/RISC resides in sites of mammalian mRNA decay known as cytoplasmic bodies. Nature Cell Biology 2005; 7, 633-636.

[22] Liu J, Rivas FV, Wohlschlegel J, Yates JR, Parker R, Hannon GJ. A role for the P-body component GW182 in microRNA function. Nature Cell Biology 2005; 7, 1261-1266.

[23] Eulalio A, Behm-Ansmant I, Schweizer D, and Izaurralde E. P-Body formation is a consequence, not the cause, of RNA-mediated gene silencing. Molecular and Cellular Biology 2007; 27, 3970–3981.

[24] Hwang HW, Wentzel EA, Mendell JT. A hexanucleotide element directs microRNA nuclear import. Science 2007; 315, 97–100.

[25] Földes-Papp Z, König K, Studier H, Bückle R, Breunig HG, Uchugonova A, Kostner GM. Trafficking of Mature miRNA-122 into the Nucleus of Live Liver Cells. Current Pharmaceutical Biotechnology 2009; 10, 569-578.

[26] Valadi H, Ekström K, Bossios A, Sjöstrand M, Lee JJ, Lötvall JO. Exosome-mediated transfer of mRNAs and microRNAs is a novel mechanism of genetic exchange between cells. Nature Cell Biology 2007; 9, 654–659.

[27] Davis BN, Hilyard AC, Nguyen PH, Lagna G, Hata A. Induction of microRNA-221 by platelet-derived growth factor signaling is critical for modulation of vascular smooth muscle phenotype. Journal of Biological Chemistry 2009; 284, 3728-3738

[28] Saito Y, Liang G, Egger G, Friedman JM, Chuang JC, Coetzee GA, Jones PA. Specific activation of microRNA-127 with downregulation of the proto-oncogene BCL6 by chromatin-modifying drugs in human cancer cells. Cancer Cell 2006; 9, 435-443

[29] Scott GK, Mattie MD, Berger CE, Benz SC, Benz CC. Rapid alteration of microRNA levels by histone deacetylase inhibition. Cancer Research 2006; 66,1277-1281.

[30] Yanaihara N, Caplen N, Bowman E, Seike M, Kumamoto K, Yi M, Stephens RM, Okamoto A, Yokota J, Tanaka T, Calin GA, Liu CG, Croce CM, Harris CC. Unique microRNA molecular profiles in lung cancer diagnosis and prognosis. Cancer Cell 2006; 9, 189-198.

[31] Lu J, Getz G, Miska EA, Alvarez-Saavedra E, Lamb J, Peck D, Sweet-Cordero A, Ebert BL, Mak RH, Ferrando AA, Downing JR, Jacks T, Horvitz HR, Golub TR. MicroRNA expression profiles classify human cancers. Nature 2005; 435, 834-838.

[32] Volinia S, Calin GA, Liu CG, Ambs S, Cimmino A, Petrocca F, Visone R, Iorio M, Roldo C, Ferracin M, Prueitt RL, Yanaihara N, Lanza G, Scarpa A, Vecchione A, Negrini M, Harris CC, Croce CM. A microRNA expression signature of human solid tumors defines cancer gene targets. Proceedings of the National Academy of Sciences of the United States of America 2006; 103, 2257-2261.

[33] Esquela-Kerscher A, Slack FJ. Oncomirs-microRNAs with a role in cancer. Nature Reviews Cancer 2006; 6, 259–269.

[34] Zhang B, Pan X, Cobb GP, Anderson TA. microRNAs as oncogenes and tumor suppressors. Developmental Biology. 2007; 302 (1), 1–12.

[35] Calin GA, Sevignani C, Dumitru CD, Hyslop T, Noch E, Yendamuri S, Shimizu M, Rattan S, Bullrich F, Negrini M, Croce CM. Human microRNA genes are frequently located at fragile sites and genomic regions involved in cancers. Proceedings of the National Academy of Sciences of the United States of America 2004; 101, 2999–3004.

[36] Hernando E. microRNAs and cancer: Role in tumorigenesis, patient classification and therapy. Clinical and Translation Oncology 2007; 9, 155–160.

[37] Yanaihara N, Caplen N, Bowman E, Seike M, Kumamoto K, Yi M, Stephens RM,Okamoto A, Yokota J, Tanaka T, Calin GA, Liu CG, Croce CM, Harris CC. Unique microRNA molecular profiles in lung cancer diagnosis and prognosis. Cancer Cell 2006; 9, 189-198.

[38] Yu SL, Chen HY, Chang GC, Chen CY, Chen HW, Singh S, Cheng CL, Yu CJ, Lee YC, Chen HS, Su TJ, Chiang CC, Li HN, Hong QS, Su HY, Chen CC, Chen WJ, Liu CC, Chan WK, Chen WJ, Li KC, Chen JJ, Yang PC. MicroRNA Signature predicts survivaland relapse in lung cancer. Cancer Cell 2008; 13, 48-57.

[39] Schetter AJ, Leung SY, Sohn JJ, Zanetti KA, Bowman ED, Yanaihara N, Yuen ST, Chan TL, Kwong DL, Au GK, Liu CG, Calin GA, Croce CM, Harris CC. MicroRNA expression profiles associated with prognosis and therapeutic outcome in colon adenocarcinoma. Journal of the American Medical Association 2008; 299, 425-436.

[40] Karube Y, Tanaka H, Osada H, Tomida S, Tatematsu Y, Yanagisawa K, Yatabe Y, Takamizawa J, Miyoshi S, Mitsudomi T, Takahashi T. Reduced expression of Dicer associated with poor prognosis in lung cancer patients. Cancer Science 2005; 96, 111–115.

[41] Merritt WM, Lin YG, Han LY, Kamat AA, Spannuth WA, Schmandt R, Urbauer D, Pennacchio LA, Cheng JF, Nick AM, Deavers MT, Mourad-Zeidan A, Wang H, Mueller P, Lenburg ME, Gray JW, Mok S, Birrer MJ, Lopez-Berestein G, Coleman RL, Bar-Eli M, Sood AK. Dicer, Drosha, and outcomes in patients with ovarian cancer. New England Journal of Medicine 2008; 359, 2641–2650.

[42] Kim MS, Oh JE, Kim YR, Park SW, Kang MR, Kim SS, Ahn CH, Yoo NJ, Lee SH. Somatic mutations and losses of expression of microRNA regulation-related genes AGO2 and TNRC6A in gastric and colorectal cancers. Journal of Pathology 2010; 221(2), 139-146.

[43] Christofori G. New signals from the invasive front. Nature 2006; 441, 444–450.

[44] Gupta GP, Massague J. Cancer metastasis: building a framework. Cell 2006; 127, 679–695.

[45] Hess KR, Varadhachary GR, Taylor SH, Wei W, Raber MN, Lenzi R, Abbruzzese JL. Metastatic patterns in adenocarcinoma. Cancer 2006; 106, 1624–1633.

[46] Fidler IJ, Kripke ML. Metastasis results from preexisting variant cells within a malignant tumor. Science 1977; 197, 893–895.

[47] Liotta LA, Kohn EC. The microenvironment of the tumour-host interface. Nature 2001; 411, 375–379.

[48] Ramaswamy S, Ross KN, Lander ES, Golub TR. A molecular signature of metastasis in primary solid tumors. Nature Genetics 2003; 33, 49–54.

[49] Stein U, Walther W, Arlt F, Schwabe H, Smith J, Fichtner I, Birchmeier W, Schlag PM. MACC1, a newly identified key regulator of HGF-MET signaling, predicts colon cancer metastasis. Nature Medicine 2009; 15, 59–67.

[50] Guo C, Sah JF, Beard L, Willson JK, Markowitz SD, Guda K. The noncoding RNA, miR-126, suppresses the growth of neoplastic cells by targeting phosphatidylinositol 3 kinase

signaling and is frequently lost in colon cancers. Genes Chromosomes Cancer 2008; 47, 939–946.

[51] Hynes RO. Integrins: Bidirectional, allosteric signaling machines. Cell 2002; 110, 673–687.

[52] Biancone L, Araki M, Araki K, Vassalli P, Stamenkovic I. Redirection of tumor metastasis by expression of E-selectin in vivo. Journal of Experimental Medicine 1996; 183, 581–587.

[53] Yang J, Weinberg RA. Epithelial-mesenchymal transition: At the crossroads of development and tumor metastasis. Developmental Cell 2008; 14, 818–829.

[54] Carmeliet P. Mechanisms of angiogenesis and arteriogenesis. Nature Medicine 200; 6, 389-395.

[55] Sethi N, Kang Y. Unravelling the complexity of metastasis - molecular understanding and targeted therapies. Nature Reviews Cancer 2011; 11(10), 735-748.

[56] Kang Y, Siegel PM, Shu W, Drobnjak M, Kakonen SM, Cordón-Cardo C, Guise TA, Massagué J. A multigenic program mediating breast cancer metastasis to bone. Cancer Cell 2003; 3 (6), 537–549.

[57] Bos PD, Zhang XH, Nadal C, Shu W, Gomis RR, Nguyen DX, Minn AJ, van de Vijver MJ, Gerald WL, Foekens JA, Massagué J. Genes that mediate breast cancer metastasis to the brain. Nature 2009; 459, 1005–1009.

[58] Minn AJ, Gupta GP, Siegel PM, Bos PD, Shu W, Giri DD, Viale A, Olshen AB, Gerald WL, Massagué J. Genes that mediate breast cancer metastasis to lung. Nature 2005; 436, 518–524.

[59] Cook LM, Hurst DR, Welch DR. Metastasis suppressors and the tumor microenvironment. Seminars in Cancer Biology 2011; 21, 113–122.

[60] Smith SC, Theodorescu D. Learning therapeutic lessons from metastasis suppressor proteins. Nature Reviews Cancer 2009; 9, 253–264.

[61] Steeg PS, Bevilacqua G, Kopper L, Thorgeirsson UP, Talmadge JE, Liotta LA, Sobel ME. Evidence for a novel gene associated with low tumor metastatic potential. Journal of the National Cancer Institute 1998; 80, 200–204.

[62] Lopez-Camarillo C, Marchat LA, Arechaga-Ocampo E, Perez-Plasencia C, Del Moral-Hernandez O, Castaneda-Ortiz EJ, Rodriguez-Cuevas S. MetastamiRs: Non-Coding MicroRNAs Driving Cancer Invasion and Metastasis. International Journal of Molecular Sciences 2012; 13(2), 1347-79.

[63] Hurst DR, Edmonds MD, Welch DR. Metastamir: The field of metastasis-regulatory microRNA is spreading. Cancer Research 2009; 69, 7495–749.

[64] Jemal A, Siegel R, Xu J, Ward E. Cancer statistics 2010. CA a Cancer Journal for Clinicians. 2010; 60, 277–300.

[65] Shi XB, Tepper CG, White RW, Krichevsky AM, Gabriely G. MicroRNAs and prostate cancer. Journal of Cellular and Molecular Medicine 2008; 5A, 1456–1465.

[66] Li T, Li D, Sha J, Sun P, Huang Y. MicroRNA-21 directly targets MARCKS and promotes apoptosis resistance and invasion in prostate cancer cells. Biochemistry and Biophysics Research Communications 2009; 383, 280–285.

[67] Watahiki A, Wang Y, Morris J, Dennis K, O'Dwyer HM, Gleave M, Gout PW, Wang Y. MicroRNAs associated with metastatic prostate cancer. PLoS One 2011; 6(9):e24950

[68] Gandellini P, Folini M, Longoni N, Pennati M, Binda M, Colecchia M, Salvioni R, Supino R, Moretti R, Limonta P, Valdagni R, Daidone MG, Zaffaroni N. MiR-205 exerts tumor-suppressive functions in human prostate through down-regulation of protein kinase C-epsilon. Cancer Research 2009; 69, 2287–2295.

[69] Peng X, Guo W, Liu T, Wang X, Tu X, Xiong D, Chen S, Lai Y, Du H, Chen G, Liu G, Tang Y, Huang S, Zou X. Identification of miRs-143 and -145 that is associated with bone metastasis of prostate cancer and involved in the regulation of EMT. PLoS One 2011; 6(5):e20341.

[70] Yang L, Belaguli N, Berger DH. MicroRNA and colorectal cancer. World Journal of Surgery 2009; 33, 638–646.

[71] Schetter AJ, Harris CC. Alterations of microRNAs contribute to colon carcinogenesis. Seminars in Oncology 2011; 38, 734–742.

[72] Dews M, Homayouni A, Yu D, Murphy D, Sevignani C, Wentzel E, Furth EE, Lee WM, Enders GH, Mendell JT, Thomas-Tikhonenko A. Augmentation of tumor angiogenesis by a MYC-activated microRNA cluster. Nature Genetics 2006; 38, 1060–1065.

[73] Ma L, Teruya-Feldstein J, Weinberg RA. Tumour invasion and metastasis initiated by microRNA-10b in breast cancer. Nature 2007; 449, 682–688.

[74] Yang J, Mani SA, Donaher JL, Ramaswamy S, Itzykson RA, Come C, Savagner P, Gitelman I, Richardson A, Weinberg R.A. Twist, a master regulator of morphogenesis, plays an essential role in tumor metastasis. Cell 2004; 117, 927–939.

[75] Botas J. Control of morphogenesis and differentiation by HOM/Hox genes. Current Opinion in Cell Biology 1993; 5, 1015–1022.

[76] Makiyama K, Hamada J, Takada M, Murakawa K, Takahashi Y, Tada M, Tamoto E, Shindo G, Matsunaga A, Teramoto K, Komuro K, Kondo S, Katoh H, Koike T, Moriuchi T. Aberrant expression of HOX genes in human invasive breast carcinoma. Oncology Reports 2005; 13, 673–679.

[77] Ma L, Reinhardt F, Pan E, Soutschek J, Bhat B, Marcusson EG, Teruya-Feldstein J, Bell GW, Weinberg RA. Therapeutic silencing of miR-10b inhibits metastasis in a mouse mammary tumor model. Nature Biotechnology 2010; 28, 341–347.

[78] Huang Q, Gumireddy K, Schrier M, le Sage C, Nagel R, Nair S, Egan DA, Li A, Huang G, Klein-Szanto AJ, Gimotty PA, Katsaros D, Coukos G, Zhang L, Puré E, Agami R. The microRNAs miR-373 and miR-520c promote tumour invasion and metastasis. Nature Cell Biology 2008; 10, 292–210.

[79] Tavazoie SF, Alarcon C, Oskarsson T, Padua D, Wang Q, Bos PD, Gerald WL, Massague J. Endogenous human microRNAs that suppress breast cancer metastasis. Nature 2008; 451, 147–152.

[80] Oskarsson T, Acharyya S, Zhang XH, Vanharanta S, Tavazoie SF, Morris PG, Downey RJ, Manova-Todorova K, Brogi E, Massagué J. Breast cancer cells produce tenascin C as a metastatic niche component to colonize the lungs. Nature Medicine 2011; 17, 867–874.

[81] Bhaumik D, Scott GK, Schokrpur S, Patil CK, Campisi J, Benz CC. Expression of microRNA-146 suppresses NF-kappaB activity with reduction of metastatic potential in breast cancer cells. Oncogene 2008; 27, 5643–5647

[82] Hurst DR, Edmonds MD, Scott GK, Benz CC, Vaidya KS, Welch DR. Breast cancer metastasis suppressor 1 up-regulates miR-146, which suppresses breast cancer metastasis. Cancer Research 2009; 69, 1279–1283.

[83] Valastyan S, Reinhardt F, Benaich N, Calogrias D, Szász AM, Wang ZC, Brock JE, Richardson AL, Weinberg RA. A pleiotropically acting microRNA, miR-31, inhibits breast cancer metastasis. Cell 2009; 137, 1032–1046.

[84] Li XF, Yan PJ, Shao ZM. Downregulation of miR-193b contributes to enhance urokinase-type plasminogen activator (uPA) expression and tumor progression and invasion in human breast cancer. Oncogene 2009; 28, 3937–3948.

[85] Dykxhoorn DM, Wu Y, Xie H, Yu F, Lal A, Petrocca F, Martinvalet D, Song E, Lim B, Lieberman J. MiR-200 enhances mouse breast cancer cell colonization to form distant metastases. PLoS One 2009; 4:e7181.

[86] Vetter G, Saumet A, Moes M, Vallar L, Le Béchec A, Laurini C, Sabbah M, Arar K, Theillet C, Lecellier CH, Friederich E. MiR-661 expression in SNAI1-induced epithelial to mesenchymal transition contributes to breast cancer cell invasion by targeting Nectin-1 and StarD10 messengers. Oncogene 2010; 29, 4436–4448.

[87] Tonini T, Rossi F, Claudio PP. Molecular basis of angiogenesis and cancer. Oncogene 2003; 22, 6549-6556.

[88] Dery, MA, Michaud MD, Richard DE. Hypoxia-inducible factor 1: regulation by hypoxic and non-hypoxic activators. The International Journal of Biochemistry and Cell Biology 2005; 37, 535-540.

[89] Kulshreshtha R, Ferracin M, Negrini M, Calin GA, Davuluri RV, Ivan M. Regulation of microRNA expression: the hypoxic component. Cell Cycle 2007; 6, 1426-1431.

[90] Zagorska A, Dulak J. HIF-1: the knowns and unknowns of hypoxia sensing. Acta biochimica Polonica 2004; 51, 563-585.

[91] Devlin C, Greco S, Martelli F, Ivan M. miR-210: More than a silent player in hypoxia. IUBMB life 2011; 63, 94-100.

[92] Kulshreshtha R, Davuluri RV, Calin GA, Ivan M. A microRNA component of the hypoxic response. Cell Death and Differentiation 2008; 15, 667-671.

[93] Hua Z, Lv Q, Ye W, Wong CK, Cai G, Gu D, Ji Y, Zhao C, Wang J, Yang BB, Zhang Y. MiRNA-directed regulation of VEGF and other angiogenic factors under hypoxia. PloS one 2006; 1:e116.

[94] Loscalzo J. The cellular response to hypoxia: tuning the system with microRNAs. The Journal of Clinical Investigation 2010: 120, 3815-3817.

[95] Zhou X, Ruan J, Wang G, Zhang W. Characterization and identification of microRNA core promoters in four model species. PLoS Computational Biology 2007; 3:e37.

[96] Ivan M, Harris AL, Martelli F, Kulshreshtha R. Hypoxia response and microRNAs: no longer two separate worlds. Journal of Cellular and Molecular Medicine 2008; 12, 1426-1431.

[97] Kuehbacher A, Urbich C, Zeiher AM, Dimmeler S. Role of Dicer and Drosha for endothelial microRNA expression and angiogenesis. Circulation Research 2007; 101, 59-68.

Chapter 4

Genetic Profiling: Searching for Novel Genetic Aberrations in Glioblastoma

Pouya Jamshidi and Clark C. Chen

Additional information is available at the end of the chapter

http://dx.doi.org/10.5772/53387

1. Introduction

Glioblastoma multiforme (GBM) is the most common primary brain tumors and remains one of the deadliest of human cancers [1]. The incidence of this cancer is fairly low, with 2-3 cases per 100,000 people in Europe and North America. GBM is slightly more common in whites than in blacks, Latinos, and Asians, with a slight male predominance - M:F ratio of 3:2 [2]. The overall prognosis for GBM has changed little in the past two decades, despite major improvements in neuroimaging, neurosurgery, radiation treatment techniques, adjuvant chemotherapy, and supportive care. Without treatment, the median survival is approximately 3 months [3]. The current standard of care involves maximal surgical resection followed by concurrent radiation and chemotherapy with the DNA alkylating agent temozolomide [4]. Despite this aggressive regimen, the median survival remains approximately 14 months. Thus, meaningful strategies for therapeutic intervention are desperately needed.

The most reliable evidence suggests that glioblastomas originate from cells that give rise to glial cells [5, 6]. The World Health Organization (WHO) classifies these glial-derived tumors into four major categories, namely WHO grade I-IV. The higher grade signifies patho-histologic features of increased malignancy. WHO grade IV glioma is synonymous with glioblastoma [7].

Rigorous scientific investigations over the past three decades indicate that glioblastomas, similar to other cancers, are the stem from collection of genetic alterations. These alterations can present in a variety of forms, including epigenetic alterations, point mutations, translocations, amplification or deletions – resulting in gene modifications. The genetic alteration results in either activation or inactivation of specific gene functions that may contribute to the process of carcinogenesis [8]. Those genes, that when activated, contribute to the development of cancer are often termed proto-oncogenes. The mutated forms of these genes are referred to as oncogenes. Conversely, genes that when inactivated contribute to carcinogenesis are generally termed tumor suppressor genes. Although it is well established that central nervous system (CNS) carcinogenesis requires multiple deregulations of the normal cellular circuitry, the exact number and nature of genetic alterations and deregulated signaling pathways required for tumorigenesis remains subject of ongoing scientific investigations [9].

1.1. Cancer genomic era

The current decade will likely be remembered, in the history of cancer research, as the decade of cancer genomics. The marriage of technology and annotated specimen collection has culminated to provide us with a glimpse of the complex genomic landscape that underlies cancer pathogenesis. Remarkably, these efforts have demonstrated true collaborative spirits between clinicians and basic science researchers with common goals of furthering translational science.

The Cancer Genome Atlas (TCGA) constitutes the largest of the genomic efforts. It is a comprehensive and coordinated effort to accelerate our understanding of the molecular basis of cancer through the application of genome analysis technologies, including large-scale genome sequencing. This is accomplished via cataloguing the genetic and epigenetic changes in the cancer genome, with goals of identifying those responsible for carcinogenesis. The project represents a joint effort of the National Human Genome Research Institute (NHGRI), National Cancer Institute (NCI), the U.S. Department of Health and Human Services, and collects of tumor specimen from major cancer centers spanning across the continental USA. The project aims to provide the genomic profile of 500 specimens of various cancer types using state-of-the-art platforms for sequencing, microRNA, mRNA, single- nucleotide polymorphisms (SNPs), and methylation profiling. TCGA started as a pilot project in 2006 with focus on glioblastoma as the first cancer type for study. With the success of the pilot project, TCGA has committed to expand its efforts to aggressively pursue 20 or more additional cancers. While acknowledging the importance of the TCGA in cancer research, one cannot neglect the value of the pioneering genomic efforts that, in many ways, laid the groundwork for the TCGA [10]. The knowledge to sequence the entire genomes of human tumors including glioblastoma, helps formulating new concepts and principles in tumor cell biology, and enables potential exploitation of these major advances for personalized disease management in oncology.

With advances in genomic profiling and sequencing technology, we are beginning to understand the landscape of the genetic events that accumulate during the neoplastic process. The insights gleamed from these genomic profiling has been instrumental to advancing therapeutic strategy. This chapter will aim to review the existing data with regards to chromosomal aberration, mutations, non-doing sequences, over-expressed mRNA, miRNA dysregulation and will explore the opportunities for major therapeutic developments in the cancer gemonic era.

2. Chromosomal aberration

Chromosomal aberration refers to an abnormality in the structure or number of chromosomal content of a cell. Increasingly, cancer is recognized as a heterogeneous collection of diseases whose initiation and progression are prompted by the aberrant function of genes that govern DNA repair, genome stability, cell proliferation, cell death, adhesion, invasion, angiogenesis in complex cell and tissue microenvironment [11, 12]. In addition to high-resolution chromosome banding and advanced chromosomal imaging technologies, chromosome aberrations in cancer cells can be analyzed with an increasing number of large-scale, comprehensive genomic and molecular genetic technologies. These growing technologies include fluorescence in situ hybridization (FISH) [13, 14], spectral karyotyping (SKY) [13], comparative genomic hybrizidation (CGH) [15, 16], and other high-throughput methods that detects loss of heterzygosity (LOH) [17, 18], in cancer cells such as a new single nucleotide polymorphism arrays (SNP Chips) [19] that detect comprehensive genome-wide copy number changes. With the use of comprehensive molecular technologies, the discovery of the recurrent chromosomal aberrations in cancer is proceeding at a very promising pace. To date, glioblastoma has been subjected to the most extensive genomic profiling of any cancer [20]. Studies carried out over the past three decades suggest that glioblastomas, like other cancers, arise secondary to the accumulation of genetic alterations. These alterations can present as epigenetic modifications, point mutations, translocations, amplifications, or deletions, and modify gene function in ways that dysregulate cellular signaling pathways leading to the cancer phenotype [11, 21]. While the exact number and nature of genetic alterations and deregulated signaling pathways required for tumorigenesis remains an issue of debate, [9] it is now well understood that central nervous system (CNS) carcinogenesis requires multiple disruptions to the normal cellular circuitry [22, 23].

Amongst chromosomal aberrations, amplifications and deletions can be distinguished when considering glioblastoma genesis [24]. Conversely, the reports of incidental translocation are rare in glioblastoma [25]. Thus we will mainly focus our review on chromosomal aberrations that present as amplification or deletion and discuss their contribution in the development of glioblastoma.

2.1. Amplification

Amplification of the epidermal growth factor receptor (EGFR) gene is a distinguishing feature in primary glioblastoma [26-28] Moreover, it is now evident that the type of genetic alterations involving EGFR in glioblastoma are distinct from those observed in other EGFR-altered cancers, such as non-small-cell lung cancer (NSCLC). In glioma, focal EGFR amplification occurs at an extremely high level (>20 copies) [20]. Focal (limited to a few Mb) and broader (from several Mbs to entire chromosomes) copy number alterations (CNAs) that include the EGFR gene may have different molecular consequences [27]. Focal amplification of EGFR correlates with EGFR over-expression or mutations and deletions in the EGFR gene, and subsequent activation of the PI3K/AKT pathway [27, 29]. Up-regulated

PI3K/ AKT signaling has been associated with poor prognosis [30]. Evidence of RTK/RAS/PI3K activation has been reported in 88% of tumors, including contributions from unexpected mutations or deletions in NF1 (18%) and PIK3R1, which encodes the p85a regulatory subunit of PIK3CA [20].

Furthermore, amplification of the entire chromosome 7 containing EGFR, MET [22] and its ligand HGF has been found to correlate with activation of the MET axis [20, 27]. EGFR amplification is reported to appear as double minutes (small fragments of extra-chromosomal DNA), and extra copies of EGFR have also been found inserted into different loci on chromosome 7 [31]. Additionally ~50% of EGFR-amplified cells harbor the EGFRvIII mutant, which is an intragenic gene rearrangement generated by an in-frame deletion of exons 2–7 that encode part of the extracellular region [20]. Remarkably, gain of chromosome 7 and amplification of EGFR have been found more frequently in short-term survivors [26, 32], however to date EGFR alterations are not thought to be of prognostic importance in glioblastoma [28, 32, 33].

Amplification of 12q13-15, where the oncogenes CDK4 and MDM2 are located, results in the disruption of both the retinoblastoma (RB) and p53 pathways [22, 27, 34, 35] Specifically, p53 signaling pathway has been reported to be impaired in 87% of the samples through CDKN2A deletion (49%), MDM2 (14%) and MDM4 (7%) amplification, and mutation and deletion of TP53 (35%) [20]. Pathway inactivating mutations in the RB pathway were described in glioblastomas prior to the large-scale genomic efforts [23, 36, 37] and the TCGA validated these results and demonstrated that mutations and gene amplifications disrupting RB function are found in approximately 68–80% of glioblastomas, signifying the critical importance of evading anti-growth signals [21]. RB signaling has been reported to be impaired in 78% of the samples through CDKN2 family deletion; amplification of CDK4 (18%), CDK6 (1%), and CCND2 (2%); and mutation or deletion of RB1 (11%) [20]. Additionally, Genome-Wide Association Studies (GWAS) revealed that single nucleotide polymorphisms (SNPs) in the CDKN2A and CDKN2B have been identified as risk factors for glioma growth [21] [38, 39]. Moreover, the genes encoding the receptor tyrosine kinases KIT, KDR, and PDGFRA, adjacently located on chromosome 4q12, are frequently found to be (co)amplified [40]. Nearly 30% of human gliomas show expression patterns that are correlated with PDGFR signaling [41]. For instance, PDGFRA amplification is found in 15% of all tumors [30, 42]. Of those PDGFRA amplified tumors harboring gene amplification, 40% harbor an intragenic deletion, termed PDGFRAD8, 9 [43], in which an in-frame deletion of 243 base pairs (bp) of exons 8 and 9 leads to a truncated extracellular domain [44]. Point mutations in PDGFRA are associated with amplification but, unlike EGFR, happen rarely. Elevated AKT phosphorylation has been observed in up to 85% of glioblastoma cell lines and patient samples [45]. RTK-independent activation of this pathway in glioblastoma can occur via mutation or amplification of PIK3CA (p110a) [46, 47], and PIK3CD (p110d) is also overexpressed in some gliomas [48]. Other amplified regions containing oncogenes, for example AKT3 [22, 49] and CCND2 [22, 27].

Over-expression of c-Myc is frequently observed in different tumor types, including glioblastoma, and usually results from chromosome translocation involving the c-Myc genes in addition to gene amplification [50]. In a study it was reported that during multistep carcinogenesis using fibroblast lineages transfected with SV40 LT, expression levels of c-Myc and Sp1 associate with the levels of telomerase activity in different stages of transformation [51]. Transcriptional regulation of hTERT is thought to be the chief mechanism of telomerase regulation. Cooperative action of c-Myc and Sp1 is required for full activation of hTERT promoter. Sp1 is also a key molecule that binds to GC-rich sites on the core promoter and activates hTERT transcription [51]. In the core promoter, multiple E-boxes and Sp1 binding sites are located. C-Myc binds to these E-boxes through heterodimer formation with Max proteins and activates transcription of hTERT [52, 53]. This is a direct effect of c-*myc* that does not require *de novo* protein synthesis. Mad proteins are antagonists of c-Myc and switching from Myc/Max binding to Mad/Max binding decreases promoter activity of hTERT [51, 54-56]. Thus, up-regulation of these critical transcription factors may, at least in part, be involved in telomerase activation during carcinogenesis [57].

Amplified Region	Gene of Interest	References
1q	AKT3	[22, 49]
3q	PIK3CA	[22, 23, 27]
4q	PDGFR	[22, 34]
7p	EGFR, MET, HGF, CDK6	[22, 23, 27, 34, 35]
8q	c-MYC	[50]
12q	CDK4, MDM2	[22, 27, 35]

Table 1. Genes frequently identified to be amplified in glioblastoma

2.2. Deletions

Loss of heterozygosity LOH of chromosome 10q is the most common genomic alteration found in both primary and secondary glioblastomas [28, 35] and is associated with poor prognosis [26, 28]. Different regions are frequently lost at chromosome 10, including the regions containing PTEN, MGMT [28, 58], and ANXA7, an EGFR inhibitor [59]. PTEN directly antagonizes PI3K signaling and is one of the most frequently altered genes in cancer. It undergoes genomic loss, mutation, or epigenetic inactivation in 40%–50% of gliomas, resulting in high levels of PI3K activity and downstream signaling [60]. In addition, AKT activation due to PTEN loss likely contributes to RTK inhibitor insensitivity in glioblastoma [29, 61]. Another frequently deleted inhibitor of EGFR signaling is NFKBIA, which is located on chromosome 14; this deletion is also linked to poor survival [62]. Furthermore, loss of chromosome 9p, which contains a variety of tumor-suppressor genes, including CDKN2A, CDKN2B, and PTPRD, is frequently seen [28, 34, 63], especially in short-term survivors [26, 32]. CDKN2A and CDKN2B encode three important cell cycle proteins, p14ARF and p16INK4A, and p15INK4B [26-28, 34, 64], which are involved in the RB and P53 pathways. Deletion of CDKN2A and CDKN2B is often accompanied by deletion of CDKN2C on chromosome 1p32, which encodes another cell cycle protein p18INK4C [64]. LOH of chromosome 1p is found in both primary and secondary glioblastomas [65]. Longstanding hypothesis about the location of tumor suppressor gene at 1p has recently been advanced by identification of the suggested candidate genes CIC and FUPB1 [66]. Co-deletion of 1p and 19q is frequently seen in oligodendrogliomas and is, in those, associated with prolonged survival [32] and translocations [67]. Although this co-deletion has been observed in glioblastomas, no similar association has been identified elsewhere. Isolated LOH 19q is frequently observed in secondary glioblastoma [26, 65] and may be a marker of longer survival [26]. Moreover >50% of oligodendrogliomas has been reported to display loss of heterozygosity (LOH) at chromosomes 1p and 19q [68], although the targets of these deletions are still unclear.

Frequent allelic losses on 22q indicating the presence of tumor suppressor genes have been found in primary and secondary glioblastomas [69]. LOH of 22q identified two sites of minimally deleted regions at 22q12.3–13.2 and 22q13.31 in primary glioblastomas and in most of the secondary glioblastomas. The affected shared deletion of 22q12.3 is the region in which the human tissue inhibitor of metalloproteinases-3 (TIMP-3) is located. As its name implies, expression of TIMP-3 inhibits metalloprotease activity and impair glioblastoma migration and invasiveness [70]. Expectedly, deletion of TIMP-3 enhances glioblastoma invasiveness [69].

It is important to note that the various deletions and amplifications do not exist in isolation. For instance, NFKBIA deletions and EGFR amplifications are essentially mutually exclusive events, suggesting that these events serve redundant functions in glioblastoma pathogenesis [62]. Systematic analysis of the patterns of co-occurrence of the various deletions and amplifications revealed genomic regions with synergistic tumor-promoting relationships [71]. Analysis of the general patterns of co-occurring and mutually exclusive regions in glioblastomas suggests common pathways that are disrupted during carcinogenesis. Targeting these pathways in the context of the genetic landscape of the glioblastoma constitutes one therapeutic strategy.

Deleted Region	Gene of Interest	References
9p	CDKN2A, 2B	[22, 27, 35]
10q	PTEN, MGMT, ANXA7	[22, 23, 34, 35]
13q	RB	[22, 34]
17p	P53, NF1	[22, 23, 34]
19q	BAX	[34, 65]
22q	TIMP3	[69]

Table 2. Genes frequently identified to be deleted in glioblastoma

3. Mutations

The abnormal behaviors demonstrated by cancer cells are thought to be the result of a series of mutations in key regulatory genes. A detailed understanding of the genomic lesions underlying cancer will facilitate the identification of the cellular pathways and networks perturbed by genomic mutations, improve cancer diagnosis through molecular classification, enhance the selection of therapeutic targets for drug development, promote the development of faster and more efficient clinical trials using agents targeted to specific genomic abnormalities, and create markers for early detection and prevention. Results from the genomic profiling efforts and a number of studies over the past three decades have revealed that nearly all glioblastomas harbor activating mutations in genes that play instrumental role in growth signaling cascades, evading apoptosis, insensitivity to antigrowth signals. In addition to amplifications and deletions, genes implicated in glioblastoma can be affected by somatic mutations. Point mutations include base substitutions, deletions, or insertions in coding regions and splice sites. Large-scale mutation analysis has identified mutations activating oncogenes and others inactivating tumor-suppressor genes in glioblastoma.

It was previously thought that glioblastoma arises from the acquisition of a defined set of mutations that occur in a particular temporal order. This model is largely grounded on the framework established in colon cancer, where a series of genetic alterations characterizes different phases of neoplastic progression [72]. This hypothesis is supported by the observation that Grade II astrocytomas typically harbor mutations in p53; Grade III astrocytomas harbor activating mutations/amplifications of CDKN2A (p16Ink4a); and Grade IV astrocytomas harbor mutations in PTEN and EGFR [73]. This data was interpreted to suggest that glioblastoma results from sequential inactivation of the p53, RB, and RTK/PI3K axes. While such a paradigm may hold true for a subset of the secondary glioblastomas, the picture emerging from the genomic characterization of primary glioblastomas reveals a much more dynamic process [22, 23]. The profile of somatic mutations in different glioblastomas is highly variable. These results suggest that most glioblastomas, primary or secondary, evolve along a multitude of pathways in response to differing selective pressures to achieve the phenotypes described by Hanahan and Weinberg [74].

Aberrant centrosome behavior, such as centrosome amplification, has been associated with mutation of *TP53* and has been proposed as a primary source of genetic instability in human tumors. Mutations in "common" cancer genes, for example TP53 and PTEN, are very frequent in glioblastomas, but are not of prognostic importance [22, 23, 28, 32, 33, 75]. On the other hand PTEN loss has been shown clinically to confer resistance to EGFR inhibitors in patients harboring EGFRvIII expressing glioblastoma in part due to its activation of downstream AKT [29, 76] as well as loss of its RTK degradation function [76].

There are several lines of evidence that point to the importance of the p53 axis in glioblastoma pathogenesis. There is a body of literature associating p53 pathway inactivation to glioblastoma genesis [37, 77]. It must be noted that these studies implicate p53 pathway inactivation only in a subset of glioblastomas. The TCGA effort and the effort by Parsons et al. [22, 23] enhanced the literature by demonstrating that the p53 axis is more broadly impaired in glioblastomas than previously thought. Mutations that inactivate this axis are found in greater than 70% of all glioblastoma specimens as reported by both studies. This understanding has led to more accurate modeling of glioblastoma by combined inactivation of p53 and PTEN [78].

There are a number of mutations that are thought be glioblastoma specific, even though they may be seen in only a subgroup of tumor cells. The EGFRvIII mutant lacks 267 amino acids in the extracellular part, resulting in a constitutively activated receptor that no longer requires its ligand EGF to signal downstream [79]. Despite the well-recognized proproliferative functions of EGFRvIII, its expression in human glioblastoma is heterogeneous and is most often observed only in a subpopulation of cells [80]. Recent observations support a model of functional heterogeneity in which a minority of EGFRvIII-expressing cells not only drive their own intrinsic growth, but also potentiate the proliferation of adjacent wild-type EGFR-expressing cells in a paracrine fashion through the cytokine co-receptor gp130 [81]. EGFRvIII expression may be linked to differentiation and/ or development. EGFR point mutations have also been identified in glioblastoma, in the extracellular domain, whereas they are predominantly found in the kinase domain in other tumor types, such as lung cancer [82]. *EGFR* mutations have recently been identified as clinically significant, due to their association with striking responses in subsets of patients treated with targeted therapeutic agents. [83, 84].

The PI3K signaling pathway is dysregulated in many cancers [85], including glioblastomas. A number of investigations have reported activating mutations in the RTK–PI3K pathway [43, 86], validating the importance of this pathway in glioblastoma pathogenesis. Mutations in PIK3CA and PIK3R1, coding for the PI3K catalytic subunit p110a and regulatory subunit P85a, have been described [22, 23]. RTK-independent activation of this pathway in glioblastoma can occur via mutation of PIK3CA (p110a) [46, 47] or through recurrent mutations in the gene encoding the p85a regulatory subunit PIK3R1. This will likely drive PIK3CA activation through decreased SH2 domain-mediated inhibition [87]. In the TCGA report [22] activating mutations in the RTK–PI3K pathways are reported in 88% of the 206 glioblastomas sequenced.

Although mutations in the RAS genes constitute a fairly rare phenomenon in glioblastoma (>5%) [88], inactivating mutations and deletions have been identified in their inhibitory tumor suppressor gene NF1 [22]. The protein encoded by neurofibromatosis 1 (NF1) functions to catalyze the exchange of GTP for GDP in Ras - preventing cell proliferation. While it is reported that NF1 patients are predisposed to gliomagenesis [89], inactivating mutations in NF1 was not discovered in glioblastoma until recently [22, 23, 90, 91]. The TCGA results indicated that approximately 20% of glioblastomas harbor loss of function mutations in NF1 [22, 23] and more significantly, mutations in NF1 appear to define a particular subtype of glioblastoma.

The majority of malignant brain tumors, including glioblastoma, demonstrate inactivating mutations in either the p53 and/or retinoblastoma (RB) pathways [92-95]. In addition to their adverse cellular functions, these two pathways are most directly involved in cell cycling regulations during times of cell repair or cell growth.

The *TP53* tumor suppressor gene, located on 17p13, is frequently mutated or deleted in gliomas [96, 97]. P53 is a short-lived transcription factor that can execute diverse cellular programs, such as cell cycle arrest, DNA repair, apoptosis, autophagy, differentiation, senescence and self- renewal [98, 99]. It facilitates DNA repair by halting the cell cycle for repair enzymes to work, or if the damage is too great, it induces cell death. The retinoblastoma (Rb, 13q14) pathway is also a key cell cycle regulatory complex at the G1 checkpoint. *CDKN2A,* located on 9p21 and deleted in many cancers, encodes the p16 protein, a key inhibitor of the cell cycle via Rb pathway signaling. Homozygous deletion of p16 has been reported to be associated with WHO grade III or IV gliomas [7, 100]. Gliomas often display mutations in the ARF- MDM2-p53 and p16INK4A-CDK4-RB tumor suppressor pathways [101, 102]. Primary glioblastoma often exhibits loss of the INK4A/ARF tumor suppressor gene locus along with PTEN mutation and EGFR amplification/mutation, and secondary glioblastoma shows frequent mutations of TP53 [58].

The relevance of p53 to the treatment and outcome of patients with high-grade glioma has remained controversial. Some studies have shown that p53 status, assayed either by expression or mutation analysis, is correlated with relatively good outcome [103, 104], while others have demonstrated no prognostic impact in anaplastic gliomas and GBM [105, 106]. Also, *MDM2* amplification, although infrequent, has been shown by some to be predictive of poor outcome [103, 107], whereas others have observed no prognostic value [108]. P53 status might cooperate with other prognostic variables; for example, *TP53* mutation has been linked to low *MGMT* mRNA expression [109], although this does not correlate with *MGMT* promoter methylation [110]. Loss of *CDKN2A, CDKN2B,* or *RB* or *CDK4* amplification, disrupting the Rb pathway, has been shown in anaplastic astrocytoma to associate with decreased survival [111, 112]. Conversely, p16 appears to be associated with improved survival in patients treated with chemotherapy and radiation [113]. Overall, it appears that the prognostic impact of p53 and Rb aberrations is at best marginal.

Comprehensive analysis of genomic data in glioblastoma revealed recurrent mutations in the R132 residue of isocitrate dehydrogenase 1 (IDH1) and is involved in energy metabolism [23]. IDH1/2 is mutated in grade II and III gliomas as well as the secondary glioblastomas that arise from prior low-grade tumors, with most mutations found in the IDH1 gene. IDH1 mutations have been predominantly identified in secondary glioblastomas and low-grade gliomas, with mutations in more than 70% of cases [23, 114-118]. Patients with IDH1 mutated primary glioblastomas are generally younger and have longer median survival and wild-type EGFR. Because these are characteristics of secondary glioblastomas, it is hypothesized that these are in fact secondary glioblastomas for which no histological evidence of evolution from a less malignant glioma is found. Significantly, these mutations usually occur at conserved residues and are virtually never homozygous. While only 3%–7% of primary glioblastomas harbor IDH1 mutations, the majority (50%–80%) of secondary glioblastomas express mutant IDH1. Thus, IDH1 could be used to differentiate primary from secondary glioblastomas [116]. In addition, 3% of the tumors that express wild-type IDH1 were found to express IDH2 R172 mutations [117-120], although this mutation in IDH2 has only been documented in a single glioblastoma in the literature [121].

Studies on the downstream biological effects of IDH1/2 mutation expression have focused largely on the inhibition of α-KG-dependent dioxygenases by 2-HG, as IDH mutations result in a novel function to catalyze α-ketoglutarate (α-KG) to 2-hydroxyglutarate (2-HG)

[122]. The wild-type IDH1 normally functions as a homodimer that converts isocitrate to α-ketoglutarate [120]. Biochemical depiction of the R132 mutated IDH1 revealed that it functions to inhibit the process. Thus, glioblastoma harboring the R132 IDH1 mutation harbor decreased levels of α-KG. It is imperative to note that α-KG dependent dioxygenases is a diverse group of enzymes controls a broad range of physiological processes, including hypoxic sensing, histone demethylation, demethylation of hypermethylated DNA, fatty acid metabolism, and collagen modification, among others [123]. Several studies have provided evidence to demonstrate that several of these functions are influenced by IDH1/2 mutation expression.

Mutational and epigenetic profiling of patients specimen has revealed that IDH1 mutations closely associated with a specific hyper-methylation signature. The hyper-methylation state may be caused in part by the 2-HG-mediated inhibition of the α-KG-dependent TET2 enzyme [124, 125]; the resultant decrease in 5-hydroxymethylcytosine was also observed in glioblastoma specimens [124]. Moreover, expression of IDH1 mutations is thought to induce global DNA hyper-methylation [126]. Thus it is suggested that IDH1 mutations may lead to dysregulated epigenetic processes. 2-HG inhibits histone demethylases and TET 5-methylcytosine hydroxylases, thought to be involved in epigenetic control. This suggests that mutations in IDH1 change the expression of a potentially large number of genes [124].

Most lower-grade gliomas harbor IDH1 mutations; although grade I pilocytic astrocytomas usually express wild-type IDH1; 60%–80% of grade II and III astrocytomas, oligodendrogliomas, and oligoastrocytomas express mutant IDH1, with the R132H mutation representing the majority of mutations observed. Given that mutations in IDH1 are an early event in gliomagenesis [127], this may suggest widespread modification of epigenetic regulator as the key mechanism in gliomagenesis in IDH1 mutated tumors. Furthermore, it might explain the extensive and fundamental differences between mutated and wild-type IDH1 glioblastoma. It has been reported that global expression profiles of IDH1 mutant glioblastomas more closely resembled lineage-committed neural precursors, whereas wild-type counterparts appear to resemble neural stem cells [128].

Independent glioblastoma studies have pointed to IDH1 mutations as an objective positive prognostic marker [23, 114, 115, 120]. Reports of the association between IDH1 mutations and favorable prognosis hold promise for biomarker development [23, 42, 120], although these correlations await validation in prospective clinical trials. Thorough understanding of mutant IDH biology and the mutant status of the IDH1/2 genes may serve as a key prognostic indicator. Specifically, patients with anaplastic astrocytoma [23, 115, 120, 121] and glioblastoma harboring mutant IDH1 demonstrate a significantly longer overall survival compared with wild-type IDH1 counterparts and are younger at presentation. Similar survival benefit has also been observed in grade II gliomas. [115] Furthermore, a comprehensive genomic and clinical analysis of glioblastomas harboring mutant and wild-type IDH1 suggests that, while histo-pathologically similar, these tumors may represent disease processes far more unique than has been appreciated. Specifically, IDH1 mutant tumors display less contrast enhancement, less peritumoral edema, larger initial size, greater cystic components, and a greater likelihood of frontal lobe involvement compared with wild-type tumors [128].

A frequently encountered critique of genomic sequencing effort involves the following. The first generation sequencing used to characterize the glioblastoma landscape captures the most prevalent mutations. They did not analyze the deeper heterogeneity of low prevalence mutations that have been found in several tumor types, including colon cancer [129]. Efforts to examine whether such sub-clonal diversity exist in glioblastoms using highly sensitive techniques [130] have not identified the presence of low-prevalence mutations. These results suggest that clonal expansion of select mutation in glioblastoma constitute a major mechanism of tumor expansion and that random mutagenesis through mutator phenotype does not contribute significantly to glioblastoma pathogenesis. The insights gained from the TCGA and other sequencing efforts should be viewed in this light.

4. Non-coding DNA sequences

While the identification of nucleotide alterations within the coding sequence of protooncogenes or tumor suppressor genes has significantly contributed to our understanding of carcinogenesis, there is an emerging appreciation that alterations in non-coding sequences similarly contribute to development of cancer [131]. Non-coding DNA describes components of DNA arrangements that do not participate in the coding of protein sequences. These DNA sequences may present in different forms including non-coding functional RNA, cis- and trans-regulatory elements, introns, pseudogenes, repeat sequences, transposons, and telomeres. A notable example involves the regulation of gene transcription by reversible modification of gene promoter regions a phenomenon often referred to as 'epigenetic regulation' [132]. The term 'epigenetic regulation' describes the phenomenon in which heritable changes in gene expression can occur in the absence of changes in the DNA sequences encoding for gene function. Understanding the concept that non-coding sequences play critical roles in glioblastoma pathogenesis and resistance to chemotherapy offers novel strategies for biomarker development and therapy.

The mechanism underlying epigenetic involves cytosine methylation [133] or histone modifications that, in turn, modulate the accessibility of gene promoter regions to transcriptional factors [134]. Cytosine methylation often occurs in the context of CpG di-nucleotide repeats, or CpG islands [133]. Thus promoters that harbor heavily methylated CpG islands are typically transcriptionally silenced. There are two types of promoter methylation that are particularly pertinent to glioblastoma therapy: methylation in the promoter region of the DNA repair gene, methyl-guanine methyl transferase (MGMT) and the glioma-CpG island methylator (G-CIMP) phenotype [135].

MGMT encodes an enzyme that removes alkyl adducts at the O6 position of guanine [136]. Because alkyl modification at this position is highly toxic and constitutes the primary mechanism for the tumoricidal activity of the chemotherapeutic agent TMZ, MGMT expression level correlates well with TMZ response in patients with glioblastoma [137]. The human MGMT gene possesses a CpG island that spans approximately 1000 bases around the transcriptional start site. Detailed analysis of this region revealed 108 CpG sites [138] that are methylated. Methylation of a subset of these CpGs has been associated with transcriptional silencing of MGMT [139, 140] and is associated with improved clinical outcome in patients with glioblastoma receiving TMZ therapy. Interestingly, MGMT promoter methylation is also associated with improved survival in patients who did not receive TMZ therapy [141, 142]. While the mechanism underlying this observation remains unclear, it seems likely that MGMT may participate in detoxifying the accumulation of endogenous DNA damage that is typically associated with the oncogenic state [143]. Glioblastoma cells accumulate endogenous DNA damage in the absence of DNA damaging agents [143]. These endogenous DNA damages are not unlike those induce by temozolomide or radiation in that they could trigger cell death if unrepaired. Thus, tumors with high levels of MGMT may grow more robustly since MGMT is capable of detoxifying these endogenous DNA damages. If the tumor cells grow more robustly, the patient will survive for a shorter duration. In contrast, the glioblastoma cells with low MGMT may be more susceptible to the deleterious effects of the endogenous DNA damages. These tumors may grow less robustly, resulting in longer patient survival.

The G-CIMP phenotype refers to the observation that a subset of glioblastomas exhibits concerted CpG island methylation at a large number of loci [144]. Since genes required for tumour growth are located at many of these loci, glioblastomas harboring the G-CIMP phenotype tend to be more benign. Correspondingly, patients with G-CIMP glioblastomas experienced significantly improved outcome. Understanding the concept that the patterns of CpG island methylation directly impact outcomes in patients with glioblastoma open the door to therapeutic strategies aimed at enhancing promoter methylation at select promoter loci. Importantly, recent studies suggest that promoter methylation at distinct loci may be affected by specific chromatin-modulating factors [135, 145].

While much of cellular DNA has no known biological function, many types of non-coding DNA sequences do have recognized biological functions, including the transcriptional and translational regulation of protein-coding sequences. These governing functions may include genetic switches, regulation of gene expression, transcription factors, operators, enhancers, promoters, and insulators [146-148]. Genome-wide association (GWA's) studies have uncovered a large number of cancer susceptibility regions that do not overlap protein-coding genes but rather map to non-coding intervals [132, 135]. The concept that non-coding DNA sequences regulate gene function and impact carcinogenesis has significantly expanded the repertoire of strategies available for glioblastoma therapeutics [135]. Integrating the biology of non-coding sequences in the context of mutational profile is critical in understanding tumor physiology and meaningful therapeutic development.

5. Over-expressed mRNA

Over-expression or under-expression of genes in glioblastoma compared with that in a normal brain or in low-grade gliomas may serve as an indication of genes that are involved in gliomagenesis [24]. While glioblastoma has been conceptualized as a single disease, it is widely appreciated that the term captures significant histologic heterogeneity. This heterogeneity suggests distinct subtypes with differing physiologic states that are captured under the umbrella term "glioblastoma" [21]. In fact, the genome-wide analysis of mRNA expression to identify molecular subclasses (Golub et al. 1999) has led to a fundamental shift in our understanding of glioblastoma subtypes. In fact, the identification of multiple subtypes within glioblastoma has highlighted the heterogeneity of diseases that are in the same group based on the WHO histo-pathological grade.

Primary and secondary glioblastoma subtypes are histo-pathologically indistinguishable, but differences can be demonstrated by molecular markers at the epigenetic [69], genetic [28, 35, 58], expression [149], and proteomic [150] levels. Primary glioblastomas have a greater prevalence of EGFR alterations, MDM2 duplications, PTEN mutations, and homozygous deletions of CDKN2A [28, 58]. MET amplification [35], over-expression of PDGFRA, and mutations in IDH1 and TP53 are more prevalent in secondary glioblastomas [23, 29, 58, 75, 114, 116, 118]. Moreover, the large-scale analysis has revealed the highly structured nature of glioma transcriptome and has shown correlation of tumor histology and molecular alterations with patient outcome [10, 24, 42]. While expression profiling of glioblastoma has been widely used, two fundamental studies have provided the groundwork for the classification of glioblastoma subtypes [30, 42]. The first subtype initially reported by Phillips et al. [30] and subsequently confirmed by the TCGA mRNA [42] and microRNA profiling [151]. The transcript signature resembles those of neuro-blasts and oligodendrocytes derived from fetal and adult brain cells [30]. The subtype harbors transcriptomal and clinical features that emulate those previously classified as secondary glioblastomas. Molecularly, proneural glioblastomas harbor mutations classically associated with the secondary glioblastomas [42]. Hence, grade II and III gliomas harbor transcriptomal signatures most reminiscent of the proneural subtype [30]. Clinically, this subtype typically affects younger patients, is associated with improved overall survival [30], and responds poorly to concurrent radiation/temozolomide treatment upon disease progression [42].

The second subtype that has emerged is characterized by a gene expression signature that illustrates those observed in the neural stem cells of the forebrain [30], cultured astroglial cells [152], and tissue of mesenchymal origin [30]. Thus, the subtype is termed "mesenchymal" for the latter correlation. Similar to the proneural subtype, this second subtype was initially identified by Phillips et al. [30] and subsequently confirmed by the TCGA [42]. This subtype is highly enriched for mutations inactivating NF1, suggesting a common genetic etiology. The mesenchymal signature appear driven a common transcriptional network, as expression of two key critical factors (STAT3 and CEBPb) enhance tumor aggressiveness in murine models [153].

Benefiting from unsupervised hierarchical clustering analysis, Verhaak et al. (2010) classified 200 TCGA glioblastoma samples into four subtypes, which were subsequently validated using previously published data from 260 independent samples. Large-scale expression studies are validated by reverse transcription (RT)-PCR for individual genes. Bioinformatics analysis revealed that three of the four subtypes were found to harbor distinct molecular aberrations. In particular, the proneural subtype was enriched for amplifications of PDGFRA, CDK6, CDK4, and MET; 11 out of 12 IDH1 mutations found in the TCGA samples; PIK3CA/ PIK3R1mutations; and mutation or LOH of TP53. While the mesenchymal subtype carries mutations and/or loss of NF1, TP53, and CDKN2A, the classical subtype shows amplification for EGFR and loss of PTEN. On the other hand, to date no distinguishing genetic alterations have been indicated to define the neural class from the other classes [20]. It is imperative to keep in mind that interpretations of these results are difficult due to methodological differences in profiling platforms, bioinformatic extrapolation, and specimen collection.

While the number of subtypes identified by the Verhaak et al. (2010) and Phillips et al. (2006) studies differs, the proneural and mesenchymal classifications identified using distinct methodologies and sample sets are the most robust and concordant [10]. For instance, both groups identified proneural class expression of DLL3 and OLIG2 and mesenchymal class expression of CD40 and CHI3L1/YKL-40, the latter of which appears to be a potential serum protein marker of prognosis in glioblastoma patients [154]. Both studies share the observation that patients afflicted with the mesenchymal subtype exhibit poorer clinical prognosis relative to the proneural subtype. A high level of expression of insulin-like growth factor binding proteins, for example IGFBP-2/3 [155], angiogenesic factors, such as vascular endothelial growth factor A (VEGFA) [156], and mesenchymal markers, like YKL-40/CHI3L1, are frequently seen in glioblastoma and have been associated with poor prognosis [157-159]. In contrast, NOTCH signaling genes, for example DLL3, are indicative of better survival [160].

Hence, the collection of data suggests at least two distinct subtypes that reflect essential biologic behavior [10, 30, 42] and have been validated by independent studies. In addition to promising improvement in the grading of glioblastoma, gene expression profiling has shown great promise in prognosis of this deadly tumor, as the genes represented in these subtypes could help to predict outcome in glioblastoma. For example, increased expression of mesenchymal genes such as CHI3L1/YKL-40 and LGALS3 combined with decreased expression of a proneural gene, OLIG2, are associated with typical short-termsurvival compared with longer-termsurvivors [161]. Additional studies have extended the utility of mRNA profiling by using computational network analysis to uncover the causal regulatory modules underlying particular transcriptomically defined subtypes. It is important to note that most of these subtypes have not been as rigorously validated as the proneural and the mesenchymal. The emerging literature suggests that the proneural and mesenchymal subtypes define the two poles in the spectrum of molecular glioblastoma physiology [10, 30, 42]. It remains unclear whether the other proposed subtypes constitute a "forced fit" of a set of truly heterogeneous biology, a gradation of phenotypes between the two extreme poles, or a genuine subtype whose biologic basis remains to be understood.

With genomics approaches, discoveries of common features of different types of tumor may lead to new therapeutic targets and drugs for other tumor types also. The discovery of overexpression of VEGFA and its correlation with poor prognosis in glioblastomas [156] led to trials with the angiogenesis inhibitor bevacizumab.

6. Micro-RNA (miRNA) dysregulation

Micro-RNAs (miRNA or miR) are a class of small non-coding RNAs, approximately 22 nucleotides long that are involved in post-transcriptional gene regulation [162]. Through imperfect pairing, miRNA's bind to untranslated regions of protein-coding mRNAs and function mainly as negative regulators of gene expression. Binding of miRNA often leads to mRNA degradation or inhibition of protein translation – resulting in suppression of the target proteins. A number of cellular processes are regulated by miRNAs including development, proliferation, and differentiation. Micro-RNAs play an important role in many different disorders, particularly in cancer [163]. Bioinformatic analysis predicts that a single miRNA can potentially regulate hundreds of target oncogenes or tumour suppressor proteins. The association of miRNA deregulation with pathogenesis and progression of malignant disease illustrates great potential of utilizing miRNAs as targets for therapeutic intervention. Thus, modulation of miRNA expression provides great hope for potential cancer therapy. Furthermore, since each miRNA may have more than one target, miRNA-based gene therapy offers the therapeutic appeal of targeting multiple gene networks that are controlled by a single miRNA [164]. Over 1000 miRNAs have been described in humans [165]. Bioinformatics analysis has recently revealed that miRNAs are differentially expressed in glioblastoma tissues compared to normal brain tissue [166-169]. For example, while primary glioblastomas and cell lines over-express miR-221 and miR-222, which are thought to target cell cyclin-dependent kinase inhibitors p27 and p57, set of brain-enriched miRNAs (miR-128, miR-181a, miR-181b, and miR-181c) show reduced expression [170, 171].

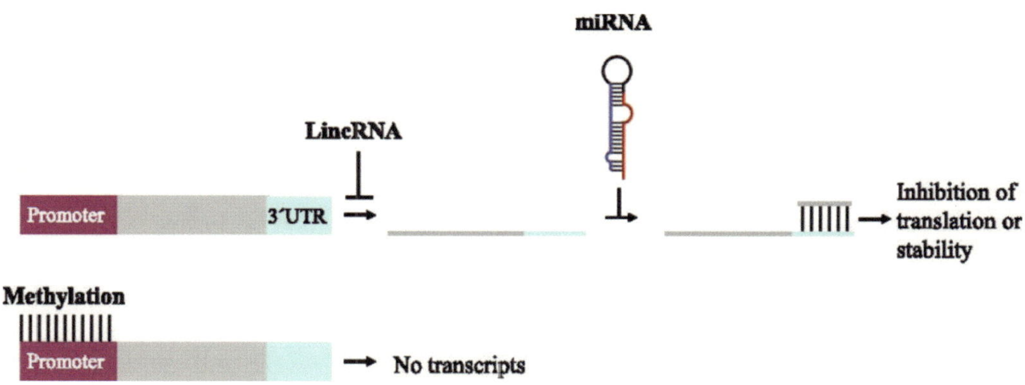

Figure 1. Gene regulation by non-coding RNAs. Figure is adapted with permission from reference [135].

Frequently up-regulated miRNAs are called onco-miRNAs and are thought to contribute to carcinogenesis. As an example miRNA-10b is known to be highly expressed in glioblastoma samples [170], suggesting an important role for miR-10b in glioblastoma tumorigenesis. Furthermore, a recent study revealed that miR-10b expression is inversely correlated with glioblastoma patient survival [172]. Notably, miR-10b was also found to be up-regulated in breast cancer, leukemia, and pancreatic cancer and promote tumor invasion and metastasis in breast cancer [173-175]. These results suggest that some miRNAs, such as miR-10b, may function as a global oncogene to trigger tumorigenesis in multiple tissues. Another example of onco-miRNA in glioblastoma is miR-26a, which is thought to target PTEN [176]. PTEN has been reported to be down-regulated in 70% of human cancers, and there are several indications that it functions as a haplo-insufficient tumor suppressor gene [177]. PTEN expression is down-regulated by several different miRNAs, and it is thought that post-transcriptional regulation is an essential player in determining PTEN abundance in cancer cells. By targeting the tumor suppressor PTEN, overexpression of miR-26a facilitates tumorigenesis [168, 176]. Furthermore, miR-26 cooperates with oncogenes CDK4 and CENTG1, forming an onco-miRNA/oncogene cluster, targeting the RB, PI3K/AKT, and JNK pathways and increasing aggressiveness in glioblastoma [168]. Over-expressed oncogenic miRNAs may be targeted by antagomirs or miRNA sponges, because over-expression of the onco-miRNAs miR-26a, miR-196, and miR-451 has been correlated with poorer survival [167].

In contrast with the onco-miRNA's, frequently down-regulated miRNA's in glioblastoma are considered tumor-suppressor miRNA's. Reduced miR-128 expression in glioblastoma and consequent reduced cell proliferation *in vitro* and in xenografts [178]. Furthermore, miR-128 regulates the expression of the complex protein Bmi-1 through binding at the *BMI-1* 3'-UTR, resulting in decreased Bmi-1 and H3K27me3 levels. In GBM-derived neurosphere cells, miR-128 over-expression has been reported to block stem cell self-renewal, indicating that miR-128 can govern the stem cell-like capabilities of a subset of GBM cells [132]. Glioblastoma tumor tissue profiling has revealed that miRNA-124 is down-regulated in glioblastoma tissue [163, 170]. Notably, miR-124 is also frequently down-regulated in other cancers, such as medulloblastoma, hepatocellular carcinoma, and oral squamous carcinoma [179, 180], suggesting that it may function as a general tumor suppressor. Moreover, miRNA-137 and miRNA-451 exhibit reduced expression in malignant glioblastoma tissues relative to normal brain tissues [181, 182].

Despite advances in biomedical science, the prognosis of glioblastoma patients remains poor. Biomarkers for this disease are needed for early detection of tumor progression. Clinical significance of miRNA expression profiles in glioblastoma has not been explored extensively. Nevertheless, 16 candidate miRNAs have been described to associate with malignant behavior of gliomas (miR-196a, miR-15b, miR-105, miR-367, miR-184, miR-196b, miR-363, miR-504, miR-302b, miR-128b, miR-601, miR-21, miR-517c, miR-302d, miR-383, miR-135b). Among them, miR-196a and miR-196b indicated the highest level of significance) [183]. Both miRNAs showed increased expression levels in glioblastomas relative to anaplastic astrocytomas and normal brain tissues. Higher level of miR-196 transcript significantly correlated with poorer survival [167, 183]. Treatment of malignant gliomas remains one of the greatest challenges facing oncologists today through a frequent resistance to both chemo- and radiotherapeutic agents [184]. Important question for management of glioblastoma patients is the possibility of predicting therapeutic outcome. The miRNA expression profiles of glioblastoma tissues have shown association of miR-181b and miR-181c with response to concomitant chemoradiotherapy with temozolomide (RT/RMZ). MiR-181b and miR-181c were significantly down-regulated in glioblastoma tissue of patients who responded to RT/TMZ in comparison to patients with progressive disease [183, 185]. In a recent study by Zhang et al. [186] genome-wide miRNA profiling of 82 glioblastomas demonstrated that miR-181d was inversely associated with patient overall survival and temozolomide (TMZ) treatment. Bioinformatics analysis of potential genes regulated by miR-181d revealed methyl-guanine-methyl-transferase (MGMT) as a downstream target. Together, these results suggest that miR-181d is a predictive biomarker for TMZ response and that its role is mediated, in part, by post-transcriptional regulation of MGMT.

The basic strategy of current miRNA-based treatment studies is either to antagonize the expression of target miRNAs with antisense technology or to restore or strengthen the function of given miRNAs to inhibit the expression of certain protein-coding gene. Unfortunately, several major challenges have to be addressed before the application of miRNA-based treatment. First, the multi-targeting nature of miRNAs gives the risk of unintended off-target effects that need to be carefully evaluated. Moreover, the expression of target gene may be governed by several different miRNAs, which may compromise the effect of miRNA-based treatment. Finally, there is still lack of miRNA delivery system with enough specificity and efficacy [183].

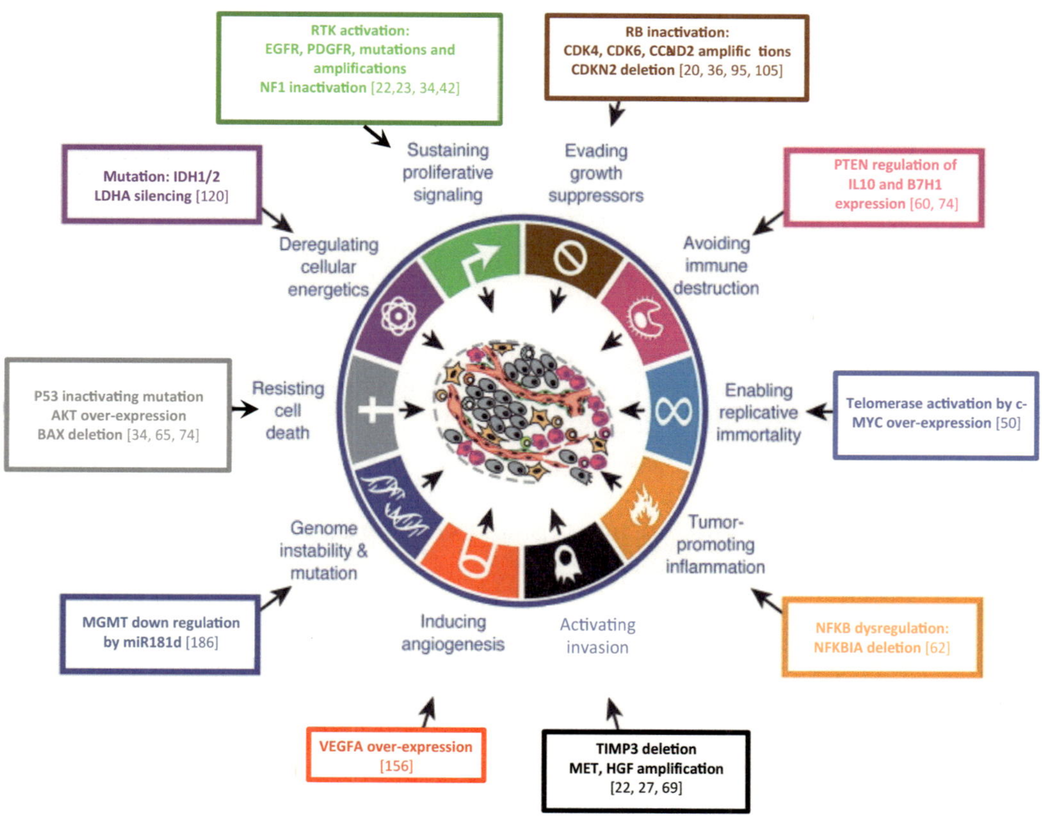

Figure 2. TCGA revealed genes that are known to contribute to the cancer phenotype, as proposed by Hanahan and Weinberg (2011). Figure is adapted with permission from reference [8].

7. Conclusion

In this chapter, we have reviewed and discussed key molecular participants glioblastoma, including chromosomal aberration, mutations, non-coding DNA sequences, over-expressed mRNA, and miRNA dysregulation. We placed our focus to explore the opportunities for major therapeutic developments in the cancer genomic era, where a more comprehensive mechanistic insight into glioblastoma pathogenesis and biology is arguably the most promising approach to discoveries of innovative treatment strategies.

Future development of tools for subtyping, biomarker development, and therapeutic strategies grounded in the genomic landscape of the particular glioblastoma will facilitate clinical trial designs. Ultimately, robust therapeutic gain can be achieved only when agents are directed toward the most vulnerable features inherent within the distinct physiologies of different glioblastoma.

Author details

Pouya Jamshidi
School of Medicine, University of California at San Diego, La Jolla, CA, USA
Center for Theoretical and Applied Neuro-Oncology, Moores Cancer Center, Health Sciences Drive, La Jolla, CA, USA

Clark C. Chen
Center for Theoretical and Applied Neuro-Oncology, Moores Cancer Center, Health Sciences Drive, La Jolla, USA
Division of Neurosurgery, University of California, San Diego Health System, Health Science Drive, La Jolla, USA

Acknowledgement

This work was supported by the American Association of Neurological Surgeons (AANS) Medical Student Summer Research Fellowship (P.J.), Doris Duke Charitable Foundation Clinical Scientist Development Award (C.C.C.), the Sontag Foundation Distinguished Scientist Award (C.C.C.), the Burroughs Wellcome Fund Career Awards for Medical Sciences (C.C.C.), and an National Cancer Institute K12 award (C.C.C.).

8. References

[1] Wen PY, Kesari S. Malignant gliomas in adults. The New England journal of medicine. 2008;359(5):492-507. Epub 2008/08/02.

[2] Jemal A, Siegel R, Xu J, Ward E. Cancer statistics, 2010. CA: a cancer journal for clinicians. 2010;60(5):277-300. Epub 2010/07/09.

[3] Walker MD, Alexander E, Jr., Hunt WE, MacCarty CS, Mahaley MS, Jr., Mealey J, Jr., et al. Evaluation of BCNU and/or radiotherapy in the treatment of anaplastic gliomas. A cooperative clinical trial. Journal of neurosurgery. 1978;49(3):333-43. Epub 1978/09/01.

[4] Stupp R, Mason WP, van den Bent MJ, Weller M, Fisher B, Taphoorn MJ, et al. Radiotherapy plus concomitant and adjuvant temozolomide for glioblastoma. The New England journal of medicine. 2005;352(10):987-96. Epub 2005/03/11.

[5] Alcantara Llaguno S, Chen J, Kwon CH, Jackson EL, Li Y, Burns DK, et al. Malignant astrocytomas originate from neural stem/progenitor cells in a somatic tumor suppressor mouse model. Cancer cell. 2009;15(1):45-56. Epub 2008/12/30.

[6] Ignatova TN, Kukekov VG, Laywell ED, Suslov ON, Vrionis FD, Steindler DA. Human cortical glial tumors contain neural stem-like cells expressing astroglial and neuronal markers in vitro. Glia. 2002;39(3):193-206. Epub 2002/08/31.

[7] Louis DN, Ohgaki H, Wiestler OD, Cavenee WK, Burger PC, Jouvet A, et al. The 2007 WHO classification of tumours of the central nervous system. Acta neuropathologica. 2007;114(2):97-109. Epub 2007/07/10.

[8] Hanahan D, Weinberg RA. Hallmarks of cancer: the next generation. Cell. 2011;144(5):646-74. Epub 2011/03/08.

[9] Stratton MR, Campbell PJ, Futreal PA. The cancer genome. Nature. 2009;458(7239):719-24. Epub 2009/04/11.

[10] Huse JT, Phillips HS, Brennan CW. Molecular subclassification of diffuse gliomas: seeing order in the chaos. Glia. 2011;59(8):1190-9. Epub 2011/03/30.

[11] Hanahan D, Weinberg RA. The hallmarks of cancer. Cell. 2000;100(1):57-70. Epub 2000/01/27.

[12] Albertson DG, Collins C, McCormick F, Gray JW. Chromosome aberrations in solid tumors. Nature genetics. 2003;34(4):369-76. Epub 2003/08/19.

[13] Schrock E, du Manoir S, Veldman T, Schoell B, Wienberg J, Ferguson-Smith MA, et al. Multicolor spectral karyotyping of human chromosomes. Science. 1996;273(5274):494-7. Epub 1996/07/26.

[14] Speicher MR, Gwyn Ballard S, Ward DC. Karyotyping human chromosomes by combinatorial multi-fluor FISH. Nature genetics. 1996;12(4):368-75. Epub 1996/04/01.

[15] Kallioniemi A, Kallioniemi OP, Sudar D, Rutovitz D, Gray JW, Waldman F, et al. Comparative genomic hybridization for molecular cytogenetic analysis of solid tumors. Science. 1992;258(5083):818-21. Epub 1992/10/30.

[16] Pinkel D, Segraves R, Sudar D, Clark S, Poole I, Kowbel D, et al. High resolution analysis of DNA copy number variation using comparative genomic hybridization to microarrays. Nature genetics. 1998;20(2):207-11. Epub 1998/10/15.

[17] Knuutila S, Autio K, Aalto Y. Online access to CGH data of DNA sequence copy number changes. The American journal of pathology. 2000;157(2):689. Epub 2000/08/10.

[18] Hampton GM, Larson AA, Baergen RN, Sommers RL, Kern S, Cavenee WK. Simultaneous assessment of loss of heterozygosity at multiple microsatellite loci using semi-automated fluorescence-based detection: subregional mapping of chromosome 4 in cervical carcinoma. Proceedings of the National Academy of Sciences of the United States of America. 1996;93(13):6704-9. Epub 1996/06/25.

[19] Zhao X, Li C, Paez JG, Chin K, Janne PA, Chen TH, et al. An integrated view of copy number and allelic alterations in the cancer genome using single nucleotide polymorphism arrays. Cancer research. 2004;64(9):3060-71. Epub 2004/05/06.

[20] Dunn GP, Rinne ML, Wykosky J, Genovese G, Quayle SN, Dunn IF, et al. Emerging insights into the molecular and cellular basis of glioblastoma. Genes & development. 2012;26(8):756-84. Epub 2012/04/18.

[21] Ng K, Kim R, Kesari S, Carter B, Chen CC. Genomic profiling of glioblastoma: convergence of fundamental biologic tenets and novel insights. Journal of neuro-oncology. 2012;107(1):1-12. Epub 2011/10/18.

[22] Comprehensive genomic characterization defines human glioblastoma genes and core pathways. Nature. 2008;455(7216):1061-8. Epub 2008/09/06.

[23] Parsons DW, Jones S, Zhang X, Lin JC, Leary RJ, Angenendt P, et al. An integrated genomic analysis of human glioblastoma multiforme. Science. 2008;321(5897):1807-12. Epub 2008/09/06.

[24] Bleeker FE, Molenaar RJ, Leenstra S. Recent advances in the molecular understanding of glioblastoma. Journal of neuro-oncology. 2012;108(1):11-27. Epub 2012/01/25.

[25] Mulholland PJ, Fiegler H, Mazzanti C, Gorman P, Sasieni P, Adams J, et al. Genomic profiling identifies discrete deletions associated with translocations in glioblastoma multiforme. Cell Cycle. 2006;5(7):783-91. Epub 2006/04/04.

[26] Burton EC, Lamborn KR, Feuerstein BG, Prados M, Scott J, Forsyth P, et al. Genetic aberrations defined by comparative genomic hybridization distinguish long-term from typical survivors of glioblastoma. Cancer research. 2002;62(21):6205-10. Epub 2002/11/05.

[27] Beroukhim R, Getz G, Nghiemphu L, Barretina J, Hsueh T, Linhart D, et al. Assessing the significance of chromosomal aberrations in cancer: methodology and application to glioma. Proceedings of the National Academy of Sciences of the United States of America. 2007;104(50):20007-12. Epub 2007/12/14.

[28] Ohgaki H, Dessen P, Jourde B, Horstmann S, Nishikawa T, Di Patre PL, et al. Genetic pathways to glioblastoma: a population-based study. Cancer research. 2004;64(19):6892-9. Epub 2004/10/07.

[29] Mellinghoff IK, Wang MY, Vivanco I, Haas-Kogan DA, Zhu S, Dia EQ, et al. Molecular determinants of the response of glioblastomas to EGFR kinase inhibitors. The New England journal of medicine. 2005;353(19):2012-24. Epub 2005/11/12.

[30] Phillips HS, Kharbanda S, Chen R, Forrest WF, Soriano RH, Wu TD, et al. Molecular subclasses of high-grade glioma predict prognosis, delineate a pattern of disease progression, and resemble stages in neurogenesis. Cancer cell. 2006;9(3):157-73. Epub 2006/03/15.

[31] Lopez-Gines C, Gil-Benso R, Ferrer-Luna R, Benito R, Serna E, Gonzalez-Darder J, et al. New pattern of EGFR amplification in glioblastoma and the relationship of gene copy number with gene expression profile. Modern pathology : an official journal of the United States and Canadian Academy of Pathology, Inc. 2010;23(6):856-65. Epub 2010/03/23.

[32] Krex D, Klink B, Hartmann C, von Deimling A, Pietsch T, Simon M, et al. Long-term survival with glioblastoma multiforme. Brain : a journal of neurology. 2007;130(Pt 10):2596-606. Epub 2007/09/06.

[33] Weller M, Felsberg J, Hartmann C, Berger H, Steinbach JP, Schramm J, et al. Molecular predictors of progression-free and overall survival in patients with newly diagnosed

glioblastoma: a prospective translational study of the German Glioma Network. Journal of clinical oncology : official journal of the American Society of Clinical Oncology. 2009;27(34):5743-50. Epub 2009/10/07.

[34] Yin D, Ogawa S, Kawamata N, Tunici P, Finocchiaro G, Eoli M, et al. High-resolution genomic copy number profiling of glioblastoma multiforme by single nucleotide polymorphism DNA microarray. Molecular cancer research : MCR. 2009;7(5):665-77. Epub 2009/05/14.

[35] Maher EA, Brennan C, Wen PY, Durso L, Ligon KL, Richardson A, et al. Marked genomic differences characterize primary and secondary glioblastoma subtypes and identify two distinct molecular and clinical secondary glioblastoma entities. Cancer research. 2006;66(23):11502-13. Epub 2006/11/23.

[36] Costello JF, Plass C, Arap W, Chapman VM, Held WA, Berger MS, et al. Cyclin-dependent kinase 6 (CDK6) amplification in human gliomas identified using two-dimensional separation of genomic DNA. Cancer research. 1997;57(7):1250-4. Epub 1997/04/01.

[37] Henson JW, Schnitker BL, Correa KM, von Deimling A, Fassbender F, Xu HJ, et al. The retinoblastoma gene is involved in malignant progression of astrocytomas. Annals of neurology. 1994;36(5):714-21. Epub 1994/11/01.

[38] Shete S, Hosking FJ, Robertson LB, Dobbins SE, Sanson M, Malmer B, et al. Genome-wide association study identifies five susceptibility loci for glioma. Nature genetics. 2009;41(8):899-904. Epub 2009/07/07.

[39] Wrensch M, Jenkins RB, Chang JS, Yeh RF, Xiao Y, Decker PA, et al. Variants in the CDKN2B and RTEL1 regions are associated with high-grade glioma susceptibility. Nature genetics. 2009;41(8):905-8. Epub 2009/07/07.

[40] Holtkamp N, Ziegenhagen N, Malzer E, Hartmann C, Giese A, von Deimling A. Characterization of the amplicon on chromosomal segment 4q12 in glioblastoma multiforme. Neuro-oncology. 2007;9(3):291-7. Epub 2007/05/17.

[41] Brennan C, Momota H, Hambardzumyan D, Ozawa T, Tandon A, Pedraza A, et al. Glioblastoma subclasses can be defined by activity among signal transduction pathways and associated genomic alterations. PloS one. 2009;4(11):e7752. Epub 2009/11/17.

[42] Verhaak RG, Hoadley KA, Purdom E, Wang V, Qi Y, Wilkerson MD, et al. Integrated genomic analysis identifies clinically relevant subtypes of glioblastoma characterized by abnormalities in PDGFRA, IDH1, EGFR, and NF1. Cancer cell. 2010;17(1):98-110. Epub 2010/02/05.

[43] Clarke ID, Dirks PB. A human brain tumor-derived PDGFR-alpha deletion mutant is transforming. Oncogene. 2003;22(5):722-33. Epub 2003/02/06.

[44] Ozawa T, Brennan CW, Wang L, Squatrito M, Sasayama T, Nakada M, et al. PDGFRA gene rearrangements are frequent genetic events in PDGFRA-amplified glioblastomas. Genes & development. 2010;24(19):2205-18. Epub 2010/10/05.

[45] Wang H, Wang H, Zhang W, Huang HJ, Liao WS, Fuller GN. Analysis of the activation status of Akt, NFkappaB, and Stat3 in human diffuse gliomas. Laboratory investigation; a journal of technical methods and pathology. 2004;84(8):941-51. Epub 2004/06/09.

[46] Gallia GL, Rand V, Siu IM, Eberhart CG, James CD, Marie SK, et al. PIK3CA gene mutations in pediatric and adult glioblastoma multiforme. Molecular cancer research : MCR. 2006;4(10):709-14. Epub 2006/10/20.

[47] Kita D, Yonekawa Y, Weller M, Ohgaki H. PIK3CA alterations in primary (de novo) and secondary glioblastomas. Acta neuropathologica. 2007;113(3):295-302. Epub 2007/01/20.

[48] Mizoguchi M, Nutt CL, Mohapatra G, Louis DN. Genetic alterations of phosphoinositide 3-kinase subunit genes in human glioblastomas. Brain Pathol. 2004;14(4):372-7. Epub 2004/12/21.

[49] Ichimura K, Vogazianou AP, Liu L, Pearson DM, Backlund LM, Plant K, et al. 1p36 is a preferential target of chromosome 1 deletions in astrocytic tumours and homozygously deleted in a subset of glioblastomas. Oncogene. 2008;27(14):2097-108. Epub 2007/10/16.

[50] Alitalo K, Koskinen P, Makela TP, Saksela K, Sistonen L, Winqvist R. myc oncogenes: activation and amplification. Biochimica et biophysica acta. 1987;907(1):1-32. Epub 1987/04/20.

[51] Kyo S, Takakura M, Taira T, Kanaya T, Itoh H, Yutsudo M, et al. Sp1 cooperates with c-Myc to activate transcription of the human telomerase reverse transcriptase gene (hTERT). Nucleic acids research. 2000;28(3):669-77. Epub 2000/01/19.

[52] Wu KJ, Grandori C, Amacker M, Simon-Vermot N, Polack A, Lingner J, et al. Direct activation of TERT transcription by c-MYC. Nature genetics. 1999;21(2):220-4. Epub 1999/02/13.

[53] Greenberg RA, O'Hagan RC, Deng H, Xiao Q, Hann SR, Adams RR, et al. Telomerase reverse transcriptase gene is a direct target of c-Myc but is not functionally equivalent in cellular transformation. Oncogene. 1999;18(5):1219-26. Epub 1999/02/18.

[54] Gunes C, Lichtsteiner S, Vasserot AP, Englert C. Expression of the hTERT gene is regulated at the level of transcriptional initiation and repressed by Mad1. Cancer research. 2000;60(8):2116-21. Epub 2000/04/29.

[55] Oh S, Song YH, Yim J, Kim TK. Identification of Mad as a repressor of the human telomerase (hTERT) gene. Oncogene. 2000;19(11):1485-90. Epub 2000/03/21.

[56] Xu D, Popov N, Hou M, Wang Q, Bjorkholm M, Gruber A, et al. Switch from Myc/Max to Mad1/Max binding and decrease in histone acetylation at the telomerase reverse transcriptase promoter during differentiation of HL60 cells. Proceedings of the National Academy of Sciences of the United States of America. 2001;98(7):3826-31. Epub 2001/03/29.

[57] Kyo S, Inoue M. Complex regulatory mechanisms of telomerase activity in normal and cancer cells: how can we apply them for cancer therapy? Oncogene. 2002;21(4):688-97. Epub 2002/02/19.

[58] Ohgaki H, Kleihues P. Genetic pathways to primary and secondary glioblastoma. The American journal of pathology. 2007;170(5):1445-53. Epub 2007/04/26.

[59] Yadav AK, Renfrow JJ, Scholtens DM, Xie H, Duran GE, Bredel C, et al. Monosomy of chromosome 10 associated with dysregulation of epidermal growth factor signaling in glioblastomas. JAMA : the journal of the American Medical Association. 2009;302(3):276-89. Epub 2009/07/16.

[60] Koul D. PTEN signaling pathways in glioblastoma. Cancer biology & therapy. 2008;7(9):1321-5. Epub 2008/10/07.

[61] Mellinghoff IK, Cloughesy TF, Mischel PS. PTEN-mediated resistance to epidermal growth factor receptor kinase inhibitors. Clinical cancer research : an official journal of the American Association for Cancer Research. 2007;13(2 Pt 1):378-81. Epub 2007/01/27.
[62] Bredel M, Scholtens DM, Yadav AK, Alvarez AA, Renfrow JJ, Chandler JP, et al. NFKBIA deletion in glioblastomas. The New England journal of medicine. 2011;364(7):627-37. Epub 2010/12/24.
[63] Veeriah S, Brennan C, Meng S, Singh B, Fagin JA, Solit DB, et al. The tyrosine phosphatase PTPRD is a tumor suppressor that is frequently inactivated and mutated in glioblastoma and other human cancers. Proceedings of the National Academy of Sciences of the United States of America. 2009;106(23):9435-40. Epub 2009/05/30.
[64] Wiedemeyer R, Brennan C, Heffernan TP, Xiao Y, Mahoney J, Protopopov A, et al. Feedback circuit among INK4 tumor suppressors constrains human glioblastoma development. Cancer cell. 2008;13(4):355-64. Epub 2008/04/09.
[65] Nakamura M, Yang F, Fujisawa H, Yonekawa Y, Kleihues P, Ohgaki H. Loss of heterozygosity on chromosome 19 in secondary glioblastomas. Journal of neuropathology and experimental neurology. 2000;59(6):539-43. Epub 2000/06/13.
[66] Bettegowda C, Agrawal N, Jiao Y, Sausen M, Wood LD, Hruban RH, et al. Mutations in CIC and FUBP1 contribute to human oligodendroglioma. Science. 2011;333(6048):1453-5. Epub 2011/08/06.
[67] Jenkins RB, Blair H, Ballman KV, Giannini C, Arusell RM, Law M, et al. A t(1;19)(q10;p10) mediates the combined deletions of 1p and 19q and predicts a better prognosis of patients with oligodendroglioma. Cancer research. 2006;66(20):9852-61. Epub 2006/10/19.
[68] Cairncross JG, Ueki K, Zlatescu MC, Lisle DK, Finkelstein DM, Hammond RR, et al. Specific genetic predictors of chemotherapeutic response and survival in patients with anaplastic oligodendrogliomas. Journal of the National Cancer Institute. 1998;90(19):1473-9. Epub 1998/10/17.
[69] Nakamura M, Ishida E, Shimada K, Kishi M, Nakase H, Sakaki T, et al. Frequent LOH on 22q12.3 and TIMP-3 inactivation occur in the progression to secondary glioblastomas. Laboratory investigation; a journal of technical methods and pathology. 2005;85(2):165-75. Epub 2004/12/14.
[70] Qi JH, Ebrahem Q, Moore N, Murphy G, Claesson-Welsh L, Bond M, et al. A novel function for tissue inhibitor of metalloproteinases-3 (TIMP3): inhibition of angiogenesis by blockage of VEGF binding to VEGF receptor-2. Nature medicine. 2003;9(4):407-15. Epub 2003/03/26.
[71] Bredel M, Scholtens DM, Harsh GR, Bredel C, Chandler JP, Renfrow JJ, et al. A network model of a cooperative genetic landscape in brain tumors. JAMA : the journal of the American Medical Association. 2009;302(3):261-75. Epub 2009/07/16.
[72] Vogelstein B, Fearon ER, Hamilton SR, Kern SE, Preisinger AC, Leppert M, et al. Genetic alterations during colorectal-tumor development. The New England journal of medicine. 1988;319(9):525-32. Epub 1988/09/01.
[73] Gladson CL, Prayson RA, Liu WM. The pathobiology of glioma tumors. Annual review of pathology. 2010;5:33-50. Epub 2009/09/10.

[74] Salk JJ, Fox EJ, Loeb LA. Mutational heterogeneity in human cancers: origin and consequences. Annual review of pathology. 2010;5:51-75. Epub 2009/09/12.

[75] Zheng H, Ying H, Yan H, Kimmelman AC, Hiller DJ, Chen AJ, et al. p53 and Pten control neural and glioma stem/progenitor cell renewal and differentiation. Nature. 2008;455(7216):1129-33. Epub 2008/10/25.

[76] Vivanco I, Rohle D, Versele M, Iwanami A, Kuga D, Oldrini B, et al. The phosphatase and tensin homolog regulates epidermal growth factor receptor (EGFR) inhibitor response by targeting EGFR for degradation. Proceedings of the National Academy of Sciences of the United States of America. 2010;107(14):6459-64. Epub 2010/03/24.

[77] Watanabe T, Yokoo H, Yokoo M, Yonekawa Y, Kleihues P, Ohgaki H. Concurrent inactivation of RB1 and TP53 pathways in anaplastic oligodendrogliomas. Journal of neuropathology and experimental neurology. 2001;60(12):1181-9. Epub 2002/01/05.

[78] Holland EC. Gliomagenesis: genetic alterations and mouse models. Nature reviews Genetics. 2001;2(2):120-9. Epub 2001/03/17.

[79] Ekstrand AJ, Sugawa N, James CD, Collins VP. Amplified and rearranged epidermal growth factor receptor genes in human glioblastomas reveal deletions of sequences encoding portions of the N- and/or C-terminal tails. Proceedings of the National Academy of Sciences of the United States of America. 1992;89(10):4309-13. Epub 1992/05/15.

[80] Nishikawa R, Sugiyama T, Narita Y, Furnari F, Cavenee WK, Matsutani M. Immunohistochemical analysis of the mutant epidermal growth factor, deltaEGFR, in glioblastoma. Brain tumor pathology. 2004;21(2):53-6. Epub 2005/02/11.

[81] Inda MM, Bonavia R, Mukasa A, Narita Y, Sah DW, Vandenberg S, et al. Tumor heterogeneity is an active process maintained by a mutant EGFR-induced cytokine circuit in glioblastoma. Genes & development. 2010;24(16):1731-45. Epub 2010/08/18.

[82] Lee JC, Vivanco I, Beroukhim R, Huang JH, Feng WL, DeBiasi RM, et al. Epidermal growth factor receptor activation in glioblastoma through novel missense mutations in the extracellular domain. PLoS medicine. 2006;3(12):e485. Epub 2006/12/21.

[83] Paez JG, Janne PA, Lee JC, Tracy S, Greulich H, Gabriel S, et al. EGFR mutations in lung cancer: correlation with clinical response to gefitinib therapy. Science. 2004; 304(5676):1497-500. Epub 2004/05/01.

[84] Lynch TJ, Bell DW, Sordella R, Gurubhagavatula S, Okimoto RA, Brannigan BW, et al. Activating mutations in the epidermal growth factor receptor underlying responsiveness of non-small-cell lung cancer to gefitinib. The New England journal of medicine. 2004;350(21):2129-39. Epub 2004/05/01.

[85] Yuan TL, Cantley LC. PI3K pathway alterations in cancer: variations on a theme. Oncogene. 2008;27(41):5497-510. Epub 2008/09/17.

[86] Soroceanu L, Kharbanda S, Chen R, Soriano RH, Aldape K, Misra A, et al. Identification of IGF2 signaling through phosphoinositide-3-kinase regulatory subunit 3 as a growth-promoting axis in glioblastoma. Proceedings of the National Academy of Sciences of the United States of America. 2007;104(9):3466-71. Epub 2007/03/16.

[87] Sun M, Hillmann P, Hofmann BT, Hart JR, Vogt PK. Cancer-derived mutations in the regulatory subunit p85alpha of phosphoinositide 3-kinase function through the

catalytic subunit p110alpha. Proceedings of the National Academy of Sciences of the United States of America. 2010;107(35):15547-52. Epub 2010/08/18.
[88] Knobbe CB, Reifenberger J, Reifenberger G. Mutation analysis of the Ras pathway genes NRAS, HRAS, KRAS and BRAF in glioblastomas. Acta neuropathologica. 2004;108(6):467-70. Epub 2004/11/02.
[89] Walker L, Thompson D, Easton D, Ponder B, Ponder M, Frayling I, et al. A prospective study of neurofibromatosis type 1 cancer incidence in the UK. British journal of cancer. 2006;95(2):233-8. Epub 2006/06/21.
[90] McGillicuddy LT, Fromm JA, Hollstein PE, Kubek S, Beroukhim R, De Raedt T, et al. Proteasomal and genetic inactivation of the NF1 tumor suppressor in gliomagenesis. Cancer cell. 2009;16(1):44-54. Epub 2009/07/04.
[91] Zhu Y, Harada T, Liu L, Lush ME, Guignard F, Harada C, et al. Inactivation of NF1 in CNS causes increased glial progenitor proliferation and optic glioma formation. Development. 2005;132(24):5577-88. Epub 2005/11/30.
[92] Kanu OO, Hughes B, Di C, Lin N, Fu J, Bigner DD, et al. Glioblastoma Multiforme Oncogenomics and Signaling Pathways. Clinical medicine Oncology. 2009;3:39-52. Epub 2009/09/25.
[93] Fulci G, Labuhn M, Maier D, Lachat Y, Hausmann O, Hegi ME, et al. p53 gene mutation and ink4a-arf deletion appear to be two mutually exclusive events in human glioblastoma. Oncogene. 2000;19(33):3816-22. Epub 2000/08/19.
[94] He J, Olson JJ, James CD. Lack of p16INK4 or retinoblastoma protein (pRb), or amplification-associated overexpression of cdk4 is observed in distinct subsets of malignant glial tumors and cell lines. Cancer research. 1995;55(21):4833-6. Epub 1995/11/01.
[95] Ishii N, Maier D, Merlo A, Tada M, Sawamura Y, Diserens AC, et al. Frequent co-alterations of TP53, p16/CDKN2A, p14ARF, PTEN tumor suppressor genes in human glioma cell lines. Brain Pathol. 1999;9(3):469-79. Epub 1999/07/23.
[96] Louis DN. The p53 gene and protein in human brain tumors. Journal of neuropathology and experimental neurology. 1994;53(1):11-21. Epub 1994/01/01.
[97] Nozaki M, Tada M, Kobayashi H, Zhang CL, Sawamura Y, Abe H, et al. Roles of the functional loss of p53 and other genes in astrocytoma tumorigenesis and progression. Neuro-oncology. 1999;1(2):124-37. Epub 2001/09/12.
[98] Vousden KH, Prives C. Blinded by the Light: The Growing Complexity of p53. Cell. 2009;137(3):413-31. Epub 2009/05/05.
[99] Zhao T, Xu Y. p53 and stem cells: new developments and new concerns. Trends in cell biology. 2010;20(3):170-5. Epub 2010/01/12.
[100] Masui K, Cloughesy TF, Mischel PS. Review: molecular pathology in adult high-grade gliomas: from molecular diagnostics to target therapies. Neuropathology and applied neurobiology. 2012;38(3):271-91. Epub 2011/11/22.
[101] Hulleman E, Helin K. Molecular mechanisms in gliomagenesis. Advances in cancer research. 2005;94:1-27. Epub 2005/08/13.
[102] Furnari FB, Fenton T, Bachoo RM, Mukasa A, Stommel JM, Stegh A, et al. Malignant astrocytic glioma: genetics, biology, and paths to treatment. Genes & development. 2007;21(21):2683-710. Epub 2007/11/03.

[103] Schiebe M, Ohneseit P, Hoffmann W, Meyermann R, Rodemann HP, Bamberg M. Analysis of mdm2 and p53 gene alterations in glioblastomas and its correlation with clinical factors. Journal of neuro-oncology. 2000;49(3):197-203. Epub 2001/02/24.

[104] Birner P, Piribauer M, Fischer I, Gatterbauer B, Marosi C, Ungersbock K, et al. Prognostic relevance of p53 protein expression in glioblastoma. Oncology reports. 2002;9(4):703-7. Epub 2002/06/18.

[105] Kraus JA, Glesmann N, Beck M, Krex D, Klockgether T, Schackert G, et al. Molecular analysis of the PTEN, TP53 and CDKN2A tumor suppressor genes in long-term survivors of glioblastoma multiforme. Journal of neuro-oncology. 2000;48(2):89-94. Epub 2000/11/18.

[106] Kraus JA, Wenghoefer M, Glesmann N, Mohr S, Beck M, Schmidt MC, et al. TP53 gene mutations, nuclear p53 accumulation, expression of Waf/p21, Bcl-2, and CD95 (APO-1/Fas) proteins are not prognostic factors in de novo glioblastoma multiforme. Journal of neuro-oncology. 2001;52(3):263-72. Epub 2001/08/25.

[107] Stark AM, Hugo HH, Witzel P, Mihajlovic Z, Mehdorn HM. Age-related expression of p53, Mdm2, EGFR and Msh2 in glioblastoma multiforme. Zentralblatt fur Neurochirurgie. 2003;64(1):30-6. Epub 2003/02/13.

[108] Newcomb EW, Cohen H, Lee SR, Bhalla SK, Bloom J, Hayes RL, et al. Survival of patients with glioblastoma multiforme is not influenced by altered expression of p16, p53, EGFR, MDM2 or Bcl-2 genes. Brain Pathol. 1998;8(4):655-67. Epub 1998/11/06.

[109] Rolhion C, Penault-Llorca F, Kemeny JL, Kwiatkowski F, Lemaire JJ, Chollet P, et al. O(6)-methylguanine-DNA methyltransferase gene (MGMT) expression in human glioblastomas in relation to patient characteristics and p53 accumulation. International ournal of cancer Journal international du cancer. 1999;84(4):416-20. Epub 1999/07/15.

[110] Criniere E, Kaloshi G, Laigle-Donadey F, Lejeune J, Auger N, Benouaich-Amiel A, et al. MGMT prognostic impact on glioblastoma is dependent on therapeutic modalities. Journal of neuro-oncology. 2007;83(2):173-9. Epub 2007/01/16.

[111] Puduvalli VK, Kyritsis AP, Hess KR, Bondy ML, Fuller GN, Kouraklis GP, et al. Patterns of expression of Rb and p16 in astrocytic gliomas, and correlation with survival. International journal of oncology. 2000;17(5):963-9. Epub 2000/10/13.

[112] Backlund LM, Nilsson BR, Liu L, Ichimura K, Collins VP. Mutations in Rb1 pathway-related genes are associated with poor prognosis in anaplastic astrocytomas. British ournal of cancer. 2005;93(1):124-30. Epub 2005/06/23.

[113] Ang C, Guiot MC, Ramanakumar AV, Roberge D, Kavan P. Clinical significance of molecular biomarkers in glioblastoma. The Canadian journal of neurological sciences Le ournal canadien des sciences neurologiques. 2010;37(5):625-30. Epub 2010/11/10.

[114] Bleeker FE, Lamba S, Leenstra S, Troost D, Hulsebos T, Vandertop WP, et al. IDH1 mutations at residue p.R132 (IDH1(R132)) occur frequently in high-grade gliomas but not in other solid tumors. Human mutation. 2009;30(1):7-11. Epub 2009/01/02.

[115] Sanson M, Marie Y, Paris S, Idbaih A, Laffaire J, Ducray F, et al. Isocitrate dehydrogenase 1 codon 132 mutation is an important prognostic biomarker in gliomas. Journal of clinical oncology : official journal of the American Society of Clinical Oncology. 2009;27(25):4150-4. Epub 2009/07/29.

[116] Nobusawa S, Watanabe T, Kleihues P, Ohgaki H. IDH1 mutations as molecular signature and predictive factor of secondary glioblastomas. Clinical cancer research : an official journal of the American Association for Cancer Research. 2009;15(19):6002-7. Epub 2009/09/17.

[117] Ichimura K, Pearson DM, Kocialkowski S, Backlund LM, Chan R, Jones DT, et al. IDH1 mutations are present in the majority of common adult gliomas but rare in primary glioblastomas. Neuro-oncology. 2009;11(4):341-7. Epub 2009/05/14.

[118] Balss J, Meyer J, Mueller W, Korshunov A, Hartmann C, von Deimling A. Analysis of the IDH1 codon 132 mutation in brain tumors. Acta neuropathologica. 2008;116(6):597-602. Epub 2008/11/06.

[119] Hartmann C, Meyer J, Balss J, Capper D, Mueller W, Christians A, et al. Type and frequency of IDH1 and IDH2 mutations are related to astrocytic and oligodendroglial differentiation and age: a study of 1,010 diffuse gliomas. Acta neuropathologica. 2009;118(4):469-74. Epub 2009/06/26.

[120] Yan H, Parsons DW, Jin G, McLendon R, Rasheed BA, Yuan W, et al. IDH1 and IDH2 mutations in gliomas. The New England journal of medicine. 2009;360(8):765-73. Epub 2009/02/21.

[121] Hartmann C, Hentschel B, Wick W, Capper D, Felsberg J, Simon M, et al. Patients with IDH1 wild type anaplastic astrocytomas exhibit worse prognosis than IDH1-mutated glioblastomas, and IDH1 mutation status accounts for the unfavorable prognostic effect of higher age: implications for classification of gliomas. Acta neuropathologica. 2010;120(6):707-18. Epub 2010/11/23.

[122] Dang L, White DW, Gross S, Bennett BD, Bittinger MA, Driggers EM, et al. Cancer-associated IDH1 mutations produce 2-hydroxyglutarate. Nature. 2009;462(7274):739-44. Epub 2009/11/26.

[123] Loenarz C, Schofield CJ. Expanding chemical biology of 2-oxoglutarate oxygenases. Nature chemical biology. 2008;4(3):152-6. Epub 2008/02/19.

[124] Xu W, Yang H, Liu Y, Yang Y, Wang P, Kim SH, et al. Oncometabolite 2-hydroxyglutarate is a competitive inhibitor of alpha-ketoglutarate-dependent dioxygenases. Cancer cell. 2011;19(1):17-30. Epub 2011/01/22.

[125] Turcan S, Rohle D, Goenka A, Walsh LA, Fang F, Yilmaz E, et al. IDH1 mutation is sufficient to establish the glioma hypermethylator phenotype. Nature. 2012;483(7390):479-83. Epub 2012/02/22.

[126] Figueroa ME, Abdel-Wahab O, Lu C, Ward PS, Patel J, Shih A, et al. Leukemic IDH1 and IDH2 mutations result in a hypermethylation phenotype, disrupt TET2 function, and impair hematopoietic differentiation. Cancer cell. 2010;18(6):553-67. Epub 2010/12/07.

[127] Watanabe T, Nobusawa S, Kleihues P, Ohgaki H. IDH1 mutations are early events in the development of astrocytomas and oligodendrogliomas. The American journal of pathology. 2009;174(4):1149-53. Epub 2009/02/28.

[128] Lai A, Kharbanda S, Pope WB, Tran A, Solis OE, Peale F, et al. Evidence for sequenced molecular evolution of IDH1 mutant glioblastoma from a distinct cell of origin. Journal of clinical oncology : official journal of the American Society of Clinical Oncology. 2011;29(34):4482-90. Epub 2011/10/26.

[129] Sepulveda AR, Jones D, Ogino S, Samowitz W, Gulley ML, Edwards R, et al. CpG methylation analysis--current status of clinical assays and potential applications in molecular diagnostics: a report of the Association for Molecular Pathology. The Journal of molecular diagnostics : JMD. 2009;11(4):266-78. Epub 2009/06/23.

[130] Milbury CA, Chen CC, Mamon H, Liu P, Santagata S, Makrigiorgos GM. Multiplex amplification coupled with COLD-PCR and high resolution melting enables identification of low-abundance mutations in cancer samples with low DNA content. The Journal of molecular diagnostics : JMD. 2011;13(2):220-32. Epub 2011/03/01.

[131] Mattick JS, Makunin IV. Non-coding RNA. Human molecular genetics. 2006;15 Spec No 1:R17-29. Epub 2006/05/03.

[132] Nagarajan RP, Costello JF. Epigenetic mechanisms in glioblastoma multiforme. Seminars in cancer biology. 2009;19(3):188-97. Epub 2009/05/12.

[133] Clark SJ, Harrison J, Frommer M. CpNpG methylation in mammalian cells. Nature genetics. 1995;10(1):20-7. Epub 1995/05/01.

[134] Turner BM. Reading signals on the nucleosome with a new nomenclature for modified histones. Nature structural & molecular biology. 2005;12(2):110-2. Epub 2005/02/11.

[135] Bartek J, Jr., Ng K, Bartek J, Fischer W, Carter B, Chen CC. Key concepts in glioblastoma therapy. Journal of neurology, neurosurgery, and psychiatry. 2012;83(7):753-60. Epub 2012/03/08.

[136] Tano K, Shiota S, Collier J, Foote RS, Mitra S. Isolation and structural characterization of a cDNA clone encoding the human DNA repair protein for O6-alkylguanine. Proceedings of the National Academy of Sciences of the United States of America. 1990;87(2):686-90. Epub 1990/01/01.

[137] Hegi ME, Liu L, Herman JG, Stupp R, Wick W, Weller M, et al. Correlation of O6-methylguanine methyltransferase (MGMT) promoter methylation with clinical outcomes in glioblastoma and clinical strategies to modulate MGMT activity. Journal of clinical oncology : official journal of the American Society of Clinical Oncology. 2008;26(25):4189-99. Epub 2008/09/02.

[138] Mikeska T, Bock C, El-Maarri O, Hubner A, Ehrentraut D, Schramm J, et al. Optimization of quantitative MGMT promoter methylation analysis using pyrosequencing and combined bisulfite restriction analysis. The Journal of molecular diagnostics : JMD. 2007;9(3):368-81. Epub 2007/06/27.

[139] Herfarth KK, Brent TP, Danam RP, Remack JS, Kodner IJ, Wells SA, Jr., et al. A specific CpG methylation pattern of the MGMT promoter region associated with reduced MGMT expression in primary colorectal cancers. Molecular carcinogenesis. 1999;24(2):90-8. Epub 1999/03/17.

[140] Watts GS, Pieper RO, Costello JF, Peng YM, Dalton WS, Futscher BW. Methylation of discrete regions of the O6-methylguanine DNA methyltransferase (MGMT) CpG island is associated with heterochromatinization of the MGMT transcription start site and silencing of the gene. Molecular and cellular biology. 1997;17(9):5612-9. Epub 1997/09/01.

[141] Hegi ME, Diserens AC, Gorlia T, Hamou MF, de Tribolet N, Weller M, et al. MGMT gene silencing and benefit from temozolomide in glioblastoma. The New England ournal of medicine. 2005;352(10):997-1003. Epub 2005/03/11.

[142] Rivera AL, Pelloski CE, Gilbert MR, Colman H, De La Cruz C, Sulman EP, et al. MGMT promoter methylation is predictive of response to radiotherapy and prognostic in the absence of adjuvant alkylating chemotherapy for glioblastoma. Neuro-oncology. 2010;12(2):116-21. Epub 2010/02/13.
[143] Nitta M, Kozono D, Kennedy R, Stommel J, Ng K, Zinn PO, et al. Targeting EGFR induced oxidative stress by PARP1 inhibition in glioblastoma therapy. PloS one. 2010;5(5):e10767. Epub 2010/06/10.
[144] Noushmehr H, Weisenberger DJ, Diefes K, Phillips HS, Pujara K, Berman BP, et al. Identification of a CpG island methylator phenotype that defines a distinct subgroup of glioma. Cancer cell. 2010;17(5):510-22. Epub 2010/04/20.
[145] Orkin SH, Hochedlinger K. Chromatin connections to pluripotency and cellular reprogramming. Cell. 2011;145(6):835-50. Epub 2011/06/15.
[146] Zheng D, Frankish A, Baertsch R, Kapranov P, Reymond A, Choo SW, et al. Pseudogenes in the ENCODE regions: consensus annotation, analysis of transcription, and evolution. Genome research. 2007;17(6):839-51. Epub 2007/06/15.
[147] Hasler J, Samuelsson T, Strub K. Useful 'junk': Alu RNAs in the human transcriptome. Cellular and molecular life sciences : CMLS. 2007;64(14):1793-800. Epub 2007/05/22.
[148] Lander ES, Linton LM, Birren B, Nusbaum C, Zody MC, Baldwin J, et al. Initial sequencing and analysis of the human genome. Nature. 2001;409(6822):860-921. Epub 2001/03/10.
[149] Tso CL, Freije WA, Day A, Chen Z, Merriman B, Perlina A, et al. Distinct transcription profiles of primary and secondary glioblastoma subgroups. Cancer research. 2006;66(1):159-67. Epub 2006/01/07.
[150] Furuta M, Weil RJ, Vortmeyer AO, Huang S, Lei J, Huang TN, et al. Protein patterns and proteins that identify subtypes of glioblastoma multiforme. Oncogene. 2004;23(40):6806-14. Epub 2004/08/03.
[151] Kim TM, Huang W, Park R, Park PJ, Johnson MD. A developmental taxonomy of glioblastoma defined and maintained by MicroRNAs. Cancer research. 2011;71(9):3387-99. Epub 2011/03/10.
[152] Gunther HS, Schmidt NO, Phillips HS, Kemming D, Kharbanda S, Soriano R, et al. Glioblastoma-derived stem cell-enriched cultures form distinct subgroups according to molecular and phenotypic criteria. Oncogene. 2008;27(20):2897-909. Epub 2007/11/27.
[153] Carro MS, Lim WK, Alvarez MJ, Bollo RJ, Zhao X, Snyder EY, et al. The transcriptional network for mesenchymal transformation of brain tumours. Nature. 2010;463(7279):318-25. Epub 2009/12/25.
[154] Iwamoto FM, Hottinger AF, Karimi S, Riedel E, Dantis J, Jahdi M, et al. Serum YKL-40 is a marker of prognosis and disease status in high-grade gliomas. Neuro-oncology. 2011;13(11):1244-51. Epub 2011/08/13.
[155] Santosh V, Arivazhagan A, Sreekanthreddy P, Srinivasan H, Thota B, Srividya MR, et al. Grade-specific expression of insulin-like growth factor-binding proteins-2, -3, and -5 in astrocytomas: IGFBP-3 emerges as a strong predictor of survival in patients with newly diagnosed glioblastoma. Cancer epidemiology, biomarkers & prevention : a publication of the American Association for Cancer Research, cosponsored by the American Society of Preventive Oncology. 2010;19(6):1399-408. Epub 2010/05/27.

[156] Godard S, Getz G, Delorenzi M, Farmer P, Kobayashi H, Desbaillets I, et al. Classification of human astrocytic gliomas on the basis of gene expression: a correlated group of genes with angiogenic activity emerges as a strong predictor of subtypes. Cancer research. 2003;63(20):6613-25. Epub 2003/10/30.

[157] Nigro JM, Misra A, Zhang L, Smirnov I, Colman H, Griffin C, et al. Integrated array-comparative genomic hybridization and expression array profiles identify clinically relevant molecular subtypes of glioblastoma. Cancer research. 2005;65(5):1678-86. Epub 2005/03/09.

[158] Hormigo A, Gu B, Karimi S, Riedel E, Panageas KS, Edgar MA, et al. YKL-40 and matrix metalloproteinase-9 as potential serum biomarkers for patients with high-grade gliomas. Clinical cancer research : an official journal of the American Association for Cancer Research. 2006;12(19):5698-704. Epub 2006/10/06.

[159] Tso CL, Shintaku P, Chen J, Liu Q, Liu J, Chen Z, et al. Primary glioblastomas express mesenchymal stem-like properties. Molecular cancer research : MCR. 2006;4(9):607-19. Epub 2006/09/13.

[160] Lee Y, Scheck AC, Cloughesy TF, Lai A, Dong J, Farooqi HK, et al. Gene expression analysis of glioblastomas identifies the major molecular basis for the prognostic benefit of younger age. BMC medical genomics. 2008;1:52. Epub 2008/10/23.

[161] Colman H, Zhang L, Sulman EP, McDonald JM, Shooshtari NL, Rivera A, et al. A multigene predictor of outcome in glioblastoma. Neuro-oncology. 2010;12(1):49-57. Epub 2010/02/13.

[162] Yogev O, Lagos D. Noncoding RNAs and cancer. Silence. 2011;2(1):6. Epub 2011/10/01.

[163] Fowler A, Thomson D, Giles K, Maleki S, Mreich E, Wheeler H, et al. miR-124a is frequently down-regulated in glioblastoma and is involved in migration and invasion. Eur J Cancer. 2011;47(6):953-63. Epub 2011/01/05.

[164] Asadi-Moghaddam K, Chiocca EA, Lawler SE. Potential role of miRNAs and their inhibitors in glioma treatment. Expert review of anticancer therapy. 2010;10(11):1753-62. Epub 2010/11/18.

[165] Filipowicz W, Bhattacharyya SN, Sonenberg N. Mechanisms of post-transcriptional regulation by microRNAs: are the answers in sight? Nature reviews Genetics. 2008;9(2):102-14. Epub 2008/01/17.

[166] le Sage C, Nagel R, Egan DA, Schrier M, Mesman E, Mangiola A, et al. Regulation of the p27(Kip1) tumor suppressor by miR-221 and miR-222 promotes cancer cell proliferation. The EMBO journal. 2007;26(15):3699-708. Epub 2007/07/14.

[167] Guan Y, Mizoguchi M, Yoshimoto K, Hata N, Shono T, Suzuki SO, et al. MiRNA-196 is upregulated in glioblastoma but not in anaplastic astrocytoma and has prognostic significance. Clinical cancer research : an official journal of the American Association for Cancer Research. 2010;16(16):4289-97. Epub 2010/07/06.

[168] Kim H, Huang W, Jiang X, Pennicooke B, Park PJ, Johnson MD. Integrative genome analysis reveals an oncomir/oncogene cluster regulating glioblastoma survivorship. Proceedings of the National Academy of Sciences of the United States of America. 2010;107(5):2183-8. Epub 2010/01/19.

[169] Kefas B, Comeau L, Floyd DH, Seleverstov O, Godlewski J, Schmittgen T, et al. The neuronal microRNA miR-326 acts in a feedback loop with notch and has therapeutic

potential against brain tumors. The Journal of neuroscience : the official journal of the Society for Neuroscience. 2009;29(48):15161-8. Epub 2009/12/04.

[170] Ciafre SA, Galardi S, Mangiola A, Ferracin M, Liu CG, Sabatino G, et al. Extensive modulation of a set of microRNAs in primary glioblastoma. Biochemical and biophysical research communications. 2005;334(4):1351-8. Epub 2005/07/26.

[171] Zhang CZ, Zhang JX, Zhang AL, Shi ZD, Han L, Jia ZF, et al. MiR-221 and miR-222 target PUMA to induce cell survival in glioblastoma. Molecular cancer. 2010;9:229. Epub 2010/09/04.

[172] Gabriely G, Yi M, Narayan RS, Niers JM, Wurdinger T, Imitola J, et al. Human glioma growth is controlled by microRNA-10b. Cancer research. 2011;71(10):3563-72. Epub 2011/04/08.

[173] Ma L, Teruya-Feldstein J, Weinberg RA. Tumour invasion and metastasis initiated by microRNA-10b in breast cancer. Nature. 2007;449(7163):682-8. Epub 2007/09/28.

[174] Calin GA, Liu CG, Sevignani C, Ferracin M, Felli N, Dumitru CD, et al. MicroRNA profiling reveals distinct signatures in B cell chronic lymphocytic leukemias. Proceedings of the National Academy of Sciences of the United States of America. 2004;101(32):11755-60. Epub 2004/07/31.

[175] Bloomston M, Frankel WL, Petrocca F, Volinia S, Alder H, Hagan JP, et al. MicroRNA expression patterns to differentiate pancreatic adenocarcinoma from normal pancreas and chronic pancreatitis. JAMA : the journal of the American Medical Association. 2007;297(17):1901-8. Epub 2007/05/03.

[176] Huse JT, Brennan C, Hambardzumyan D, Wee B, Pena J, Rouhanifard SH, et al. The PTEN-regulating microRNA miR-26a is amplified in high-grade glioma and facilitates gliomagenesis in vivo. Genes & development. 2009;23(11):1327-37. Epub 2009/06/03.

[177] Poliseno L, Salmena L, Zhang J, Carver B, Haveman WJ, Pandolfi PP. A coding-independent function of gene and pseudogene mRNAs regulates tumour biology. Nature. 2010;465(7301):1033-8. Epub 2010/06/26.

[178] Godlewski J, Nowicki MO, Bronisz A, Williams S, Otsuki A, Nuovo G, et al. Targeting of the Bmi-1 oncogene/stem cell renewal factor by microRNA-128 inhibits glioma proliferation and self-renewal. Cancer research. 2008;68(22):9125-30. Epub 2008/11/18.

[179] Li KK, Pang JC, Ching AK, Wong CK, Kong X, Wang Y, et al. miR-124 is frequently down-regulated in medulloblastoma and is a negative regulator of SLC16A1. Human pathology. 2009;40(9):1234-43. Epub 2009/05/12.

[180] Furuta M, Kozaki KI, Tanaka S, Arii S, Imoto I, Inazawa J. miR-124 and miR-203 are epigenetically silenced tumor-suppressive microRNAs in hepatocellular carcinoma. Carcinogenesis. 2010;31(5):766-76. Epub 2009/10/22.

[181] Silber J, Lim DA, Petritsch C, Persson AI, Maunakea AK, Yu M, et al. miR-124 and miR-137 inhibit proliferation of glioblastoma multiforme cells and induce differentiation of brain tumor stem cells. BMC medicine. 2008;6:14. Epub 2008/06/26.

[182] Gal H, Pandi G, Kanner AA, Ram Z, Lithwick-Yanai G, Amariglio N, et al. MIR-451 and Imatinib mesylate inhibit tumor growth of Glioblastoma stem cells. Biochemical and biophysical research communications. 2008;376(1):86-90. Epub 2008/09/04.

[183] Sana J, Hajduch M, Michalek J, Vyzula R, Slaby O. MicroRNAs and glioblastoma: roles in core signalling pathways and potential clinical implications. Journal of cellular and molecular medicine. 2011;15(8):1636-44. Epub 2011/03/26.

[184] Ziegler DS, Wright RD, Kesari S, Lemieux ME, Tran MA, Jain M, et al. Resistance of human glioblastoma multiforme cells to growth factor inhibitors is overcome by blockade of inhibitor of apoptosis proteins. The Journal of clinical investigation. 2008;118(9):3109-22. Epub 2008/08/05.

[185] Slaby O, Lakomy R, Fadrus P, Hrstka R, Kren L, Lzicarova E, et al. MicroRNA-181 family predicts response to concomitant chemoradiotherapy with temozolomide in glioblastoma patients. Neoplasma. 2010;57(3):264-9. Epub 2010/04/01.

[186] Zhang W, Zhang J, Hoadley K, Kushwaha D, Ramakrishnan V, Li S, et al. miR-181d: a predictive glioblastoma biomarker that downregulates MGMT expression. Neuro-oncology. 2012;14(6):712-9. Epub 2012/05/10.

Chapter 5

MicroRNAs in Invasion and Metastasis in Lung Cancer

Lili Jiang and Xueshan Qiu

Additional information is available at the end of the chapter

http://dx.doi.org/10.5772/55624

1. Introduction

Despite advances in diagnosis and treatment, the morbidity and mortality of lung cancer remains to mount up. The key factor of cancer associated morbidity and mortality is principally attributable to the development of metastases. Cancer cells depart their normal microenvironment from the primary tumor site through complicated and multistep processes disseminate and colonize distant organs [1]. However, the cellular and molecular machinery underlying metastasis is relatively poorly understood so far. In order to resist cancer dissemination, more effective therapeutic strategies are clearly required.

Cellular migration and invasion mechanism are commonly thought to be associated with Rho family GTPases [2-4], JAK-STAT [5-7], MAPK [8-10], Wnt [11-13], Notch pathway [14-16]. Recently, epithelial–mesenchymal transition (EMT) programs have become the focus of the mechanism of metastasis [1, 17-20]. EMT is an embryologically conserved genetic program by which epithelial cells down regulate intercellular tight junctions, loose polarity, express mesenchymal markers, and manifest a migratory phenotype [1]. In the EMT process, Rho family GTPases [21], JAK-STAT [22], MAPK [23], Wnt [24] and Notch [25] pathways may also play an important role. In recent years, emerging studies have highlighted the critical role of these pathways and their regulation by microRNAs (miRNAs) in cancer invasion and metastasis.

MiRNAs, short (18-24 nucleotides) non-coding RNAs, are derived from long transcripts pri-miRNAs and pre-miRNAs [26-30]. By targeting 3′ untranslated regions (3′UTRs) of cognate mRNAs, miRNAs post-transcriptionally regulate gene expression and induce translational repression [29, 30]. Their specificity is determined by nucleotides 2–8 at the 5′ end, termed the miRNA "seed sequence". To date, 1527 human miRNAs have been identified (Sanger miRBase 18 http://www.miRbase.org/index. shtml), forming less than 1% of all human genes, potentially regulating more than 10% of all protein coding genes [1]. Recently, miRNAs have been discovered to play important roles in the invasion and metastasis of malignant tumors. [31-33]. Understanding specific characteristics of miRNAs would probably serve as predictive markers and as therapeutic strategies for patients with metastasis.

In light of these recent discoveries, the present article discusses how invasion and EMT pathways are regulated by miRNAs. We have classified invasion programs and key proteins involved in EMT according to the signaling pathway showed above and point out validated miRNAs regulating their expression and highlight critical knowledge gaps that remain to be addressed to enable improved understanding of the molecular mechanisms behind EMT and metastasis. A list of experimentally validated miRNAs regulating key proteins involved in invasion–metastasis programs or participating in some principal pathways can be found in Figure 1.

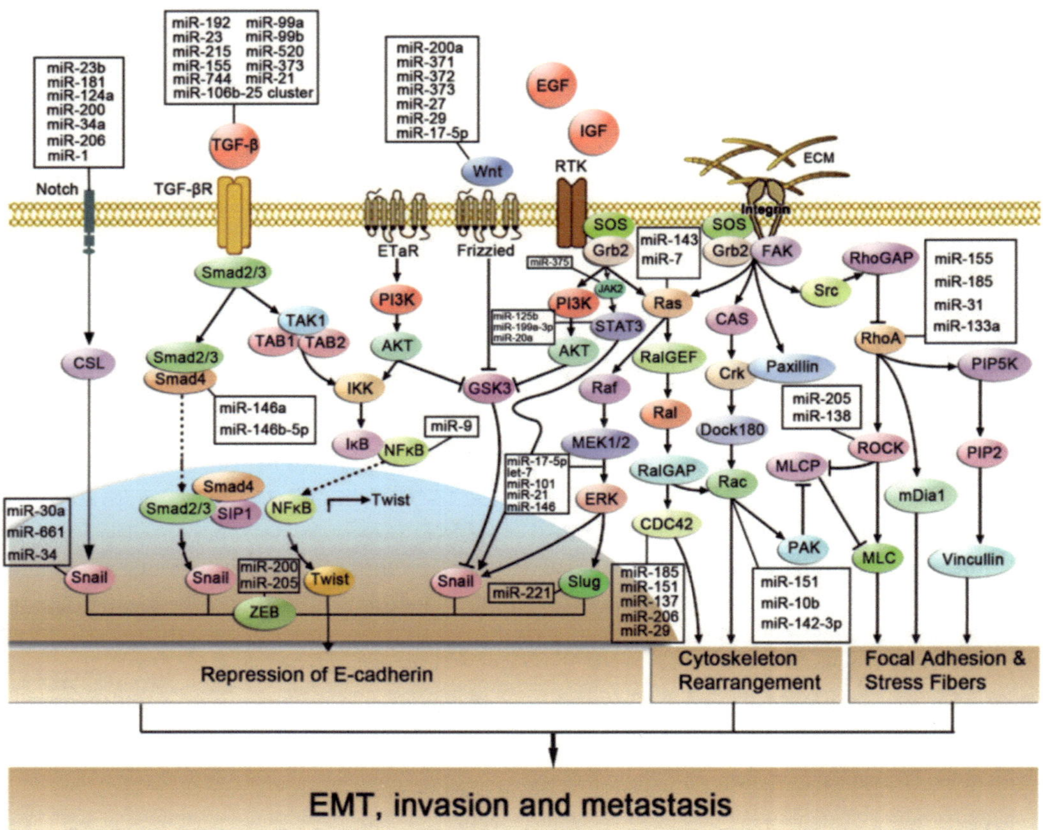

Figure 1. The experimentally validated miRNAs regulate key proteins involved in invasion–metastasis programs or participating in some principal pathways.

2. Rho family of GTPases

The Rho family of GTPases, a family of small (~21 kDa) signaling G protein, is a subfamily of the Ras superfamily [34]. In mammals, the Rho family is made of 20 members distributed into eight subfamilies: Rho, Rac, Cdc42, Rnd, RhoU/V, RhoBTB, RhoH and RhoD/F. Almost all research involves the three most common members of the Rho family: Cdc42, Rac1 and RhoA [35]. Over expression of Rho GTPases is associated with reorganization of actin cytoskeleton, which plays an important role in cell migration, invasion and metastasis that are important aspects of cancer progression [36].

Emerging studies have indicated that miRNAs participate in the Rho GTPases signaling pathway. Among the tested miRNAs, the present articles demonstrated that miR-155, miR-185, miR-31 and miR-133a are associated with RhoA in cell migration and invasion. MiR-155 may play an important role in TGF-β-induced EMT and cell migration and invasion by targeting RhoA [37]. MiR-185 is a negative regulator of RhoA and Cdc42, and could inhibit proliferation and invasion of colorectal cancer cells [38]. The Effects of miR-31 on metastasis may be associated with concurrent suppression of integrin alpha 5, radixin, and RhoA phenocopies [39]. Chiba and his colleagues reported that RhoA expression is negatively regulated by miR-133a in bronchial smooth muscle cells [40].

Moreover, some studies discussed the regulation of cell migration and invasion by miRNA may be attribute to Rho-associated serine-threonine protein kinase (ROCK), one of the best characterized downstream effectors of Rho, that is activated when it selectively binds to the active GTP-bound form of Rho [41, 42]. As with Rho, ROCK has been implicated in altering cell migration and invasion during tumor cell metastasis [43, 44]. Yu and his colleagues indicate that downregulation of miR-205 resulted in an increase in Rho-ROCKI activity, phosphorylation of the actin severing protein cofilin, and a corresponding diminution of filamentous actin [45].

A number of articles reported that some miRNAs regulate cell migration and invasion by targeting Rac and Cdc42. Recently, microRNA-142-3p, a new regulator of Rac1, suppresses the migration and invasion of hepatocellular carcinoma cells [46]. The regulation of cancer cell migration by MiR-10b may be attribute to activate Rac by targets Tiam1 [47]. MiR-151 exerts this function by directly targeting RhoGDIA, a putative metastasis suppressor in hepatocellular carcinoma (HCC), thus leading to the activation of Rac1, Cdc42 and Rho GTPases [48]. Liu and his colleagues have found that miR-137 may have a tumor suppressor function by directly targeting Cdc42 to inhibit the proliferation and invasion activities of colorectal cancer cells [49, 50]. MiR-206 may suppress invasion and migration of MDA-MB-231 cells in vitro partly via regulating actin cytoskeleton remodelling by downregulating Cdc42 [51]. MiR-29 activates p53 by targeting p85 alpha and Cdc42 [52].

In addition, MiR-21 targets the tumor suppressor Rho B and regulates proliferation, invasion positively in colorectal cancer cells [53, 54]. Jiang and his colleagues have indicated that miR-138 plays an important role in tongue squamous cell carcinoma cell migration and invasion by concurrently targeting Rho C and ROCK2 [36]. Studies on the association of Rho with miRNAs highlight the importance of miRNAs in invasion and metastasis of malignant tumors.

3. JAK-STAT

The JAK-STAT signaling pathway transmits information from chemical signals outside the cell, through the cell membrane, and into gene promoters on the DNA in the cell nucleus, which causes DNA transcription and activity in the cell. JAK, short for Janus Kinase, is a family of intracellular, nonreceptor tyrosine kinases that transduce cytokine-mediated signals via the JAK-STAT pathway. As a key component of the JAK/STAT pathway, Signal Transducer and Activator of Transcription, an important transcription factors, is activated by JAK [55, 56]. In JAK and STAT family, emerging studies have indicated that JAK2/STAT3 pathway is well-established regulators of cell migration, and has been implicated in the process of tumor cell invasion and metastasis [57].

Some studies have indicated that miRNAs participate in the JAK-STAT signaling pathway. MiR-375 may function as a tumor suppressor to regulate gastric cancer cell proliferation potentially by targeting the JAK2 oncogene [58]. MiR-125b suppresses the proliferation and migration of osteosarcoma cells through downregulation of STAT3 [59]. Transfection of precursor miR-199a-3p into osteosarcoma cell lines significantly decreased cell growth and migration. Duan and his colleagues observed decreased mTOR and STAT3 expression in miR-199a-3p transfected cells [60]. Yan and his colleagues indicated that miR-20a regulates STAT3 at the post-transcriptional level, resulting in inhibition of cell proliferation and invasion of pancreatic carcinoma [61].

4. MAPK pathway

The Mitogen Activated Protein Kinase (MAPK) pathway is a frequent event in tumorigenesis. MAPKs have been implicated in cell migration, proteinase induction, apoptosis, and angiogenesis, events that are essential for successful completion of metastasis [8]. The presence of at least six MAPK in yeast suggests that there are more in mammals: extracellular signal-regulated kinases (ERK1, ERK2), c-Jun N-terminal kinases (JNKs), p38 isoforms, ERK5, ERK3/4, ERK7/8. In vivo and in vitro studies have confirmed that three major subgroups of MAPK including ERK1/2, JNK, and p38, are specifically involved in invasion and metastasis [9, 10, 62].

Mounting studies have indicated that miRNAs participate in the MAPK signaling pathway. MiR-143 plays an important role in prostate cancer proliferation, migration and chemosensitivity by suppressing KRAS and subsequent inactivation of MAPK pathway [63]. MiR-17-5p significantly activates the p38 kinase pathway [64]. Raf kinase inhibitory protein suppresses a cascade of metastasis signalling involving LIN28 and let-7 [65]. Zhu and his colleagues found that miR-101 targets MAPK phosphatase 1 to regulate the activation of MAPKs in macrophages [66]. MiR-146a suppresses tumor growth and progression by targeting EGFR pathway and in a p-ERK-dependent manner in castration-resistant prostate cancer [67]. Liu and his colleagues indicated that miR-21 induces tumor angiogenesis through targeting PTEN, leading to activate AKT and ERK1/2 signaling pathways [68,69]. EGFR promotes lung tumorigenesis by activating miR-7 through a Ras/ERK/Myc pathway that targets the ETS2 transcriptional repressor ERF [70].

5. Wnt signaling pathway

Wnt signaling pathway controls tissue polarity and cell movement through the activation of RhoA, JNK, and nemo-like kinase (NLK) signaling cascades. The Wnt gene family is a group of developmental genes that encode cysteine-rich glycosylated proteins [71]. Aberrant activation of Wnt signaling pathway in human cancer leads to more malignant phenotypes, such as abnormal tissue polarity, invasion, and metastasis [72].

A number of studies have indicated that miRNAs participate in the Wnt signaling pathway. MiR-200a is a new tumor suppressor that can regulate the activity of the Wnt/β-catenin signaling pathway [73]. MiR-371-373 expression is induced by lithium chloride and is positively correlated with Wnt/β-catenin-signaling activity in several human cancer cell lines [74]. MiR-27 directly targeted and inhibited adenomatous polyposis coli (APC) gene expression, and activated Wnt signaling through accumulation of β-catenin [75]. Kapinas and his colleagues reported that miR-29 modulates Wnt signaling in human osteoblasts through a positive feedback loop [76]. MiR-17-5p plays an important role in breast cancer cell invasion and migration by suppressing HBP1 and subsequent activation of Wnt/β-catenin [77]. Kennell and his colleagues demonstrated that miR-8 family members play an evolutionarily conserved role in regulating the Wnt signaling pathway [78].

6. Notch signaling pathway

The Notch signaling pathway is a conserved ligand–receptor signaling pathway. Notch genes encode single-pass transmembrane proteins that can be activated by interacting with a family of its ligands. To date, four Notch receptors have been identified in mammals, including human, such as Notch-1-4. It has been well known that Notch signaling plays important roles in maintaining the balance involved in cell proliferation, survival, apoptosis, and differentiation which affects the development and function of many organs [79]. Therefore, dysfunction of Notch prevents differentiation, ultimately guiding undifferentiated cells toward malignant transformation. Indeed, many observations suggest that alterations in Notch signaling are associated with invasion and metastasis in many human cancers [14-16].

Mounting studies have indicated that miRNAs participate in the Notch signaling pathway. MicroRNA-23b is capable of inducing tolerogenic properties of dendritic cells in vitro through the inhibition of the Notch1 and NF-κB signalling pathways [80]. MicroRNA-181 promotes natural killer (NK) cell development by regulating Notch signaling [81]. MiR-124a mediates stroke-induced neurogenesis by targeting the JAG-Notch signaling pathway [82]. Pang and his colleagues demonstrated that miR-34a affected cell invasion by regulating expression of urokinase plasminogen activator through Notch [83]. MiR-206 targets Notch 3, activates apoptosis, and inhibits tumor cell migration and focus formation [84]. MiR-1 influences cardiac differentiation in Drosophila and regulates Notch signaling [85]. Some studies indicated that the ZEB1/miR-200 feedback loop controls Notch signalling in cancer cells [86, 87].

7. EMT

Several oncogenic pathways (Rho GTPases, JAK-STAT, MAPK, Wnt and Notch) may induce EMT [21-25]. In particular, the association of those pathways with EMT has been shown to activate EMT-inducing transcriptional regulators such as the members of the Snail family, the zinc finger transcription factors (ZEB), Transforming growth factor beta (TGF-β), Twist and Slug.

Members of the Snail family of transcriptional regulators, namely Snail 1 and Snail 2, have emerged as a key regulatory factor of EMT. The zinc finger transcription factors ZEB1 and ZEB2 also make a pivotal contribution to this regulation. TGF-β, a major inducer of EMT, exists in at least three isoforms called TGF-β1, TGF-β2 and TGF-β3. It cooperates with stem cell pathways like Wnt, Ras and Notch to induce EMT [88, 89]. Twist, a basic helix-loop-helix transcription factor, exists in at least two isoforms called Twist 1 and Twist 2. Twist proteins promote EMT by turning-down the expression of epithelial specific proteins, such as the E-cadherin and by up-regulating the expression of mesenchymal markers such as the N-cadherin, the vimentin and the smooth-muscle actin [90]. Slug, a zinc finger transcription factor, whose product belongs to the Snail family of developmental regulatory proteins, is transcriptional repressors of E-cadherin and induces EMT [1].

Emerging studies have indicated that miRNAs participate in the EMT. The miR-106b-25 cluster targets Smad7, activates TGF-β signaling, and induces EMT in human breast cancer [91]. MiR-27 promoted EMT by activating the Wnt pathway [92]. MiR-221/222 targeting of trichorhinophalangeal 1 (TRPS1) promotes EMT in breast cancer [93]. MiR-194 inhibits EMT of endometrial cancer cells by targeting oncogene BMI-1 [94]. Let-7d negatively modulates EMT expression and also plays a role in regulating chemo-resistant ability in oral cancer [95]. MiR-200b and miR-15b regulate chemotherapy-induced EMT in human tongue cancer cells by targeting BMI-1 [96]. Kumarswamy and his colleagues found that miR-30a targets Snail, inhibits invasion and metastasis, and is downregulated in non-small cell lung cancer (NSCLC) [97]. Vetter and his colleagues indicated that miR-661 expression in Snail 1-induced EMT contributes to breast cancer cell invasion by targeting Nectin-1 and StarD10 messengers [98]. Some studies indicated that the miR-200 family and miR-205 regulate EMT by targeting ZEB1 and SIP1 [99, 100].

8. MicroRNAs in invasion and metastasis in lung cancer

Lung cancer is the leading cause of death among the malignant tumors worldwide, and the incidence of lung cancer is increasing. Tumor invasion and metastasis are the critical steps in determining the aggressive phenotype of human cancers. Mortality of tumor patients results mainly from cancer cells spreading to distant organs. In order to resist cancer dissemination, more effective therapeutic strategies are clearly required. However, the cellular and molecular machinery, underlying invasion and metastasis by miRNA in lung cancer, is relatively poorly understood. In light of these recent discoveries, we have classified the experimentally validated miRNAs regulating the invasion and metastasis of lung cancer and showed in Figure 2.

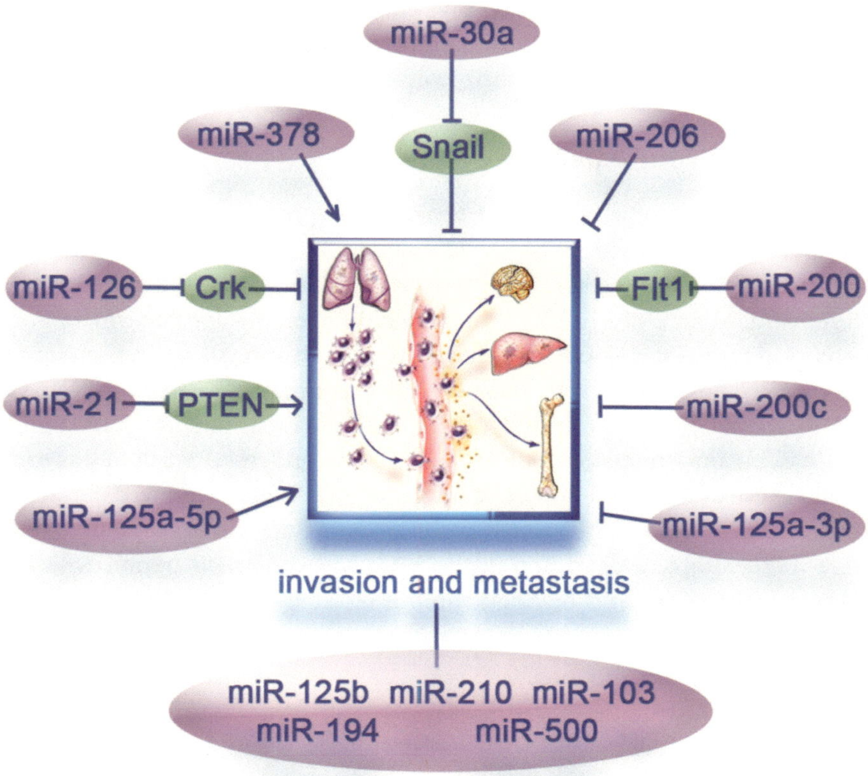

Figure 2. The experimentally validated miRNAs regulate the invasion and metastasis in lung cancer.

In light of these recent discoveries, the present article indicated that miRNAs participate in invasion and metastasis in lung cancer. Zhu and his colleagues indicated that MTA1 functions in regulating the invasive phenotype of lung cancer cells and this regulation may be through altered miRNA expression, such as miR-125b, miR-210, miR-103, miR-194 and miR-500 [101]. Hu and his colleagues reported that MiR-193b modulated proliferation, migration, and invasion of NSCLC [102]. A p53/miR-34 axis has been found that it regulates Snail1-dependent cancer cell EMT [103]. MiR-378 is associated with NSCLC brain metastasis by promoting cell migration, invasion and tumor angiogenesis [104]. MiR-30a targets Snail, inhibits invasion and metastasis, and is downregulated in NSCLC [105]. Expression level of miR-206 was inversely correlated with metastatic potential of lung cancer [106]. Roybal and his colleagues demonstrated that miR-200 Inhibits lung adenocarcinoma cell invasion and metastasis by targeting Flt1 [107]. Loss of miR-200c expression induces an aggressive, invasive, and chemoresistant phenotype in NSCLC [108]. In our previous studies, we found that hsa-miR-125a-3p and hsa-miR-125a-5p are downregulated in NSCLC and have inverse effects on invasion and migration of lung cancer cells [109]. Zhang and his colleagues reported that miR-21 post-transcriptionally downregulates the expression of tumor suppressor PTEN and stimulates growth and invasion in NSCLC [110]. Crawford and his colleagues indicated that MiR-126 alters lung cancer cell phenotype by inhibiting adhesion, migration, and invasion and the effects on invasion may be partially mediated through Crk regulation [111]. The deep mechanisms of miRNAs in invasion and metastasis which contribute to lung cancer are worthy of further investigation.

9. Conclusion and future perspective

Despite recent advances in diagnosis and treatment, lung cancer remains a leading cause of death among the malignant tumors worldwide, and the incidence of lung cancer is increasing. Even so, no improvement in prognosis has been observed if the patient presents with metastases at diagnosis. A better understanding of the mechanism of tumor cell invasion is critical for the development of more effective treatments for metastatic cancer. In recent years, emerging studies have attested to the association between miRNAs and the mechanism in critical processes during cancer dissemination, and we have summarized many of these in the present manuscript. Here, we have condensed much of this early work, and highlight key deregulated miRNAs targeting molecules involved in Rho family GTPases, JAK-STAT, MAPK, Wnt, Notch pathway and transcriptional control of EMT. In the future, a more complete dissection of the pathways controlled by miRNAs may offer new insights on metastasis, and highlight promising areas for the development of novel anti-cancer therapies.

Author details

Lili Jiang and Xueshan Qiu
Department of Pathology, the First Affiliated Hospital and College of Basic Medical Sciences, China Medical University, Shenyang, China

Lili Jiang
Department of Pathology, Medical College of Eastern Liaoning University, Dandong, China

Acknowledgement

Lili Jiang collected information and wrote the manuscript. XueShan Qiu helped with the manuscript design and gave critical review of the manuscript. We are grateful to the members of our laboratory for useful suggestions.

10. References

[1] Sreekumar R, Sayan BS, Mirnezami AH, Sayan AE. MicroRNA Control of Invasion and Metastasis Pathways. Front Genet 2011; 2: 58.
[2] Baranwal S, Alahari SK. Rho GTPase effector functions in tumor cell invasion and metastasis. Curr Drug Targets 2011; 12 (8):1194-201.
[3] Struckhoff AP, Rana MK, Worthylake RA. RhoA can lead the way in tumor cell invasion and metastasis. Front Biosci 2011; 16: 1915-26.

[4] Narumiya S, Tanji M, Ishizaki T. Rho signaling, ROCK and mDia1, in transformation, metastasis and invasion. Cancer Metastasis Rev 2009; 28 (1-2): 65-76.
[5] Lai SY, Childs EE, Xi S, Coppelli FM, Gooding WE, Wells A, Ferris RL, Grandis JR. Erythropoietin-mediated activation of JAK-STAT signaling contributes to cellular invasion in head and neck squamous cell carcinoma. Oncogene 2005; 24 (27): 4442-9.
[6] Zhao Y, Zhang J, Xia H, Zhang B, Jiang T, Wang J, Chen X, Wang Y. Stat3 is involved in the motility, metastasis and prognosis in lingual squamous cell carcinoma. Cell Biochem Funct. 2012; 30 (4): 340-6.
[7] Devarajan E, Huang S. STAT3 as a central regulator of tumor metastases. Curr Mol Med 2009; 9 (5): 626-33.
[8] Reddy KB, Nabha SM, Atanaskova N. 9. Gomes LR, Terra LF, Wailemann RA, Labriola L, Sogayar MC. Role of MAP kinase in tumor progression and invasion. Cancer Metastasis Rev 2003; 22 (4): 395-403.
[9] Del Barco Barrantes I, Nebreda AR. Roles of p38 MAPKs in invasion and metastasis. Biochem Soc Trans 2012; 40 (1): 79-84.
[10] Zhang S, Guo W, Ren TT, Lu XC, Tang GQ, Zhao FL. Arsenic trioxide inhibits Ewing's sarcoma cell invasiveness by targeting p38 (MAPK) and c-Jun N-terminal kinase. Anticancer Drugs 2012; 23 (1): 108-18.
[11] Sarkar FH, Li Y, Wang Z, Kong D. The role of nutraceuticals in the regulation of Wnt and Hedgehog signaling in cancer. Cancer Metastasis Rev 2010; 29 (3): 383-94.
[12] Huang D, Du X. Crosstalk between tumor cells and microenvironment via Wnt pathway in colorectal cancer dissemination. World J Gastroenterol 2008; 14 (12): 1823-7.
[13] Neth P, Ries C, Karow M, Egea V, Ilmer M, Jochum M. The Wnt signal transduction pathway in stem cells and cancer cells: influence on cellular invasion. Stem Cell Rev 2007; 3 (1):18-29.
[14] Asnaghi L, Ebrahimi KB, Schreck KC, Bar EE, Coonfield ML, Bell WR, Handa J, Merbs SL, Harbour JW, Eberhart CG. Notch signaling promotes growth and invasion in uveal melanoma. Clin Cancer Res 2012; 18 (3): 654-65.
[15] Bailey JM, Singh PK, Hollingsworth MA. Cancer metastasis facilitated by developmental pathways: Sonic hedgehog, Notch, and bone morphogenic proteins. J Cell Biochem 2007; 102 (4): 829-39.
[16] Wang XQ, Zhang W, Lui EL, Zhu Y, Lu P, Yu X, Sun J, Yang S, Poon RT, Fan ST. Notch1-Snail1-E-cadherin pathway in metastatic hepatocellular carcinoma. Int J Cancer 2012 131 (3):E163-72.
[17] Shih JY, Yang PC. The EMT regulator slug and lung carcinogenesis. Carcinogenesis 2011; 32 (9): 1299-304.
[18] Wells A, Chao YL, Grahovac J, Wu Q, Lauffenburger DA. Epithelial and mesenchymal phenotypic switchings modulate cell motility in metastasis. Front Biosci 2011; 16: 815-37.
[19] Savagner P. The epithelial-mesenchymal transition (EMT) phenomenon. Ann Oncol 2010; 21 Suppl 7:vii89-92.
[20] Cano CE, Motoo Y, Iovanna JL. Epithelial-to-mesenchymal transition in pancreatic adenocarcinoma. ScientificWorldJournal 2010; 10: 1947-57.

[21] Savagner P. Leaving the neighborhood: molecular mechanisms involved during epithelial-mesenchymal transition. Bioessays 2001; 23 (10): 912-23.

[22] Yadav A, Kumar B, Datta J, Teknos TN, Kumar P. IL-6 promotes head and neck tumor metastasis by inducing epithelial-mesenchymal transition via the JAK-STAT3-SNAIL signaling pathway. Mol Cancer Res 2011; 9 (12): 1658-67.

[23] Wu WS. The signaling mechanism of ROS in tumor progression. Cancer Metastasis Rev 2006; 25 (4): 695-705.

[24] Neth P, Ries C, Karow M, Egea V, Ilmer M, Jochum M. The Wnt signal transduction pathway in stem cells and cancer cells: influence on cellular invasion. Stem Cell Rev 2007; 3 (1): 18-29.

[25] Wang Z, Li Y, Kong D, Sarkar FH. The role of Notch signaling pathway in epithelial-mesenchymal transition (EMT) during development and tumor aggressiveness. Curr Drug Targets 2010; 11 (6): 745-51.

[26] Lee RC, Feinbaum RL, Ambros V. The C. elegansheterochronic gene lin-4 encodes small RNAs with antisense complementarity to lin-14. Cell 1993; 75 (5), 843-54.

[27] Lee Y, Ahn C, Han J, Choi H, Kim J, Yim J, Lee J, Provost P, Radmark O, Kim S, Kim VN. The nuclear RNase III Drosha initiates microRNA processing. Nature 2003; 425 (6956),415-9

[28] Kong W, Zhao JJ, He L&Cheng JQ. Strategies for profiling microRNA expression. J Cell Physiol 2009; 218 (1), 22-5

[29] Hutvágner G, McLachlan J, Pasquinelli AE, Bálint E, Tuschl T, Zamore PD. A cellular function for the RNA-interference enzyme Dicer in the maturation of the let-7 small temporal RNA. Science 2001; 293 (5531), 834-8.

[30] Grishok A, Pasquinelli AE, Conte D, Li N, Parrish S, Ha I, Baillie DL, Fire A, Ruvkun G, Mello CC.Genes and mechanisms related to RNA interference regulate expression of the small temporal RNAs that control C. elegans developmental timing. Cell 2001; 106 (1), 23-34.

[31] Crawford M, Brawner E, Batte K, Yu L, Hunter MG, Otterson GA, Nuovo G, Marsh CB, Nana-Sinkam SP. MicroRNA-126 inhibits invasion in non-small cell lung carcinoma cell lines. Biochem Biophys Res Commun 2008; 373 (4), 607-12.

[32] Zhu S, Wu H, Wu F, Nie D, Sheng S, Mo YY. MicroRNA-21 targets tumor suppressor genes in invasion and metastasis. Cell Res 2008; 18 (3), 350-9.

[33] Tavazoie SF, Alarcón C, Oskarsson T, Padua D, Wang Q, Bos PD, Gerald WL, Massagué J. Endogenous human microRNAs that suppress breast cancer metastasis. Nature 2008; 451 (7175), 147-52.

[34] Bustelo XR, Sauzeau V, Berenjeno IM. GTP-binding proteins of the Rho/Rac family: regulation, effectors and functions in vivo. Bioessays 2007; 29 (4): 356–370.

[35] Boureux A, Vignal E, Faure S, Fort P. Evolution of the Rho family of ras-like GTPases in eukaryotes. Mol BiolEvol 2007; 24 (1): 203–16.

[36] Rathinam R, Berrier A, Alahari SK. Role of Rho GTPases and their regulators in cancer progression. Front Biosci 2011; 16: 2561-71.

[37] Kong W, Yang H, He L, Zhao JJ, Coppola D, Dalton WS, Cheng JQ. MicroRNA-155 is regulated by the transforming growth factor beta/Smad pathway and contributes to epithelial cell plasticity by targeting RhoA. Mol Cell Biol 2008; 28 (22):6773-84.
[38] Jiang L, Liu X, Kolokythas A, Yu J, Wang A, Heidbreder CE, Shi F, Zhou X. Downregulation of the Rho GTPase signaling pathway is involved in the microRNA-138-mediated inhibition of cell migration and invasion in tongue squamous cell carcinoma. Int J Cancer 2010; 127 (3): 505-12.
[39] Valastyan S, Chang A, Benaich N, Reinhardt F, Weinberg RA. Concurrent suppression of integrin alpha5, radixin, and RhoAphenocopies the effects of miR-31 on metastasis. Cancer Res 2010; 70 (12): 5147-54.
[40] Chiba Y, Tanabe M, Goto K, Sakai H, Misawa M. Down-regulation of miR-133a contributes to up-regulation of Rhoa in bronchial smooth muscle cells. Am J RespirCrit Care Med 2009; 180 (8): 713-9.
[41] Kamai T, Tsujii T, Arai K, Takagi K, Asami H, Ito Y,Oshima H. Significant association of Rho/ROCK pathway with invasion and metastasis of bladder cancer. Clin Cancer Res 2003; 9 (7): 2632-41.
[42] Bishop AL, Hall A. Rho GTPases and their effector proteins. Biochem J 2000; 348 Pt 2:241-55.
[43] Riento K, Ridley AJ. Rocks: multifunctional kinases in cell behaviour. Nat Rev Mol Cell Biol 2003; 4 (6), 446-56.
[44] Salhia B, Rutten F, Nakada M, Beaudry C, Berens M, Kwan A,Rutka JT. Inhibition of Rho-kinase affects astrocytoma morphology, motility, and invasion through activation of Rac1. Cancer Res 2005; 65 (19), 8792-800.
[45] Yu J, Peng H, Ruan Q, Fatima A, Getsios S, Lavker RM. MicroRNA-205 promotes keratinocyte migration via the lipid phosphatase SHIP2. FASEB J 2010; 24 (10): 3950-9
[46] Wu L, Cai C, Wang X, Liu M, Li X, Tang H. MicroRNA-142-3p, a new regulator of RAC1, suppresses the migration and invasion of hepatocellular carcinoma cells. FEBS Lett 2011; 585 (9): 1322-30.
[47] Moriarty CH, Pursell B, Mercurio AM. miR-10b targets Tiam1: implications for Rac activation and carcinoma migration. J Biol Chem 2010; 285 (27): 20541-6.
[48] Luedde T. MicroRNA-151 and its hosting gene FAK (focal adhesion kinase) regulate tumor cell migration and spreading of hepatocellular carcinoma. Hepatology 2010; 52 (3): 1164-6.
[49] Liu M, Lang N, Qiu M, Xu F, Li Q, Tang Q, Chen J, Chen X, Zhang S, Liu Z, Zhou J, Zhu Y, Deng Y, Zheng Y, Bi F. miR-137 targets Cdc42 expression, induces cell cycle G1 arrest and inhibits invasion in colorectal cancer cells. Int J Cancer 2011; 128 (6): 1269-79.
[50] Chen Q, Chen X, Zhang M, Fan Q, Luo S, Cao X. miR-137 is frequently down-regulated in gastric cancer and is a negative regulator of Cdc42. Dig Dis Sci. 2011; 56 (7): 2009-16.
[51] Liu H, Cao YD, Ye WX, Sun YY. Effect of microRNA-206 on cytoskeleton remodelling by downregulating Cdc42 in MDA-MB-231 cells. Tumori 2010; 96 (5): 751-5.
[52] Park SY, Lee JH, Ha M, Nam JW, Kim VN. miR-29 miRNAs activate p53 by targeting p85 alpha and CDC42. Nat Struct Mol Biol 2009; 16 (1): 23-9.

[53] Liu M, Tang Q, Qiu M, Lang N, Li M, Zheng Y, Bi F. miR-21 targets the tumor suppressor RhoB and regulates proliferation, invasion and apoptosis in colorectal cancer cells. FEBS Lett 2011; 585 (19): 2998-3005.

[54] Connolly EC, Van Doorslaer K, Rogler LE, Rogler CE. Overexpression of miR-21 promotes an in vitro metastatic phenotype by targeting the tumor suppressor RHOB. Mol Cancer Res 2010; 8 (5): 691-700.

[55] Aaronson DS, Horvath CM. A road map for those who don't know JAK-STAT. Science 2002; 296 (5573): 1653–5.

[56] Looyenga BD, Hutchings D, Cherni I, Kingsley C, Weiss GJ, Mackeigan JP. STAT3 Is Activated by JAK2 Independent of Key Oncogenic Driver Mutations in Non-Small Cell Lung Carcinoma. PLoS One 2012; 7 (2): e30820.

[57] Devarajan E, Huang S. STAT3 as a central regulator of tumor metastases. Curr Mol Med. 2009; 9 (5): 626-33.

[58] Ding L, Xu Y, Zhang W, Deng Y, Si M, Du Y, Yao H, Liu X, Ke Y, Si J, Zhou T. MiR-375 frequently downregulated in gastric cancer inhibits cell proliferation by targeting JAK2. Cell Res 2010; 20 (7): 784-93.

[59] Liu LH, Li H, Li JP, Zhong H, Zhang HC, Chen J, Xiao T. miR-125b suppresses the proliferation and migration of osteosarcoma cells through down-regulation of STAT3. Biochem Biophys Res Commun 2011; 416 (1-2): 31-8.

[60] Duan Z, Choy E, Harmon D, Liu X, Susa M, Mankin H, Hornicek F. MicroRNA-199a-3p is downregulated in human osteosarcoma and regulates cell proliferation and migration. Mol Cancer Ther 2011; 10 (8): 1337-45.

[61] Yan H, Wu J, Liu W, Zuo Y, Chen S, Zhang S, Zeng M, Huang W. MicroRNA-20a overexpression inhibited proliferation and metastasis of pancreatic carcinoma cells. Hum Gene Ther 2010; 21 (12): 1723-34.

[62] Gomes LR, Terra LF, Wailemann RA, Labriola L, Sogayar MC. TGF-β1 modulates the homeostasis between MMPs and MMP inhibitors through p38 MAPK and ERK1/2 in highly invasive breast cancer cells. BMC Cancer 2012; 12: 26.

[63] Xu B, Niu X, Zhang X, Tao J, Wu D, Wang Z, Li P, Zhang W, Wu H, Feng N, Wang Z, Hua L, Wang X. miR-143 decreases prostate cancer cells proliferation and migration and enhances their sensitivity to docetaxel through suppression of KRAS. Mol Cell Biochem 2011; 350 (1-2): 207-13.

[64] Yang F, Yin Y, Wang F, Wang Y, Zhang L, Tang Y, Sun S. miR-17-5p Promotes migration of human hepatocellular carcinoma cells through the p38 mitogen-activated protein kinase-heat shock protein 27 pathway. Hepatology 2010; 51 (5): 1614-23.

[65] Dangi-Garimella S, Yun J, Eves EM, Newman M, Erkeland SJ, Hammond SM, Minn AJ, Rosner MR. Raf kinase inhibitory protein suppresses a metastasis signalling cascade involving LIN28 and let-7. EMBO J 2009; 28 (4): 347-58.

[66] Zhu QY, Liu Q, Chen JX, Lan K, Ge BX. MicroRNA-101 targets MAPK phosphatase-1 to regulate the activation of MAPKs in macrophages. J Immunol 2010; 185 (12): 7435-42.

[67] Xu B, Wang N, Wang X, Tong N, Shao N, Tao J, Li P, Niu X, Feng N, Zhang L, Hua L, Wang Z, Chen M. MiR-146a suppresses tumor growth and progression by targeting

EGFR pathway and in a p-ERK-dependent manner in castration-resistant prostate cancer. Prostate. 2012; 72 (11): 1171-8.
[68] Liu LZ, Li C, Chen Q, Jing Y, Carpenter R, Jiang Y, Kung HF, Lai L, Jiang BH. MiR-21 induced angiogenesis through AKT and ERK activation and HIF-1α expression. PLoS One 2011; 6 (4): e19139.
[69] Hatley ME, Patrick DM, Garcia MR, Richardson JA, Bassel-Duby R, van Rooij E, Olson EN. Modulation of K-Ras-dependent lung tumorigenesis by MicroRNA-21. Cancer Cell 2010; 18 (3): 282-93.
[70] Chou YT, Lin HH, Lien YC, Wang YH, Hong CF, Kao YR, Lin SC, Chang YC, Lin SY, Chen SJ, Chen HC, Yeh SD, Wu CW. EGFR promotes lung tumorigenesis by activating miR-7 through a Ras/ERK/Myc pathway that targets the Ets2 transcriptional repressor ERF. Cancer Res 2010; 70 (21): 8822-31.
[71] Dale TC. Signal transduction by the Wnt family of ligands. Biochem J 1998; 329 (Pt 2): 209-23.
[72] Katoh M. WNT/PCP signaling pathway and human cancer. Oncol Rep 2005; 14 (6): 1583-8.
[73] Su J, Zhang A, Shi Z, Ma F, Pu P, Wang T, Zhang J, Kang C, Zhang Q. MicroRNA-200a suppresses the Wnt/β-catenin signaling pathway by interacting with β-catenin. Int J Oncol 2012; 40 (4): 1162-70.
[74] Zhou AD, Diao LT, Xu H, Xiao ZD, Li JH, Zhou H, Qu LH. β-Catenin/LEF1 transactivates the microRNA-371-373 cluster that modulates the Wnt/β-catenin-signaling pathway. Oncogene. Oncogene. 2012; 31 (24): 2968-78.
[75] Wang T, Xu Z. miR-27 promotes osteoblast differentiation by modulating Wnt signaling. Biochem Biophys Res Commun 2010; 402 (2): 186-9.
[76] Kapinas K, Kessler C, Ricks T, Gronowicz G, Delany AM. miR-29 modulates Wnt signaling in human osteoblasts through a positive feedback loop. J Biol Chem 2010; 285 (33): 25221-31.
[77] Li H, Bian C, Liao L, Li J, Zhao RC. miR-17-5p promotes human breast cancer cell migration and invasion through suppression of HBP1. Breast Cancer Res Treat 2011; 126 (3): 565-75.
[78] Kennell JA, Gerin I, MacDougald OA, Cadigan KM. The microRNA miR-8 is a conserved negative regulator of Wnt signaling. Proc Natl Acad Sci U S A 2008; 105 (40): 15417-22.
[79] Wang Z, Li Y, Ahmad A, Azmi AS, Banerjee S, Kong D, Sarkar FH. Targeting Notch signaling pathway to overcome drug resistance for cancer therapy. Biochim Biophys Acta 2010; 1806 (2): 258-67.
[80] Zheng J, Jiang HY, Li J, Tang HC, Zhang XM, Wang XR, Du JT, Li HB, Xu G. MicroRNA-23b promotes tolerogenic properties of dendritic cells in vitro through inhibiting Notch1/NF-κB signalling pathways. Allergy 2012; 67 (3): 362-70.
[81] Cichocki F, Felices M, McCullar V, Presnell SR, Al-Attar A, Lutz CT, Miller JS. Cutting edge: microRNA-181 promotes human NK cell development by regulating Notch signaling. J Immunol 2011; 187 (12): 6171-5.

[82] Liu XS, Chopp M, Zhang RL, Tao T, Wang XL, Kassis H, Hozeska-Solgot A, Zhang L, Chen C, Zhang ZG. MicroRNA profiling in subventricular zone after stroke: MiR-124a regulates proliferation of neural progenitor cells through Notch signaling pathway. PLoS One 2011; 6 (8):e23461.

[83] Pang RT, Leung CO, Ye TM, Liu W, Chiu PC, Lam KK, Lee KF, Yeung WS. MicroRNA-34a suppresses invasion through downregulation of Notch1 and Jagged1 in cervical carcinoma and choriocarcinoma cells. Carcinogenesis 2010; 31 (6): 1037-44.

[84] Song G, Zhang Y, Wang L. MicroRNA-206 targets notch3, activates apoptosis, and inhibits tumor cell migration and focus formation. J Biol Chem 2009; 284 (46): 31921-7.

[85] Kwon C, Han Z, Olson EN, Srivastava D. MicroRNA1 influences cardiac differentiation in Drosophila and regulates Notch signaling. Proc Natl Acad Sci U S A 2005; 102 (52): 18986-91.

[86] Brabletz S, Bajdak K, Meidhof S, Burk U, Niedermann G, Firat E, Wellner U, Dimmler A, Faller G, Schubert J, Brabletz T. The ZEB1/miR-200 feedback loop controls Notch signalling in cancer cells. EMBO J 2011; 30 (4): 770-82.

[87] Vallejo DM, Caparros E, Dominguez M. Targeting Notch signalling by the conserved miR-8/200 microRNA family in development and cancer cells. EMBO J 2011; 30 (4):756-69.

[88] Fuxe J, Vincent T, Garcia de Herreros A. Transcriptional crosstalk between TGF-β and stem cell pathways in tumor cell invasion: role of EMT promoting Smad complexes. Cell Cycle 2010; 9 (12): 2363-74.

[89] Wendt MK, Allington TM, Schiemann WP. Mechanisms of the epithelial-mesenchymal transition by TGF-beta. Future Oncol 2009; 5 (8): 1145-68.

[90] Onder TT, Gupta PB, Mani SA, Yang J, Lander ES, Weinberg RA. Loss of E-cadherin promotes metastasis via multiple downstream transcriptional pathways. Cancer Res 2008; 68 (10): 3645-54.

[91] Smith AL, Iwanaga R, Drasin DJ, Micalizzi DS, Vartuli RL, Tan AC, Ford HL. The miR-106b-25 cluster targets Smad7, activates TGF-β signaling, and induces EMT and tumor initiating cell characteristics downstream of Six1 in human breast cancer. Oncogene 2012; 31(50): 5162-71.

[92] Zhang Z, Liu S, Shi R, Zhao G. miR-27 promotes human gastric cancer cell metastasis by inducing epithelial-to-mesenchymal transition. Cancer Genet 2011; 204 (9): 486-91.

[93] Stinson S, Lackner MR, Adai AT, Yu N, Kim HJ, O'Brien C, Spoerke J, Jhunjhunwala S, Boyd Z, Januario T, Newman RJ, Yue P, Bourgon R, Modrusan Z, Stern HM, Warming S, de Sauvage FJ, Amler L, Yeh RF, Dornan D. TRPS1 targeting by miR-221/222 promotes the epithelial-to-mesenchymal transition in breast cancer. Sci Signal 2011; 4 (177): ra41.

[94] Dong P, Kaneuchi M, Watari H, Hamada J, Sudo S, Ju J, Sakuragi N. MicroRNA-194 inhibits epithelial to mesenchymal transition of endometrial cancer cells by targeting oncogene BMI-1. Mol Cancer 2011; 10: 99.

[95] Chang CJ, Hsu CC, Chang CH, Tsai LL, Chang YC, Lu SW, Yu CH, Huang HS, Wang JJ, Tsai CH, Chou MY, Yu CC, Hu FW. Let-7d functions as novel regulator of epithelial-

mesenchymal transition and chemoresistant property in oral cancer. Oncol Rep 2011; 26 (4): 1003-10.

[96] Sun L, Yao Y, Liu B, Lin Z, Lin L, Yang M, Zhang W, Chen W, Pan C, Liu Q, Song E, Li J. MiR-200b and miR-15b regulate chemotherapy-induced epithelial-mesenchymal transition in human tongue cancer cells by targeting BMI1. Oncogene 2012; 31 (4): 432-45.

[97] Kumarswamy R, Mudduluru G, Ceppi P, Muppala S, Kozlowski M, Niklinski J, Papotti M, Allgayer H. MicroRNA-30a inhibits epithelial-to-mesenchymal transition by targeting Snai1 and is downregulated in non-small cell lung cancer. Int J Cancer. 2012; 130 (9): 2044-53.

[98] Vetter G, Saumet A, Moes M, Vallar L, Le Béchec A, Laurini C, Sabbah M, Arar K, Theillet C, Lecellier CH, Friederich E. miR-661 expression in SNAI1-induced epithelial to mesenchymal transition contributes to breast cancer cell invasion by targeting Nectin-1 and StarD10 messengers. Oncogene 2010; 29 (31): 4436-48.

[99] Gregory PA, Bert AG, Paterson EL, Barry SC, Tsykin A, Farshid G, Vadas MA, Khew-Goodall Y, Goodall GJ. The miR-200 family and miR-205 regulate epithelial to mesenchymal transition by targeting ZEB1 and SIP1. Nat Cell Biol 2008; 10 (5): 593-601.

[100] Xiong M, Jiang L, Zhou Y, Qiu W, Fang L, Tan R, Wen P, Yang J. The miR-200 family regulates TGF-β1-induced renal tubular epithelial to mesenchymal transition through Smad pathway by targeting ZEB1 and ZEB2 expression. Am J Physiol Renal Physiol 2012; 302 (3): F369-79.

[101] Zhu X, Zhang X, Wang H, Song Q, Zhang G, Yang L, Geng J, Li X, Yuan Y, Chen L. MTA1 gene silencing inhibits invasion and alters the microRNA expression profile of human lung cancer cells. Oncol Rep. 2012; 28 (1): 218-24.

[102] Hu H, Li S, Liu J, Ni B. MicroRNA-193b modulates proliferation, migration, and invasion of non-small cell lung cancer cells. Acta Biochim Biophys Sin. 2012; 44 (5): 424-30.

[103] Kim NH, Kim HS, Li XY, Lee I, Choi HS, Kang SE, Cha SY, Ryu JK, Yoon D, Fearon ER, Rowe RG, Lee S, Maher CA, Weiss SJ, Yook JI. A p53/miRNA-34 axis regulates Snail1-dependent cancer cell epithelial-mesenchymal transition. J Cell Biol. 2011; 195 (3): 417-33.

[104] Chen LT, Xu SD, Xu H, Zhang JF, Ning JF, Wang SF. MicroRNA-378 is associated with non-small cell lung cancer brain metastasis by promoting cell migration, invasion and tumor angiogenesis. Med Oncol 2012; 29 (3):1673-80

[105] Kumarswamy R, Mudduluru G, Ceppi P, Muppala S, Kozlowski M, Niklinski J, Papotti M, Allgayer H. MicroRNA-30a inhibits epithelial-to-mesenchymal transition by targeting Snai1 and is downregulated in non-small cell lung cancer. Int J Cancer. 2012; 130 (9): 2044-53.

[106] Wang X, Ling C, Bai Y, Zhao J. MicroRNA-206 is associated with invasion and metastasis of lung cancer. Anat Rec 2011; 294 (1): 88-92.

[107] Roybal JD, Zang Y, Ahn YH, Yang Y, Gibbons DL, Baird BN, Alvarez C, Thilaganathan N, Liu DD, Saintigny P, Heymach JV, Creighton CJ, Kurie JM. miR-200

Inhibits lung adenocarcinoma cell invasion and metastasis by targeting Flt1/VEGFR1. Mol Cancer Res 2011; 9 (1): 25-35.

[108] Ceppi P, Mudduluru G, Kumarswamy R, Rapa I, Scagliotti GV, Papotti M, Allgayer H. Loss of miR-200c expression induces an aggressive, invasive, and chemoresistant phenotype in non-small cell lung cancer. Mol Cancer Res 2010; 8 (9): 1207-16.

[109] Jiang L, Huang Q, Zhang S, Zhang Q, Chang J, Qiu X, Wang E. Hsa-miR-125a-3p and hsa-miR-125a-5p are downregulated in non-small cell lung cancer and have inverse effects on invasion and migration of lung cancer cells. BMC Cancer 2010; 10: 318.

[110] Zhang JG, Wang JJ, Zhao F, Liu Q, Jiang K, Yang GH. MicroRNA-21 (miR-21) represses tumor suppressor PTEN and promotes growth and invasion in non-small cell lung cancer (NSCLC). Clin Chim Acta 2010; 411 (11-12): 846-52.

[111] Crawford M, Brawner E, Batte K, Yu L, Hunter MG, Otterson GA, Nuovo G, Marsh CB, Nana-Sinkam SP. MicroRNA-126 inhibits invasion in non-small cell lung carcinoma cell lines. Biochem Biophys Res Commun. 2008; 373 (4): 607-12.

Chapter 6

The Importance of Cancer Cell Lines as *in vitro* Models in Cancer Methylome Analysis and Anticancer Drugs Testing

Daniela Ferreira, Filomena Adega and Raquel Chaves

Additional information is available at the end of the chapter

http://dx.doi.org/10.5772/53110

1. Introduction

Cancer is a molecularly heterogeneous disease [1] and one of the major causes of death worldwide. The existence of various types of tumours with different histopathologies, genetic and epigenetic variations, and clinical outcomes [2], difficult the understanding of this disease, the mechanisms of action of chemotherapeutics and the creation of novel therapies.

The advances in the cancer pathobiology study has its origin on the availability of different types of experimental model systems that review the various forms of this disease [2], allowing the knowledge of genetics and epigenetics alterations and anticancer drugs testing. Studies of cancer rely on the use of primary tumours [1, 3], paraffin-embedded samples [1], cancer cell lines [1, 3, 4], xenografts [2, 5, 6], tumour primary cell cultures [3, 4] and/or genetically engineered mice [2]. Each of these diverse models are used for different studies, mainly because certain types of manipulations for the genetic and DNA methylation analysis and drug testing are ethically, and in practice, difficult to perform in animals. Cell lines emerge as a feasible alternative to overcome these issues, being at the same time easy to manipulate [3] and molecularly characterize (e.g. genetic and/or epigenetically). This cell model is exceptional for the fundamental study of the cellular pathways and for disclosing critical genes involved in cancer. Nevertheless, a detailed characterization is fundamental before its use. This characterization provides important insights about the complexity of the polygenetic etiology of cancer and the biological mechanisms involved in this disease [1] reinforcing its value as models for its study [1, 7]. Also the characterization of cancer cell lines is essential for the development of new anticancer drugs, understanding the action mechanisms and the resistance/sensitivity patterns of chemotherapeutics already in use in cancer treatment and the development of more targeted anticancer drugs.

2. Cancer cell lines as a model for cancer study

Cancer cell lines have been widely used for research purposes and proved to be a useful tool in the genetic approach, and its characterization shows that they are, in fact, an excellent model for the study of the biological mechanisms involved in cancer [1]. Examples are shown in table 1. The use of cancer cell lines allowed an increment of the information about the deregulated genes and signalling pathways in this disease [2, 8]. Furthermore, the use of the cell model was in the origin of the development and testing of anticancer drugs presently used [8-10], and in the development of new therapies [1, 10, 11], but also as an alternative to transplantable animal tumours in chemotherapeutics testing [12]. In fact, the use of the appropriate *in vitro* model in cancer research is crucial for the investigation of genetic, epigenetic and cellular pathways [1], for the study of proliferation deregulation, apoptosis and cancer progression [2], to define potential molecular markers [3] and for the screening and characterization of cancer therapeutics [10, 13]. The results of the research in cancer cell lines are usually extrapolated to *in vivo* human tumours [3] and its importance as models for drug testing and translational study have been recognized by many biomedical and pharmaceutical companies [8].

Cancer cell line	Species		Morphology
HeLa	*Homo sapiens*	Cervix adenocarcinoma	Epithelial
MCF-7	*Homo sapiens*	Breast adenocarcinoma	Epithelial
U87MG	*Homo sapiens*	Glioblastoma-astrocytoma	Epithelial
HT-29	*Homo sapiens*	Colon adenocarcinoma	Epithelial
A549	*Homo sapiens*	Lung carcinoma	Epithelial
HEP-G2	*Homo sapiens*	Hepatocellular carcinoma	Epithelial
K-562	*Homo sapiens*	Chronic myeloid leukaemia	Lymphoblast
Cos7	*Cercopithecus aethiops*	SV40 transformed - kidney	Fibroblast
PC3	*Homo sapiens*	Prostate adenocarcinoma	Epithelial
A375	*Homo sapiens*	Malignant melanoma	Epithelial

Table 1. Examples of some widely used cancer cell lines with origin in different cell types. These data were obtained from the European Collection of Cell Cultures (ECCC) and American Type Culture Collection (ATCC).

In spite of the essential role of cancer cell lines in biomedical research, there is a debate among the scientific community on the fact whether they are or not representative of the original tumour [5, 14]. Some authors agree with the idea that there is a high, but not perfect, genomic similarity between the original tumour and the cancer cell line derived from it [8, 13, 15-17]. Cancer cell lines maintain the tumour-specific chromosome abnormalities in the first passages [15], show the same morphologic and molecular characteristics of the primary tumour [16] and, in general, maintain the expression of the "hallmarks of cancer", with exception of angiogenesis that requires the presence of stromal tissues [8]. As an example, Tomlinson and colleagues (1998) compared a breast primary tumour and a cell line originated from that tumour. These authors reported the same *BRCA1* mutation and an identical pattern of allelic loss in multiple *loci*, indicating that the cell line preserves numerous characteristics of the original tumour [17]. Also the data from Finlay and Bagulay (1984) demonstrated that the cancer cell lines have a similar response to anticancer drugs when compared to the original tumour [18].

The fact that a large number of long-established cancer cell lines were originated from aggressive and metastatic tumours [4, 5], restrict the study of cancer progression and of drug therapies development. Cancer cell lines derived from earlier stage and lower grade disease seems to be the more promising models. In comparative studies made between cancer cell lines derived from earlier stage tumours and the original tumour tissues showed good concordance in several parameters, including the state of P53 (100%) and ERBB2 (93%) [4]. This shows that this type of cells are more representative of the original tumour [4], reflecting more accurately the events that occur in cancer cells *in vivo* [5].

While cancer cell lines retain many genetic, epigenetic and gene expression features [3], they are genetically more complex than the tumour itself [13]. The differences between cancer cell lines and the respective tumours may be explained by the prior selection of initial cells and the *in vitro* Darwinian evolution [3]. Cancer cell lines typically present extensive chromosomal rearrangements, oncogene mutations, allelic loss and gene amplifications. This can lead to a loss of phenotypic properties and additional molecular changes during the cell culturing for long times [14], including modifications in some cellular pathways [3].

There are numerous reasons for the use of cancer cell lines as an experimental model for the study of cancer [2]. They have many intrinsic advantages for cancer research and for new therapeutic approaches, increasing their value [8]. Some of the advantages (table 2) of this model are listed below:

- Easiness to handle and manipulate [2-4]. This is an important and, in some cases an exclusive characteristic of this model [8]. Cell lines can be genetically/epigenetically manipulated using demethylation agents [1, 19], siRNA [20], expression vectors [10] and pharmacologically manipulated using cytostatics [13].
- High homogeneity [2-4]. The heterogeneity of solid tumours difficult their analysis and cancer cell lines allow the analysis of a homogeneous population of tumour cells [21]. This homogeneity can be seen as a disadvantage because of the natural heterogeneity of the tumour. However, this can be overcome using a panel of cancer cell lines representative of the heterogeneity observed in the primary tumours [2].
- High degree of similarity with the initial tumour [17]. Cancer cell lines are pure populations of tumour cells and they represent these cells without the complexity of the *in vivo* environment (stromal and inflammatory cells). This can be seen also as a disadvantage [8].
- Large number and variety of cancer cell lines available [8], although poorly characterized [5].
- Immediate accessibility to the scientific community [1, 8].

- Unlimited auto-replicative source, in continuous cell lines [4].
- Easy substitution of contaminated cultures for the respective frozen cell lines [4].
- Reproducibility of results in the correct conditions [3].

Nevertheless, some disadvantages or limitations (table 2) must be taken into account:

- Some cell lines may have cross contamination with HeLa cells. A large number of cancer cell lines in the cell banks (the most used) have been reported as contaminated with HeLa cells [3, 4, 8].
- Genomic instability [3, 4] which may cause differences between the original tumour and the respective cell line [3]. The genotypic and phenotypic drift is more common in continuous cultures, especially the ones deposited in cell banks for many years. The phenotypic changes can occur by the appearance of subpopulations selected from more competitive clones [3, 4]. This can be partially solved (in more recent cancer cell lines) limiting the number of passages and using frozen cells with few passages [3].
- Culture conditions, that can change the morphology, the gene expression and several cellular pathways [3].
- Infections with mycoplasma that can change the culture properties [3].
- Difficulty in the establishment of long-term cancer cell lines of certain types of tumours [22].
- Cell culture environment is different from that of the original tumour [2].
- Loss of the natural heterogeneity of the tumour [2].

Advantages of the use of cancer cell lines	Disadvantages of the use of cancer cell lines
• **Easy to handle and manipulate [2-4].** • **High homogeneity [2-4].** • **High degree of similarity with the initial tumour [17].** • **High variety available [8].** • **Immediate accessibility [1, 8].** • **Unlimited auto-replicative source [4].** • **Easy substitution [4].** • **Reproducibility of results [3].**	• Cross contamination with HeLa cells [3, 4, 8]. • Loss of heterogeneity [2]. • Genomic instability [3, 4]. • Possibility of modifying the characteristics of the cells [3]. • Infections with mycoplasma [3]. • Difficulty in the establishment of long-term cancer cell lines [22]. • Different environment of the tumour [2].

Table 2. Advantages and disadvantages of the use of cancer cell lines as models in cancer research.

Some of these problems can be solved by the conjugation with other type of models. Primary cell cultures (derived directly from the tumours) are a viable tool as they maintain some of the heterogeneity of the original tumour. However, the tissue environment is lost and some studies cannot be performed in this model, as those that need several passages [3, 4]. Fresh tumour samples obtained by surgery [3] or tumour samples embedded in paraffin [1] can also be used for the study of cancer biology. These models represent the state of the tumour *in vivo* with its heterogeneity, but only at a specific evolutionary moment of the tumour. This sample is limited in amount and the genetic manipulation is almost impossible [3]. The xenografts models (nude mice) are used for testing the tumorigenicity and metastatic ability of cancer cell lines. They constitute a model for drug testing, providing the *in vivo* microenvironment for human tumour original cells [2, 3]. However, the immunocompromised mice have a limitation *per se* by the important role of inflammation in cancer [2, 3]. Animal models, with spontaneous or induced tumours [3], have the advantage of providing a historical sequence of the tumour and have been used in the pathobiology research of cancer and for testing new therapeutics *in vivo*. Besides the ethical problem, this model also holds the difficulty in extrapolating the data to the human counterpart [22]. Another animal model is the genetically engineered mice for cancer that may reproduce human *in vivo* models [3]. This model is important for elucidating the regulatory mechanisms of cancer initiation and progression, however it cannot recapitulate all the aspects of the cancer [2] and also have limitations regarding genetic manipulation.

In fact, all the experimental models for cancer research present advantages and disadvantages and none of them is completely representative of the phenotype of the tumour [2, 3]. Nevertheless, cancer cell lines are adequate models for the research of this disease. They provide adequate models for the study of the origin of cancers by the presence of initiating cells or cancer stem cells [2, 3] and for drug testing in a first approach [2]. Some cancer cell lines can be used for screening RNAi (RNA interference) libraries and other small molecules as a way to study interacting pathways in the initiation and survival of the tumour [2]. The phenotype and genotype evolutionary study, under selective pressure, can be done in cancer cell lines, to understand the cancer progression until metastasis [3]. The use of a panel of various subtypes of cancer cell lines increases the importance of this model in disclosing the signalling pathways involved in therapeutic response [2]. Cancer cell lines are also an excellent tool for the genetic and epigenetic study of cancer, being the genomic and methylomic profiling of each cancer cell line crucial for cancer research and their use in anticancer drug testing.

2.1. The importance of the molecular characterization of cancer cell lines

A cancer cell line is more valuable as an *in vitro* model for cancer research if it is properly molecularly characterized [1, 7]. In Figure 1 this aspect is patent as we can observe an increasing of works regarding cell lines characterization which is accompanied by an increasing number of papers published concerning the use of cancer cell lines as models for cancer research. This type of analysis will allow a more detailed study of the genetic/epigenetic events (e.g. disclose critical cancer genes and DNA methylation alterations) and cellular pathways associated with oncogenesis [21], in the understanding of the microevolutionary progression of the tumour [1] (when the molecular profiling is done in different passages [15]) and unveil the molecular patterns associated with resistance/sensitivity to anticancer drugs [10, 15]. Specifically, the tumour transcriptional profiling and the DNA methylation patterns (i.e. that result in gene expression alterations) can be useful as a first approach in the development of new anticancer targeted therapeutics [9].

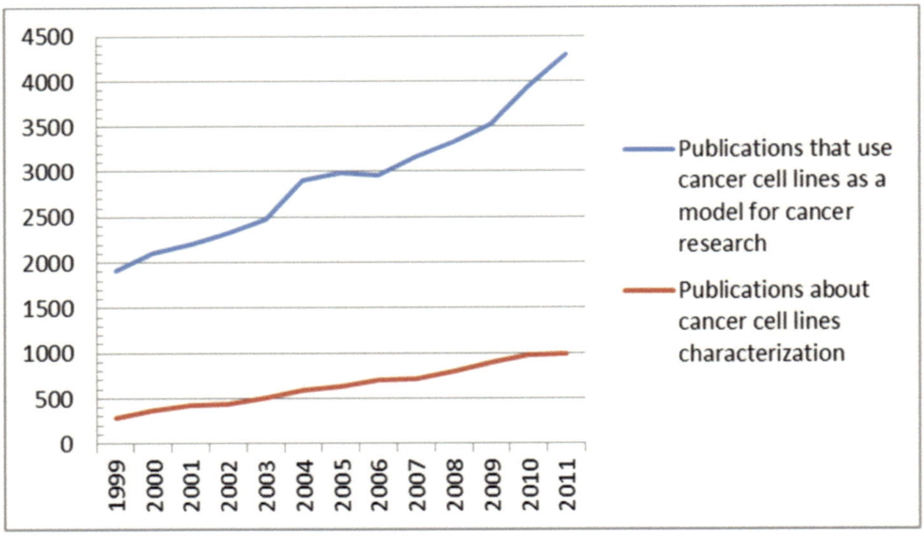

Figure 1. Number of publications regarding: cancer cell lines as models for cancer research (blue line) and cancer cell lines characterization (red line). These data were obtained from the papers indexed in the free resource PubMed (National Center for Biotechnology Information, at the U.S. National Library of Medicine, located at the National Institutes of Health).

The molecular characterization of cell lines molecular characterization can be done at different and complementary platforms - cytogenomic [1, 5, 15], genomic [1, 8], epigenomic [1, 15], transcriptomic [1, 13, 23] and proteomic [24]. In addition, the characterization of the cells morphology [21, 25], the growth rate by the doubling time measurement [25, 26], the growth curve [25] and the tumorigenic capacity in athymic nude mice by transplantation of cancer cells to the mice (xenotransplant) [21, 25, 26] should be held. It is also important to characterize cancer cell lines regarding their anchorage independency (soft agarose assay) [11, 26, 27] that can be significant for studying the interaction of drugs with the cells [28] and at their metastatic migration potential and invasiveness capacity, that can be useful for determining the genes and pathways involved in metastasis [26, 29].

The identification and characterization of chromosomal rearrangements allows the detection of breakpoints and chromosome abnormalities that can be related with deregulation of cancer genes. The characterization of chromosomal instability is also crucial because it can be caused by errors in the DNA damage checkpoints, in the DNA repair pathways and in the mitotic segregation [1].

Also the characterization of DNA amplification is important, as the overexpression of genes can be involved in the oncogenic process, as *ERBB2* in some types of breast cancer [1] or other genes that can be druggable targets like kinases [13].

Cell lines molecular profiling that disclose alterations in the cell cycle regulators and other signalling molecules is important [15, 28] and can be useful for targeting anticancer drugs for cell cycle defects. The fact that tumour cells with these alterations are more sensitive to anticancer agents highlight the importance of the characterization of cancer cell lines to molecules as P53, RB, MDM-2, CDKs, cyclins, apoptotic regulator proteins [28] and the respective genes.

Recently, Louzada and colleagues (2012) performed a genetic and cytogenetic characterization of two rat sister cancer cell lines commercially available, at the levels of morphology, ploidy and identification of clonal chromosome rearrangements and breakpoint regions. They also analysed the expression profile of two oncogenes and the influence of global demethylation in the expression of these genes [1], and realized that these two sister cell lines are a good *in vitro* cell model for *Erbb2*.

As referred, the molecular characterization of cancer cell lines is important for anticancer drug testing [16], for the definition of chemosensitivity and resistance pattern [10] and their correlation with candidate cancer genes [10]. As an example, a research from Hakazaki and colleagues (2006) on the characterization of a cancer cell line (FPS-1) derived from an undifferentiated pleomorphic sarcoma (UPS) reported upregulation of the Epidermal growth factor receptor (*EGFR*) and cyclooxygenase-2 (*COX-2*) genes, indicating the use of this cell line for the development of drugs that act on these genes or in its cellular pathways [16]. Fang and colleagues (2009), when characterizing cell lines derived from malignant peripheral nerve sheath tumours (MPNST) from patients with metastatic and recurrent disease, identified genes associated with the metastatic potential, indicating some therapeutic approaches targeted for these genes [15]. Finally, a pharmacological and molecular characterization was made in a panel of 60 different types of human cancer cell lines (NCI60) created for the development of anticancer drugs and included DNA, RNA, proteins, chromosome and functional profiling, allowing a better interpretation of the results of anticancer drug tests [30].

The molecular profiling of cancer cell lines also enables an easier assessment of cancer types and subtypes, defining which cell lines are more suitable for the different investigations [13], which in turn, enhances the screening and study of anticancer drugs. Recently, Kao and colleagues (2009) did a characterization of commercially available breast cancer cell lines at the gene expression levels and respective gene copy number variation. They were able to correlate the cancer cell lines with recognized molecular subtypes of breast cancer, concluding which is the most adequate cell line for the study of each tumour subtype [13].

Cancer cell lines must be characterized not only in the first passages, but also during their progression, in different passages [15]. The use of cancer cell lines that were characterized many years ago [4, 31] and the contamination of the cell lines deposited in cell banks with HeLa cells are a problem in cancer research [4, 8] that requires efforts in their molecular profiling. The problem of the lack of characterization of cancer cell lines that are used for many years [4] was highlighted by Osborne and colleagues (1987) in a study that demonstrated that one of the most used breast cancer cell line (MCF-7) showed different molecular characteristics according to the lab origin [31]. This fact shows the importance of the characterization of these models, that are in cell banks for many years, accumulating, in the meantime, a high number of mutations [4, 8]. The existence of a large number of cell lines deposited in cell banks contaminated with HeLa cells, the first established cancer cell line, is a serious problem [4, 8] verified after the appearance of molecular methods as DNA fingerprinting, that showed cross-contaminations in about 18% of the cell lines deposited in the German Cell Line Bank [4, 8, 32]. The generation of databases with the molecular characterization of cell lines and with the identification of its contaminants [8] is essential for the use of cell lines as credible models. Also the scientific journals, at medium-term, should require the profiling of these lines before the publication of any data [4, 8].

2.2. Methodologies for cancer cell lines molecular profiling

Several methodologies can be used for a proper molecular characterization of cancer cell lines, therefore, the selection and combination of the appropriate methods is essential.

For the cytogenetic profiling, the study of imbalances or rearrangements at the chromosomal level is initially done using G-banding karyotyping [1, 7, 15, 16, 33]. The identification of breakpoint regions and/or clonal chromosome rearrangements can be further achieved by FISH (Fluorescent *in situ* Hybridization), usually using chromosome painting and BAC/PAC clones [1]. FISH can also be used for the identification of oncogenes amplification [1, 34, 35]. Nevertheless, the resolution of such analyses in the detection of DNA gains and losses might be increased using CGH (Comparative Genomic Hybridization) that allows detecting from 10-20 Mb with metaphase chromosomes down to 200 bp with high-density array-CGH using BAC or oligonucleotide arrays [5, 15, 34, 36, 37]. CGH can be useful in detecting gene imbalances allowing the identification of new important genes that can then be up or downregulated in cancer cell lines [34].

The DNA molecular profiling is possible with the use of DNA fingerprinting [4, 21], RFLP (Restriction Fragment Length Polymorphism), probes chromosome-specific [15, 21], STR (short tandem repeats) profiling [4] or gene sequencing [36]. Techniques such as RT-qPCR (Real-Time Reverse Transcriptase Quantitative PCR) [1, 16, 33, 38, 39], RNA-FISH [1], cDNA microarrays and whole genome DNA microarrays [5, 10, 13, 34, 40] can be used for gene expression profiling of cancer cell lines. RT-qPCR and RNA-FISH (allows single cell analysis) are complementary methods that permit the expression quantification of cancer genes [1]. Whole-genome DNA microarrays techniques are useful for the analysis of the expression profile genome-wide [10, 13] and copy number variations [13] or for the expression analysis of a specific fraction of the genome like promoters, codifying regions, SNPs (Single Nucleotide Polymorphisms), spliced exons or a panel of pre-selected genes related with specific diseases as cancer. For the study of the protein expression level, the most widely used methods are immunohistochemistry [11, 13, 15, 16, 35, 38, 41] and western blotting [13, 16].

2.2.1. Next generation sequencing technologies in cancer cell lines

Although the referred methodologies have been successfully used in the characterization of cancer cell lines, recently, new promising strategies for analysis of genetic and epigenetic alterations have emerged, providing a large amount of information at low cost. These are based in Next Generation Sequencing (NGS), which allows the sequencing of almost all coding regions (and at a low-extension, non-coding sequences) of both the genome and the methylome [42, 43]. The NGS platforms have the power of sequencing massively-parallel short-read DNA [42] with a high-throughput at a low cost [44], substituting some techniques as the Sanger traditional sequencing [45] and microarrays [42]. Incredibly, NGS can produce up to 1 billion of sequences *per* instrument in four days. However, these results are highly dependent on the analysis with refined bioinformatics programs, and the large amount of information makes the data treatment sometimes difficult [42, 45].

NGS is responsible for the recent increase of epigenetic studies, transforming the resolution of the characterization at the epigenetic level [42, 43, 46], and have allowed the construction of the first map of the human methylome [43]. The genome-wide DNA methylation profiling can be done by array-based or sequencing-based (NGS) with the combination of bisulfite conversion (that transforms the unmethylated cytosines into uracil, preserving the methylated cytosines) or immunoprecipitation of the methylated DNA (MeDIP) [42, 47]. The single-nucleotide resolution of these platforms provides information about the methylation of each cytosine, which is an important mark in oncogenesis. An example of the use of genome-wide DNA methylation immunoprecipitation-sequencing for the methylome profiling in cancer cell lines was made recently by Ruike and colleagues (2010) and their data indicate breast cancer cell lines as being globally hypomethylated and with numerous hypermethylated sequences [48]. For the study of epigenetics genome-wide, a technology that combines chromatin-immunoprecipitation (ChIP) and NGS technologies has been used [42]. The ChIP methodology is based on DNA and proteins interactions and together with NGS platforms (ChIP-Seq) is used to analyse histones' modifications genome-wide, as methylation [42,43].

The development of high-throughput DNA sequencing and whole-genome platforms for the analysis of the transcriptome, methylome, microRNAs and copy number changes is essential for the advance in cancer cell lines profiling. While the use of these platforms for cancer cell lines profiling is only at the beginning, these techniques have already proved its value in the identification of copy number alterations, mutations detection or different methylation patterns of genes [8].

3. Methylome analysis in cancer

Besides the genetic alterations (as point mutations, deletions, translocations or amplifications), it is now settled that imbalances in the DNA methylation patterns are key processes in tumour formation and progression [1, 49]. Thus, the profiling of cancer cell line models must also be done at the epigenetic level, and more particularly, at the DNA methylation level [5], that leads to heritable alterations of gene expression that do not involve alterations in the sequence of DNA [5, 50, 51]. As can be observed in Figure 2, the methylation analysis in cancer cell lines is still very scarce.

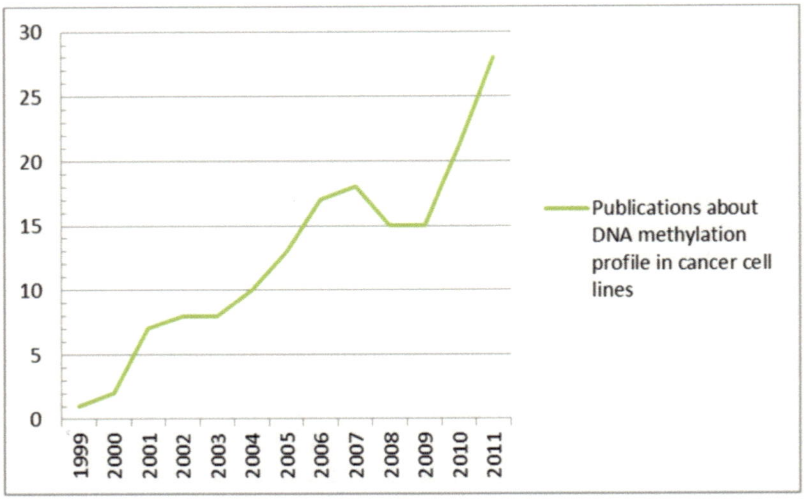

Figure 2. Number of publications regarding cancer cell lines characterization at the DNA methylation level (green line). These data were obtained from the papers indexed in the free resource PubMed (National Center for Biotechnology Information, at the U.S. National Library of Medicine, located at the National Institutes of Health).

The methylation of DNA is a chemical modification catalyzed by DNA methyltransferases (DNMT1, DNMT3A, DNMT3B) [51-53], involving the covalent addiction of a methyl group (CH_3) to the carbon in the 5-position of the cytosine ring [50-52], normally in a CpG dinucleotide context. CpG dinucleotide can be grouped in CpG islands in the promoter region of the genes [50, 53].

DNA methylation plays a crucial role in several epigenetic events of normal cells, as genomic imprinting, X chromosome inactivation, retroelement silencing, etc [53], being at the same time important in DNA repair, genomic stability and in the regulation of chromatin structure [50].

Recently, the role of DNA methylation in cancer has been an important subject of research [47, 51, 54], because we are now aware that the disruption of the methylome is an important hallmark of the oncogenic process [54], both the initiation and progression [47]. Depending on the pattern of the modification, the genome damage can result in the (over)expression or silencing of a gene [51, 53], predisposing cells to cancer [51]. The aberrant methylation can begin early in tumorigenesis and can induce most of the pathways modifications in cancer, as loss of cell cycle control and apoptosis signalling, alteration of transcription factors function, disruption of cell-cell or cell-substratum interaction, among others [55]. This deregulation can affect different types of genes as tumour suppressor genes, oncogenes and cancer-associated viral genes [50]. The cancer genome is characterized by a global genomic hypomethylation and a dense hypermethylation of CpG islands in the regulator regions of genes [50, 51, 54].

DNA hypermethylation is the most studied epigenetic alteration in cancer [51]. It can be important as a tool for cancer diagnostic, as a biomarker of malignant cells, as a prognostic factor [49, 54], and it may represent a good target for future therapy [54]. When aberrant methylation occurs in the promoter region of tumour suppressor genes, it may lead to its silencing [50, 51, 56] and loss of protein function [1]. Thus, the role of aberrant hypermethylation in cancer is easily understood for the transcriptional silencing of important genes in the cancer prevention [49]. The methylation profile is different for different types of tumours, suggesting specificity [54, 56]. However, it is unknown how this framework acts to "decide" which genes and when are they methylated [51, 56]. This profiling can be vital for the premature detection of cancer in sensitive and specific methylation markers and for the identification of important pathways as therapeutic targets [56]. The hypermethylation profiling was already done in different types of tumours, in cancer cell lines (table 3) and in fresh tumours leading to the identification of methylated genes cancer-specific and in different types of cancer [56]. A high concordance was observed between the fresh tumours and the respective cell lines, making them good models for the study of cancer methylome. Hypermethylation can influence the development and preservation of a cell-specific phenotype for the specific silencing of gene sets [5]. The genes that are most susceptible to hypermethylation include genes involved in all the cellular pathways [54]: in cell cycle regulation (*P16INK4a* [51, 52, 54, 56], *P15INK4a* [51, 53], *PRB* [51, 52], *P14ARF* [51, 54]), in DNA repair (*MLH1* [53, 54] *BRCA1* [47, 51, 54, 56], *MGMT* [51, 52, 54]), in apoptosis (*APAF-1* [53, 54], *DAPK* [51, 54]), and in differentiation, angiogenesis, metastasis and drug resistance [51]. For instance, the hypermethylation can affect the P16INK4α/PRB/CDK4 pathway by the hypermethylation of *P16INK4a* which is an inhibitor of the cell cycle, allowing the cell to escape from cellular senescence and continue to proliferate [54]. There are other genes that have shown to be hypermethylated across different types of cancer as *RASSF1A* (tumour suppressor gene Ras association domain family member 1) [47, 51, 56-58] and *P16INK4a* (cyclin-dependent kinase inhibitor) [51, 52, 56, 59-61] and genes that are hypermethylated in specific types of cancers, such as *GSTP1* that is methylated in 90% of prostate cancer but unmethylated in other types [51, 56], or *BRCA1* hypermethylated in breast and ovarian cancers [47, 51, 56, 62], among others.

Gene	Methylation status in cancer	Disease	Cancer Cell Line	Reference
P16INK4a	hypermethylated	Variety of cancers (e.g. Colon, Breast, Renal, Prostate and Lung cancers, Leukaemia and Melanoma)	Variety of cancer cell lines from Colon cancer, Breast cancer, Renal cancer, Prostate cancer, Lung cancer Leukaemia and Melanoma	[63, 64]
RASSF1A	hypermethylated	Variety of cancers (e.g. Leukaemia, Colon, Breast, Ovarian, Lung, Prostate, Renal	Variety of cancer cell lines from Leukaemia, Colon cancer, Breast cancer, Ovarian cancer, Lung	[57, 58, 63, 64]

Gene	Methylation status in cancer	Disease	Cancer Cell Line	Reference
		and CNS (central nervous system) cancers and Melanoma)	cancer, Prostate cancer, Renal cancer, CNS cancer and Melanoma.	
P15INK4a	hypermethylated	Leukaemia, Lung and Breast cancers	Cancer cell lines from Leukaemia, Lung cancer and Breast cancer	[63, 64]
P14ARF	hypermethylated	Colon, Breast and Renal cancers and Leukaemia	Cancer cell lines from Colon cancer, Breast cancer, Renal cancer and Leukaemia	[63, 64]
MLH1	hypermethylated	Colon cancer	Colon cancer cell lines	[63, 64]
BRCA1	hypermethylated	Breast cancer	Breast cancer cell lines	[65]
MGMT	hypermethylated	Leukaemia, Colon, Renal, Breast and Lung cancers and Melanoma, CNS cancer	Cancer cell lines from Leukaemia, Colon cancer, Renal cancer, Breast cancer, Lung cancer, Melanoma and CNS cancer	[63, 64]
DAPK	hypermethylated	Leukaemia, Lung, Colon, CNS, Prostate and Breast cancer and Melanoma	Cancer cell lines from Leukemia, Lung cancer, Colon cancer, CNS cancer, Prostate cancer, Breast cancer and Melanoma	[63, 64]
GSTP1	hypermethylated	Prostate, Breast and Lung cancers	Cancer cell lines from Prostate cancer, Breast cancer and Lung cancer	[64, 66]
NM23-H1	hypermethylated	MPNST	MPNST cancer cell lines	[15]
DSC3	hypermethylated	Breast cancer	Breast cancer cell lines	[67]
MASPIN	hypermethylated	Breast cancer	Breast cancer cell lines	[67]
c-MYC	hypomethylated	Gastric and Colon cancer	Gastric and Colon cancer cell lines	[68]

Table 3. Examples of genes displaying an alterated methylation status in cancer cell lines.

The information available about hypermethylation in cancer is much higher than the one concerning hypomethylation [51]. However, both conditions may lead to loss of cell cycle control and apoptosis signals, change in the function of transcription factors, genomic instability, among many other effects [55]. Unlike the hypermethylation, the global hypomethylation in cancer occurs more frequently in highly and moderately repeated DNA sequences but can also be seen in single-copy sequences [49]. These single copy-sequences can be oncogenes, like *c-MYC* [49, 51, 54] (table 3), and these can be also associated with tumour initiation and/or progression [49]. But generally, the global genome hypomethylation promotes cancer progression by the induction of chromosome instability [51, 54, 56], loss of imprinting [54, 56] and reactivation of transposable elements [51, 54]. Thus, the aberrant hypomethylation pattern, which occurs early in tumorigenesis, can be also used as a biomarker [49], highlighting the importance of its analysis in cancer cells.

Unlike the genetic, the methylation modifications are reversible [3, 50], making this event excellent for analysis in cancer cell lines and a promising target for therapy. The study of DNA methylation in cancer cell lines has been accomplished using demethylating agents, such as 5-Azacytidine (5-AZA) and its deoxy derivative 5-Aza-2'deoxycytidine (decitabine), that cause global genome demethylation [1, 5, 19, 51, 67]. These demethylating agents are used in epigenetic therapy, restoring the hypomethylation state by the inversion of the gene silencing induced by hypermethylation [1, 51]. These drugs are based in a cytosine analogue that are incorporated in the DNA (decitabine) after phosphorylation or in both the DNA and RNA (5-AZA), inhibiting DNMTs (DNA methyltransferases) to methylate the DNA, leading to a decrease of the DNA methylation level [51, 53]. Although the numerous studies on these demethylating agents, their exact mechanism of action and effects in tumour cells remains arguable [1, 52, 69, 70].

These drugs, used as chemotherapeutic agents in certain types of cancers [50, 52-54, 69], are also used to screen for changes in gene expression thought to be regulated by methylation in cell lines [1, 5, 15, 53, 54, 56]. These demethylating agents that act as DNMTs inhibitors have shown the ability to reactivate epigenetically silenced tumour suppressor genes in cancer cell lines. Thus, these drugs can also be used as molecular research tools for the induction of DNA demethylation in cancer cell lines [53, 69]. In fact, they have been used in many research works for the analysis of the methylation profile before and after cells treatment, allowing the identification of epigenetically altered genes [1, 15, 53]. For instance, the transcriptional profile of cancer cell lines of esophageal squamous cell carcinoma (ESCC) treated with 5-azacytidine allowed the identification of various putative tumour suppressor genes that are hypermethylated in these cells [53]. Fang and colleagues (2009) proved that the loss of expression of *NM23-H1*, which is related with metastatic progression, in cell lines from MPNST, can be associated with the methylation of CpG islands in the promoter region of this gene, making this a reversible process by the use of demethylation agents as anticancer drugs [15]. Another study of demethylation in breast cancer cell lines verified the transcriptional reactivation of desmocollin 3 (*DSC3*) and *MASPIN*, that are tumour suppressor genes frequently silenced in breast cancer [67]. Louzada and colleagues (2012), alternatively, analysed the effect of decitabine in the expression of two genes in rat breast cancer cell lines and their results showed a decrease of *Erbb2* expression (initially overexpressed in these cells), showing that this gene is epigenetically regulated [1]. Although these demethylation agents are excellent tools for the methylome profiling of cancer cell lines, another kind of methylation studies have been done using antisense RNA [35, 54] and interference RNA for depleting DNMTs [20, 67].

The DNA methylation profiling is difficult to perform in the majority of models, but it is extremely simple to perform in cancer cell lines, enhancing their value as cell models for the study of the methylome and to understand the relationship between the genetic and the epigenetic profiles with the effectiveness of anticancer drugs. The use of cancer cell lines as models for the methylome analysis was highlighted in a work comparing the transcriptional profiling after the treatment with decitabine in *in vitro* and *in vivo* revealing similar results, what validates the use of this model [53]. Other methylome studies performed in cancer cell lines in an epigenome-wide way were performed through the use of recent technologies as NGS. In 2010, Ruike and colleagues made a methylation profiling in breast cancer cell lines using MeDIP-seq that revealed important insights about the aberrant patterns of DNA methylation in these cell lines, allowing a more extensive study about the methylome during carcinogenesis and the correlation between the morphological changes and the observed methylome alterations [48]. These recent technologies allow the study of the methylome in cancer in an unprecedented way [47], but this type of studies are still in the beginning [47].

The methylome profiling is essential for the early cancer detection, prognostic and treatment [50, 51, 55], for the development of new epigenetic therapies [54], for distinguishing tumour types and subtypes using molecular biomarkers and predict the chemotherapy response [51, 54, 55]. But the use of cancer cell lines for the study of DNA methylation alterations in cancer is controversial. Although some authors consider it a good model, that have shown similar results in the methylome profile when comparing the results *in vivo* and *in vitro* [53]; there are others, instead, believing that this type of studies should be made in non-cultured cells due to the *in vitro* culture environment [49, 50]. Nevertheless, the problems in the association of the epigenetic profiles with cancer, when using other models (difficulties in manipulation, sample selection, sample size, data integration, among others [50]), can be, in part, solved with the use of cancer cell lines. Thus, it is crucial to analyse the relationship between methylation in cancer and the resistance/sensitivity to anticancer drugs in well-characterized cancer cell lines, making possible the detection of potential drug targets and drug resistance markers [47].

4. Drug testing in cancer cell lines

Drug testing in cancer cell lines is usually one of the initial steps in drug development. It allows the access of a large number of potential drugs before committing to large scale expensive *in vivo* clinical trials.

The use of cancer cell lines for cytotoxicity evaluation has been made by many researchers for many years, having clinical predictive value [2, 18], consistent with the expected from the original tumour. Different cancer cell lines display diverse responses to cytotoxic anticancer drugs, as colon cancer cell lines are more resistant to DNA intercalating-drugs and breast cancer or leukaemia cell lines are more sensitive [18]. Copeland and colleagues (2007) tested the cytotoxicity of an anticancer drug in different prostate cancer cell lines derived from prostate cancer subtypes, and confirmed that this drug is more efficient for prostate androgen-independent cancer. In this study they proposed this chemotherapeutic drug for the treatment of metastatic prostate cancer [71], that should, however, be more studied in cancer cell lines for the determination of the action mechanism.

The testing of anticancer drugs using cancer cell lines over other models presents other advantages than just cytotoxicity evaluation tests, because it permits to analyse the action of drugs, combinations of them and the screening for resistance/sensitivity [72], with the concomitant discovery of specific markers [10]. The identification of epigenetic or genetic alterations in specific sequences allows to specifically target the drug in order to achieve a therapeutic outcome and identify new potential druggable targets.

The fact that cancer cells have the oncogenic pathway activated makes these cells less dependent of extracellular regulators. Cancer cell lines also have this pathway activated [3], retaining the genomic deregulation of transcription of the primary tumour [24], but, at the same time, also have a more simple transcriptome by the loss of unneeded functions [3], making this one of the best models for anticancer drug testing (single drugs or in combination) [2, 3, 6, 10, 18, 24, 71]. This is valid not only in a first approach, but also for understanding drugs' mechanisms of action [10, 73], the resistance/sensitivity of some types of cancer to different drugs [10, 24, 72, 74], for the discovery of biomarkers for anticancer drugs response (resistance/sensitivity markers) [10, 75, 76], or for the research of signalling pathways associated with the therapeutic response [2, 24], among others. Nevertheless, even if a cancer cell line comes from the same subtype of tumour, it must be well-characterized before its use in anticancer drug testing due to the fact that similar cell lines may present different signatures from each other, although retaining the same signature of the original tumour [3, 24]. An example are cancer cell lines derived from the same subtype of tumour as thyroid papillary carcinomas B-CPAP and TPC-1, displaying different oncogenic pathways modified, maintaining that from the original tumour [3]. Others than cancer cell line models, will always be needed for the validation of the data, being the clinical trials mandatory before the use of any drug in a clinical approach.

The use of cell line panels is a useful tool for anticancer drug testing. The development of these cancer cell lines panels was initiated for the panel NCI60 (panel US National Cancer Institute with 60 cancer cell lines) in order to overcome the use of animal models for the test of antineoplastic drugs [12]. Afterwards, Nakatsu and colleagues (2005) established a panel of 45 cancer cell lines (JFCR-45) from different origins (breast, liver and stomach) to determine genes related with chemosensitivity to anticancer drugs. They also tried to understand the mechanisms of action of these drugs for their classification. This research, that involved an integrated bioinformatic approach using cDNA arrays, revealed many candidate genes associated with sensitivity to chemotherapeutic drugs. For the correct identification of these genes, they transfected each one in the different cell lines and discover that the overexpression of *HSPA1A* and *JUN* genes increased the sensitivity to mitomycin C, suggesting that these genes play a role in the response to this anticancer drug. The genes discovered in this study can be used as predictive markers of sensitivity to chemotherapeutic drugs, which is crucial for a higher effectiveness of the treatment [10]. Recently, Garnett and colleagues (2012) screened a panel of several hundred cancer cell lines (representing much of the tissue-type and genetic diversity of human cancers) with 130 drugs under clinical and preclinical investigation and verified that the cancer genes mutated are related with the cellular response to the most commonly used drugs, making this systematic pharmacogenomic profiling in cancer cell lines a powerful biomarker discovery platform to guide rational cancer therapeutic strategies [75]. The use of a cell line panel with subtypes of cancer cell lines for studying the signalling pathways involved in the therapeutic response was made by Neve and colleagues (2006) that used Herceptin® (Trastuzumab) immunotherapy in a system of cancer cell lines ERBB2+, that do not respond to this therapy, to identify the molecular signature associated with this phenotype [24]. Thus, the use of cancer cell line panels seems to be a powerful system for underlying the molecular mechanisms of anticancer drug response [2].

The existence of databases with detailed genetic and pharmacologic information from cancer cell lines allows the generation of genetic predictions of drug response in the preclinical setting. An example is Cancer Cell Line Encyclopedia (CCLE, launched by Novartis), a database that contains genes' expression profiling, massively parallel sequencing and chromosomal copy number data from almost a thousand human cancer cell lines. The integration of the pharmacologic profiles of anticancer drugs with the data from the cell lines deposited in CCLE allowed Barrentina and colleagues (2012) to identify genetic, lineage, and gene-expression-based predictors of drug sensitivity [76]. However, the problem of working with cancer cell lines characterized too many years ago or not characterized at all, will definitely difficult data interpretation or even lead to misinterpretations.

The availability of molecular modelling tools, such as QSAR (Quantitative Structure - Activity Relationships), giving insights about the molecular interactions of the compounds studied with proteins involved in signalling pathways [77], or docking methods that predict the strength of association or binding affinity between a drug to a particular target [78], are also fundamental tools that should be considered in drug testing studies.

The characterization of cancer cell lines about the state of cell cycle checkpoints [15, 28], regulatory cell cycle proteins [28] and the presence of Multidrug Resistance Domains (MDR) [72], are also essential in anticancer drug testing. The effect of anticancer drugs in cancer cell lines must be screened on cell cycle progression, checkpoint signalling pathways and cell proliferation, making important the characterization of these parameters in cancer cell lines before their use as models. For instance, the characterization of several cell lines from head and neck squamous cell carcinoma (HNSCC) allowed to disclose that most of them lack the checkpoint function by loss of P53 and RB functions and their upstream and downstream regulation pathways (e.g. MDM2 and CDK6, respectively) [28]. Cell cycle profiling (progression and checkpoints regulators) of cancer cell lines is thus a valuable tool in the development of chemotherapeutic agents as therapeutic targets [28, 79]. In the case of antimitotic drugs, the analysis of Microtubules (MTs) and centrosomal proteins [72] should also be considered.

One of the more successful anticancer drug targets are microtubules. These form a highly dynamic structure constituted by polymers of α and β-tubulin essential for the development and maintenance of cellular morphology, protein trafficking in the cell, cell signalling and proper chromosome segregation during mitosis [72, 80]. Their importance in mitosis by their mitotic spindle assembly and dynamics required for proper chromosome segregation make the microtubules an excellent target for antimitotic therapy [72]. At the moment, three different groups of MT-targeted anticancer drugs are widely used for chemotherapy: *Vinca* alkaloids (e.g. vinblastine) [72, 73], taxanes (e.g. paclitaxel - Taxol®) [10, 28, 72] and colchicine [72]. These antimitotic drugs bind to different binding sites in β-tubulin, exhibit different behaviours and are used for different types of cancer. These drugs act by suppression of the MT dynamics, leading to mitotic blocking and cell death by apoptosis [72]. However, the exact mechanism of action of these drugs, the resistance/sensitivity mechanisms and the combination of these drugs with others is an incomplete research field, and cancer cell lines can be excellent models for the study of these drugs as long as they are well-characterized.

Coleman and colleagues (2002) used cancer cell lines from HNSCC for determination of the mechanism of action of two drugs combination, paclitaxel and carboplatin. They concluded that the paclitaxel activity is related with the increase of cyclin B1/CDC2 activity, BCL-2 phosphorylation and mitotic block, affecting the cells in mitosis. However, their study proved that the efficiency in the inhibition of cell proliferation was higher when combining these two drugs, allowing the use of this combination in other models [28]. In other work, the sensitivity of tumour cells to paclitaxel in the absence of PLK1 (polo-like kinase 1) was studied in breast cancer cell lines [81]. PLK1 play a key role in different stages of mitosis and its overexpression is a negative prognostic indicator [81, 82]. The use of antisense oligonucleotides for PLK1 depletion leaded to the conclusion that the presence of these antisense oligos increase the response to paclitaxel [81]. Huang and colleagues (2004) studied the apoptosis induction of *Vinca* alkaloids in cancer cell lines. The type of analysis performed by these authors, as the use of glucocorticoids to inhibit mitotic arrest caused by *Vinca* alkaloids or transfection with antisense oligonucleotides are difficult to perform in other types of models. Moreover, this study revealed another signalling pathway (NF-κB/IκB) that might be related with apoptosis induction by this antimitotic drug [73].

As referred, drug resistance is a major problem in cancer chemotherapy [80, 83]. The study of the mechanisms that lead to a resistant cell can involve a diversity of molecules. Although there is no complete understanding about what leads to cell resistance to certain types of drugs, some of them are already known. Multidrug Resistance is a mechanism of drug efflux that can be caused by the upregulation of *MDR1* gene, leading to an increase of membrane transporters as p-glycoprotein (P-GP) [40, 72, 83]. However, it is not completely understood, and the apoptotic pathway also has influence in the resistance to anticancer drugs [28, 40, 83]. The resistance to paclitaxel was related with upregulation of antiapoptotic BCL-2 family members as BCL-2 e BCL-XL [40]. The resistance of tumour cells to paclitaxel and also to other antimitotic drugs can also be attributed to differences in the expression of tubulin isotypes, point mutations or post-translational modifications in β-tubulin residues that modify the binding site [40, 72, 80], binding of MT-regulatory proteins [72], decrease of CDK (cyclin-dependent kinase) level, which cause a mitotic delay, overexpression of the microtubule associated protein tau mRNA and decrease in affinity of targeted drugs to the target (MTs) [40]. Anticancer drug resistance can also be related with other tubulin forms or other proteins in the centrosome in interphase or mitotic spindle poles in mitosis, but it clearly exists a need for much more research in this field [72]. The use of cancer cell lines for resistance/sensitivity studies is imperative, neverless, their poor characterization can lead to problems in the data interpretation. Nakayama and colleagues (2009) used breast cancer cell lines and xenograft models for the discovery of characteristics related with the sensitivity or resistance to paclitaxel. They deduced that the *in vitro* response to paclitaxel do not predict exactly the sensitivity to this drug *in vivo* (80%) [40]. However they used cancer cell lines like MCF7 that were established many years ago and need to be properly characterized, as already mentioned. An altered response to certain compounds can also occur by the clonal variants of cancer cell lines and the xenograft may exhibit a cellular environment that can modify the response [5]. More importantly, they concluded that the decrease of CDK1 (cyclin-dependent kinase) is related with tumour cells' resistance and that the increase of CDK2 is required for the increase of sensitivity. Thus, analysis of CDKs can predict clinically the sensitivity to paclitaxel [40]. Nakatsu and colleagues (2005) also used cancer cell lines for the identification of genes related with the sensitivity to paclitaxel (and other anticancer drugs). With their work, they found that the genes related with tubulin-binder and cytoskeleton-related as *VIL2* (encoding ezrin) and *ACTB* (encoding h-actin) are related with the paclitaxel chemosensitivity, proposing these genes as predictor markers for anticancer drug efficacy [10]. In other work using cancer cell lines as models for paclitaxel resistance analysis, the cells were transformed into resistant by the progressive increase of the drug [80]. The profiling of cancer cell lines paclitaxel-resistants' can allow the identification of resistance mechanisms [72].

The knowledge of the specific composition of MT regulatory proteins or other regulatory proteins and different tubulin isotypes of cancer cell lines, and the way these interfere with the effectiveness of MT-targeted drugs, can be helpful for a better clinical application of these drugs and for the development of molecularly targeted drugs by its combination, overcoming the MDR [72, 83] and the side effects as neuropathy. For this, it is essential to understand the exact mechanism of action of antimitotic drugs, the relation of drug-induced mitotic block and cell death and the interaction of these drugs with centrosomes and the mitotic spindle pole (where other types of tubulin exist). Another question is why some antimitotic drugs as taxanes are efficient in some tumours as breast, ovarian and lung, but are inefficient in kidney, colon cancers, sarcomas and others of the same group of MT-targeted drugs, like *Vinca* alkaloids are more efficient in hematologic malignancies and ineffective against solid tumours [72].

The use of different types of well-characterized cancer cell lines at the genome and methylome levels can allow the study of the mechanisms of antimitotic drugs and if the mechanism of resistance are related with the methylation pattern. Thus, the characterization of cancer cell lines at the DNA methylation level and the combination of these antimitotic drugs with 5'AZA may be a straightforward strategy to understand the mechanism of action of such drugs and testing their combination.

The profiling of cancer cell lines at the DNA methylation level is also important for the prediction of chemotherapeutic response [51]. Hypermethylation of the promoter regions of some genes, as of the DNA repair gene *MGMT* that happens in glioma, increases the sensitivity to alkylating agents as carmustine (BiCNU®) [51, 54]. Arnold and colleagues (2003) analysed hypermethylated colorectal cancer cell lines after exposure to a demethylating drug and found that the hypermethylation of the gene *MLH1* was reverted by these type of drugs, decreasing the resistance to the anticancer drug fluorouracil (5-FU) [84]. Shen and colleagues (2007) in a work performed in the NCI60 panel of cancer cell lines were able to elaborate a list of methylation markers to predict the anticancer drug response [63]. These works highlight the fact that methylation/demethylation studies performed in cell lines definitely provide a powerful system model for the definition of new candidate strategies to overcome the problem of drug resistance in the treatment of cancer. The exact mechanism of action of demethylating agents or the patterns of resistance and sensitivity are unclear and it is extremely important to understand the molecular changes induced by these drugs to increase their effectiveness [69, 85].

As already mentioned, in cell lines, demethylating drugs, as azacytidine and decitabine cause global demethylation of DNA by the inhibition of DNMTs, reverting the gene silencing induced by hypermethylation [51-53, 69]. The use of such demethylating drugs can cause inhibition of cell proliferation and G2 arrest [85] but can also lead to the reestablishment of proliferation control and apoptotic sensitivity [69]. In spite of the oversight of information about the azanucleosides, these anticancer drugs are currently used in the treatment of myelodysplastic syndrome (MDS) and other types of leukaemia [51-53, 85]. However, it is essential an improved knowledge on the mechanisms of action of these epigenetic drugs at the molecular level and the cellular pathways that they influence, as well as the identification and validation of response predictor markers [69] for the application of these drugs in more cancer types and with conjugation with other anticancer drugs.

The development of treatments that accomplish a specific reversion of DNA methylation modifications without interfering in the normal epigenetic events required for the cellular function [53] has stimulated the research of other inhibitors of DNMTs [51, 53]. The use of cancer cell lines allows the testing of other potential demethylating agents with the purpose to observe the effect of such drugs in tumour cells. Other demethylating agents as hydralazine and procainamide (cardiovascular drugs) in breast cancer cell lines cause demethylation and expression reestablishment of *ER*, *RARβ*, and *P16INK4a* [86]. Alternative inhibitors of DNMTs that have focused the researchers attention are *DNMT* antisense and siRNA [51, 53]. It was proved in colon and bladder cancer cell lines that an antisense oligodeoxynucleotide as MG98 is a *DNMT1* antisense inhibitor that cleaves its mRNA resulting in the demethylation and replacement of the normal expression of *P16INK4a* [87]. The siRNA can be designed as an inhibitor of DNMTs, but can also be used as a target for the proteins involved in the regulation of the methylated gene [51].

So, the characterization of both the genome and methylome of cancer cell lines allows the discovery of targets to anticancer drugs and to create more targeted drugs for certain types of cancer, providing the development of new therapies [35], as the use of siRNA, or the combination of new or already existing ones.

The use of siRNA in cancer therapy is a new research field and promises to silence critical cancer genes, as oncogenes [88]. The use of cell lines was essential for the discovery of this potential specific gene cancer therapy by the suppression of expression of these genes [89] and blocking of the biological processes that comprise the hallmarks of cancer [88]. The major problem of using siRNAs as anticancer therapeutics does not rely in their design or mechanism of action, but in their delivery. To overcome this problem, nanoparticles [88, 90] (lipid, organic or inorganic) have been used for degradation protection, facilitating the cell transfection and allowing the delivery in the right place [88]. Presently, some siRNAs that use nanoparticles as delivery vehicles are in clinical trials [88, 90], however, at the moment, none have been approved [88]. A siRNA against *PLK1* is in conclusion of phase I of clinical trials in different types of cancer [88] (http://www.clinicaltrials.gov/ct2/show/record/NCT01437007) and good results are expected because of the importance of this protein in mitosis and in the maintenance of genome stability [82]. Another siRNA that is in a clinical trial phase with successful results is a siRNA for the depletion of M2 subunit of Ribonuclease reductase (RRM2) in solid tumours [88, 90, 91] (http://www.clinicaltrials.gov/ct2/show/NCT00689065), decreasing the proliferation of cancer cells *in vitro* and *in vivo* [91]. The mutation of *K-RAS* is associated with one third of the human cancers and is a resistance factor of many cancers to therapy. The depletion of this protein is an excellent target for cancer treatment, leading cancer cells to apoptosis. A phase I of a clinical trial is being carried out for this target (siG12D LODER (Local Drug EluteR)) in patients with pancreas adenocarcinoma, since most of the pancreas cancer cells have *K-RAS* mutated [88] (http://www.clinicaltrials.gov/ct2/show/NCT01188785). Although none siRNAs are yet available for cancer treatment, it is expected that in the near future they could be used as cancer therapeutic agents.

The identification of more cancer-type related genes, DNA methylation profiles and altered cellular pathways in cancer cell lines is crucial for understanding drugs' mechanisms of action and its resistance patterns, and for developing and testing new targeted anticancer drugs.

5. Conclusion

In conclusion, well-characterized cancer cell lines at the molecular level are excellent models for the study of the altered cellular pathways, critical genes and methylome in cancer, and for anticancer drug testing. Although we have now a reasonable knowledge of the genome of this model, we are still in the beginning of knowing its methylome. The recent technologies are very useful for this molecular profiling, which is absolutely required before the use of any cancer cell line in a research program. The study of the methylome in cancer using cell models is essential, since epigenetic modifications can occur early in oncogenesis, being the DNA methylation pattern a good target for chemotherapy. The molecular cancer cell lines profiling is also essential for the development of new anticancer drugs and for understanding the mechanism of action and the patterns involved in cell resistance to chemotherapeutics already used in the treatment of cancer. Moreover, cancer cell lines profiling can be a powerful tool for the identification of genes' alterations or pathways cancer-related and for the discovery of putative drug targets.

Nomenclature

In the present work the nomenclature for human genes and proteins was the one recommended by HGNC (HUGO Gene Nomenclature Committee). For mouse and rat, we followed the one suggested by MGI (Mouse Genome Informatics).

Author details

Daniela Ferreira, Filomena Adega and Raquel Chaves*
Institute for Biotechnology and Bioengineering, Centre of Genomics and Biotechnology, University of Trás-os-Montes and Alto Douro (IBB/CGB-UTAD), Quinta de Prados, Vila Real, Portugal

Acknowledgement

This work was supported by a research position on Animal Genomics of the "Sistema Científico e Tecnológico Nacional - Ciência 2007" and a PhD grant SFRH/BD/80446/2011, from the Science and Technology Foundation (FCT) from Portugal.

6. References

[1] Louzada S, Adega F, Chaves R. Defining the sister rat mammary tumor cell lines HH-16 cl.2/1 and HH-16.cl.4 as an in vitro cell model for Erbb2. PloS one 2012;7(1) e29923.
[2] Vargo-Gogola T, Rosen JM. Modelling breast cancer: one size does not fit all. Nature reviews Cancer 2007;7(9) 659-672.
[3] van Staveren WC, Solis DY, Hebrant A, Detours V, Dumont JE, Maenhaut C. Human cancer cell lines: Experimental models for cancer cells in situ? For cancer stem cells? Biochimica et biophysica acta 2009;1795(2) 92-103.
[4] Burdall SE, Hanby AM, Lansdown MR, Speirs V. Breast cancer cell lines: friend or foe? Breast cancer research : BCR 2003;5(2) 89-95.

---

* Corresponding Author

[5] Lacroix M, Leclercq G. Relevance of breast cancer cell lines as models for breast tumours: an update. Breast cancer research and treatment 2004;83(3) 249-289.

[6] Leonetti C, Scarsella M, Zupi G, Zoli W, Amadori D, Medri L, Fabbri F, Rosetti M, Ulivi P, Cecconetto L *et al.* Efficacy of a nitric oxide-releasing nonsteroidal anti-inflammatory drug and cytotoxic drugs in human colon cancer cell lines in vitro and xenografts. Molecular cancer therapeutics 2006;5(4) 919-926.

[7] Engel LW, Young NA, Tralka TS, Lippman ME, O'Brien SJ, Joyce MJ. Establishment and characterization of three new continuous cell lines derived from human breast carcinomas. Cancer research 1978;38(10) 3352-3364.

[8] Gazdar AF, Girard L, Lockwood WW, Lam WL, Minna JD. Lung cancer cell lines as tools for biomedical discovery and research. Journal of the National Cancer Institute 2010;102(17) 1310-1321.

[9] Ruhe JE, Streit S, Hart S, Wong CH, Specht K, Knyazev P, Knyazeva T, Tay LS, Loo HL, Foo P *et al.* Genetic alterations in the tyrosine kinase transcriptome of human cancer cell lines. Cancer research 2007;67(23) 11368-11376.

[10] Nakatsu N, Yoshida Y, Yamazaki K, Nakamura T, Dan S, Fukui Y, Yamori T. Chemosensitivity profile of cancer cell lines and identification of genes determining chemosensitivity by an integrated bioinformatical approach using cDNA arrays. Molecular cancer therapeutics 2005;4(3) 399-412.

[11] Pfragner R, Behmel A, Hoger H, Beham A, Ingolic E, Stelzer I, Svejda B, Moser VA, Obenauf AC, Siegl V *et al.* Establishment and characterization of three novel cell lines - P-STS, L-STS, H-STS - derived from a human metastatic midgut carcinoid. Anticancer research 2009;29(6) 1951-1961.

[12] Shoemaker RH. The NCI60 human tumour cell line anticancer drug screen. Nature reviews Cancer 2006;6(10) 813-823.

[13] Kao J, Salari K, Bocanegra M, Choi YL, Girard L, Gandhi J, Kwei KA, Hernandez-Boussard T, Wang P, Gazdar AF *et al.* Molecular profiling of breast cancer cell lines defines relevant tumor models and provides a resource for cancer gene discovery. PloS one 2009;4(7) e6146.

[14] Wistuba, II, Behrens C, Milchgrub S, Syed S, Ahmadian M, Virmani AK, Kurvari V, Cunningham TH, Ashfaq R, Minna JD *et al.* Comparison of features of human breast cancer cell lines and their corresponding tumors. Clinical cancer research : an official journal of the American Association for Cancer Research 1998;4(12) 2931-2938.

[15] Fang Y, Elahi A, Denley RC, Rao PH, Brennan MF, Jhanwar SC. Molecular characterization of permanent cell lines from primary, metastatic and recurrent malignant peripheral nerve sheath tumors (MPNST) with underlying neurofibromatosis-1. Anticancer research 2009;29(4) 1255-1262.

[16] Hakozaki M, Hojo H, Sato M, Tajino T, Yamada H, Kikuchi S, Abe M. Establishment and characterization of a new cell line, FPS-1, derived from human undifferentiated pleomorphic sarcoma, overexpressing epidermal growth factor receptor and cyclooxygenase-2. Anticancer research 2006;26(5A) 3393-3401.

[17] Tomlinson GE, Chen TT, Stastny VA, Virmani AK, Spillman MA, Tonk V, Blum JL, Schneider NR, Wistuba, II, Shay JW *et al.* Characterization of a breast cancer cell line

derived from a germ-line BRCA1 mutation carrier. Cancer research 1998;58(15) 3237-3242.

[18] Finlay GJ, Baguley BC. The use of human cancer cell lines as a primary screening system for antineoplastic compounds. European journal of cancer & clinical oncology 1984;20(7) 947-954.

[19] Leone G, Voso MT, Teofili L, Lubbert M. Inhibitors of DNA methylation in the treatment of hematological malignancies and MDS. Clin Immunol 2003;109(1) 89-102.

[20] Kawasaki H, Taira K. Induction of DNA methylation and gene silencing by short interfering RNAs in human cells. Nature 2004;431(7005) 211-217.

[21] Anglard P, Trahan E, Liu S, Latif F, Merino MJ, Lerman MI, Zbar B, Linehan WM. Molecular and cellular characterization of human renal cell carcinoma cell lines. Cancer research 1992;52(2) 348-356.

[22] Bright RK, Vocke CD, Emmert-Buck MR, Duray PH, Solomon D, Fetsch P, Rhim JS, Linehan WM, Topalian SL. Generation and genetic characterization of immortal human prostate epithelial cell lines derived from primary cancer specimens. Cancer research 1997;57(5) 995-1002.

[23] Trojan L, Schaaf A, Steidler A, Haak M, Thalmann G, Knoll T, Gretz N, Alken P, Michel MS. Identification of metastasis-associated genes in prostate cancer by genetic profiling of human prostate cancer cell lines. Anticancer research 2005;25(1A) 183-191.

[24] Neve RM, Chin K, Fridlyand J, Yeh J, Baehner FL, Fevr T, Clark L, Bayani N, Coppe JP, Tong F *et al.* A collection of breast cancer cell lines for the study of functionally distinct cancer subtypes. Cancer cell 2006;10(6) 515-527.

[25] Li SJ, Ren GX, Jin WL, Guo W. Establishment and characterization of a rabbit oral squamous cell carcinoma cell line as a model for in vivo studies. Oral oncology 2011;47(1) 39-44.

[26] Hughes L, Malone C, Chumsri S, Burger AM, McDonnell S. Characterisation of breast cancer cell lines and establishment of a novel isogenic subclone to study migration, invasion and tumourigenicity. Clinical & experimental metastasis 2008;25(5) 549-557.

[27] Djojosubroto M, Bollotte F, Wirapati P, Radtke F, Stamenkovic I, Arsenijevic Y. Chromosomal number aberrations and transformation in adult mouse retinal stem cells in vitro. Investigative ophthalmology & visual science 2009;50(12) 5975-5987.

[28] Coleman SC, Stewart ZA, Day TA, Netterville JL, Burkey BB, Pietenpol JA. Analysis of cell-cycle checkpoint pathways in head and neck cancer cell lines: implications for therapeutic strategies. Archives of otolaryngology--head & neck surgery 2002;128(2) 167-176.

[29] Albini A, Benelli R, Noonan DM, Brigati C. The "chemoinvasion assay": a tool to study tumor and endothelial cell invasion of basement membranes. The International journal of developmental biology 2004;48(5-6) 563-571.

[30] Ikediobi ON, Davies H, Bignell G, Edkins S, Stevens C, O'Meara S, Santarius T, Avis T, Barthorpe S, Brackenbury L *et al.* Mutation analysis of 24 known cancer genes in the NCI-60 cell line set. Molecular cancer therapeutics 2006;5(11) 2606-2612.

[31] Osborne CK, Hobbs K, Trent JM. Biological differences among MCF-7 human breast cancer cell lines from different laboratories. Breast cancer research and treatment 1987;9(2) 111-121.

[32] MacLeod RA, Dirks WG, Matsuo Y, Kaufmann M, Milch H, Drexler HG. Widespread intraspecies cross-contamination of human tumor cell lines arising at source. International journal of cancer Journal international du cancer 1999;83(4) 555-563.

[33] Dangles-Marie V, Pocard M, Richon S, Weiswald LB, Assayag F, Saulnier P, Judde JG, Janneau JL, Auger N, Validire P *et al*. Establishment of human colon cancer cell lines from fresh tumors versus xenografts: comparison of success rate and cell line features. Cancer research 2007;67(1) 398-407.

[34] Forozan F, Mahlamaki EH, Monni O, Chen Y, Veldman R, Jiang Y, Gooden GC, Ethier SP, Kallioniemi A, Kallioniemi OP. Comparative genomic hybridization analysis of 38 breast cancer cell lines: a basis for interpreting complementary DNA microarray data. Cancer research 2000;60(16) 4519-4525.

[35] Bieche I, Onody P, Laurendeau I, Olivi M, Vidaud D, Lidereau R, Vidaud M. Real-time reverse transcription-PCR assay for future management of ERBB2-based clinical applications. Clinical chemistry 1999;45(8 Pt 1) 1148-1156.

[36] Elstrodt F, Hollestelle A, Nagel JH, Gorin M, Wasielewski M, van den Ouweland A, Merajver SD, Ethier SP, Schutte M. BRCA1 mutation analysis of 41 human breast cancer cell lines reveals three new deleterious mutants. Cancer research 2006;66(1) 41-45.

[37] Urban AE, Korbel JO, Selzer R, Richmond T, Hacker A, Popescu GV, Cubells JF, Green R, Emanuel BS, Gerstein MB *et al*. High-resolution mapping of DNA copy alterations in human chromosome 22 using high-density tiling oligonucleotide arrays. Proceedings of the National Academy of Sciences of the United States of America 2006;103(12) 4534-4539.

[38] de Cremoux P, Tran-Perennou C, Brockdorff BL, Boudou E, Brunner N, Magdelenat H, Lykkesfeldt AE. Validation of real-time RT-PCR for analysis of human breast cancer cell lines resistant or sensitive to treatment with antiestrogens. Endocrine-related cancer 2003;10(3) 409-418.

[39] Kadota M, Yang HH, Gomez B, Sato M, Clifford RJ, Meerzaman D, Dunn BK, Wakefield LM, Lee MP. Delineating genetic alterations for tumor progression in the MCF10A series of breast cancer cell lines. PloS one 2010;5(2) e9201.

[40] Nakayama S, Torikoshi Y, Takahashi T, Yoshida T, Sudo T, Matsushima T, Kawasaki Y, Katayama A, Gohda K, Hortobagyi GN *et al*. Prediction of paclitaxel sensitivity by CDK1 and CDK2 activity in human breast cancer cells. Breast cancer research : BCR 2009;11(1) R12.

[41] Rhodes A, Borthwick D, Sykes R, Al-Sam S, Paradiso A. The use of cell line standards to reduce HER-2/neu assay variation in multiple European cancer centers and the potential of automated image analysis to provide for more accurate cut points for predicting clinical response to trastuzumab. American journal of clinical pathology 2004;122(1) 51-60.

[42] Hurd PJ, Nelson CJ. Advantages of next-generation sequencing versus the microarray in epigenetic research. Briefings in functional genomics & proteomics 2009;8(3) 174-183.

[43] Ku CS, Naidoo N, Wu M, Soong R. Studying the epigenome using next generation sequencing. Journal of medical genetics 2011;48(11) 721-730.

[44] Goya R, Sun MG, Morin RD, Leung G, Ha G, Wiegand KC, Senz J, Crisan A, Marra MA, Hirst M *et al.* SNVMix: predicting single nucleotide variants from next-generation sequencing of tumors. Bioinformatics 2010;26(6) 730-736.

[45] Ross JS, Cronin M. Whole cancer genome sequencing by next-generation methods. American journal of clinical pathology 2011;136(4) 527-539.

[46] Hirst M, Marra MA. Next generation sequencing based approaches to epigenomics. Briefings in functional genomics 2010;9(5-6) 455-465.

[47] Huang Y, Nayak S, Jankowitz R, Davidson NE, Oesterreich S. Epigenetics in breast cancer: what's new? Breast cancer research : BCR 2011;13(6) 225.

[48] Ruike Y, Imanaka Y, Sato F, Shimizu K, Tsujimoto G. Genome-wide analysis of aberrant methylation in human breast cancer cells using methyl-DNA immunoprecipitation combined with high-throughput sequencing. BMC genomics 2010;11 137.

[49] Ehrlich M. DNA methylation in cancer: too much, but also too little. Oncogene 2002;21(35) 5400-5413.

[50] Verma M. Epigenome-Wide Association Studies (EWAS) in Cancer. Current genomics 2012;13(4) 308-313.

[51] Das PM, Singal R. DNA methylation and cancer. Journal of clinical oncology : official journal of the American Society of Clinical Oncology 2004;22(22) 4632-4642.

[52] Oki Y, Aoki E, Issa JP. Decitabine--bedside to bench. Critical reviews in oncology/hematology 2007;61(2) 140-152.

[53] Mund C, Brueckner B, Lyko F. Reactivation of epigenetically silenced genes by DNA methyltransferase inhibitors: basic concepts and clinical applications. Epigenetics : official journal of the DNA Methylation Society 2006;1(1) 7-13.

[54] Esteller M, Herman JG. Cancer as an epigenetic disease: DNA methylation and chromatin alterations in human tumours. The Journal of pathology 2002;196(1) 1-7.

[55] Baylin SB, Esteller M, Rountree MR, Bachman KE, Schuebel K, Herman JG. Aberrant patterns of DNA methylation, chromatin formation and gene expression in cancer. Human molecular genetics 2001;10(7) 687-692.

[56] Shames DS, Girard L, Gao B, Sato M, Lewis CM, Shivapurkar N, Jiang A, Perou CM, Kim YH, Pollack JR *et al.* A genome-wide screen for promoter methylation in lung cancer identifies novel methylation markers for multiple malignancies. PLoS medicine 2006;3(12) e486.

[57] Dammann R, Yang G, Pfeifer GP. Hypermethylation of the cpG island of Ras association domain family 1A (RASSF1A), a putative tumor suppressor gene from the 3p21.3 locus, occurs in a large percentage of human breast cancers. Cancer research 2001;61(7) 3105-3109.

[58] Burbee DG, Forgacs E, Zochbauer-Muller S, Shivakumar L, Fong K, Gao B, Randle D, Kondo M, Virmani A, Bader S *et al.* Epigenetic inactivation of RASSF1A in lung and breast cancers and malignant phenotype suppression. Journal of the National Cancer Institute 2001;93(9) 691-699.

[59] Woodcock DM, Linsenmeyer ME, Doherty JP, Warren WD. DNA methylation in the promoter region of the p16 (CDKN2/MTS-1/INK4A) gene in human breast tumours. British journal of cancer 1999;79(2) 251-256.
[60] Goto T, Mizukami H, Shirahata A, Sakata M, Saito M, Ishibashi K, Kigawa G, Nemoto H, Sanada Y, Hibi K. Aberrant methylation of the p16 gene is frequently detected in advanced colorectal cancer. Anticancer research 2009;29(1) 275-277.
[61] Shaw RJ, Liloglou T, Rogers SN, Brown JS, Vaughan ED, Lowe D, Field JK, Risk JM. Promoter methylation of P16, RARbeta, E-cadherin, cyclin A1 and cytoglobin in oral cancer: quantitative evaluation using pyrosequencing. British journal of cancer 2006;94(4) 561-568.
[62] Esteller M, Silva JM, Dominguez G, Bonilla F, Matias-Guiu X, Lerma E, Bussaglia E, Prat J, Harkes IC, Repasky EA *et al*. Promoter hypermethylation and BRCA1 inactivation in sporadic breast and ovarian tumors. Journal of the National Cancer Institute 2000;92(7) 564-569.
[63] Shen L, Kondo Y, Ahmed S, Boumber Y, Konishi K, Guo Y, Chen X, Vilaythong JN, Issa JP. Drug sensitivity prediction by CpG island methylation profile in the NCI-60 cancer cell line panel. Cancer research 2007;67(23) 11335-11343.
[64] Paz MF, Fraga MF, Avila S, Guo M, Pollan M, Herman JG, Esteller M. A systematic profile of DNA methylation in human cancer cell lines. Cancer research 2003;63(5) 1114-1121.
[65] Guendel I, Carpio L, Pedati C, Schwartz A, Teal C, Kashanchi F, Kehn-Hall K. Methylation of the tumor suppressor protein, BRCA1, influences its transcriptional cofactor function. PloS one 2010;5(6) e11379.
[66] Millar DS, Ow KK, Paul CL, Russell PJ, Molloy PL, Clark SJ. Detailed methylation analysis of the glutathione S-transferase pi (GSTP1) gene in prostate cancer. Oncogene 1999;18(6) 1313-1324.
[67] Wozniak RJ, Klimecki WT, Lau SS, Feinstein Y, Futscher BW. 5-Aza-2'-deoxycytidine-mediated reductions in G9A histone methyltransferase and histone H3 K9 di-methylation levels are linked to tumor suppressor gene reactivation. Oncogene 2007;26(1) 77-90.
[68] Luo J, Li YN, Wang F, Zhang WM, Geng X. S-adenosylmethionine inhibits the growth of cancer cells by reversing the hypomethylation status of c-myc and H-ras in human gastric cancer and colon cancer. International journal of biological sciences 2010;6(7) 784-795.
[69] Stresemann C, Lyko F. Modes of action of the DNA methyltransferase inhibitors azacytidine and decitabine. International journal of cancer Journal international du cancer 2008;123(1) 8-13.
[70] Kimura S, Kuramoto K, Homan J, Naruoka H, Ego T, Nogawa M, Sugahara S, Naito H. Antiproliferative and antitumor effects of azacitidine against the human myelodysplastic syndrome cell line SKM-1. Anticancer research 2012;32(3) 795-798.
[71] Copeland RL, Jr., Das JR, Bakare O, Enwerem NM, Berhe S, Hillaire K, White D, Beyene D, Kassim OO, Kanaan YM. Cytotoxicity of 2,3-dichloro-5,8-dimethoxy-1,4-

naphthoquinone in androgen-dependent and -independent prostate cancer cell lines. Anticancer research 2007;27(3B) 1537-1546.

[72] Jordan MA, Wilson L. Microtubules as a target for anticancer drugs. Nature reviews Cancer 2004;4(4) 253-265.

[73] Huang Y, Fang Y, Wu J, Dziadyk JM, Zhu X, Sui M, Fan W. Regulation of Vinca alkaloid-induced apoptosis by NF-kappaB/IkappaB pathway in human tumor cells. Molecular cancer therapeutics 2004;3(3) 271-277.

[74] Tozawa K, Oshima T, Kobayashi T, Yamamoto N, Hayashi C, Matsumoto T, Miwa H. Oxaliplatin in treatment of the cisplatin-resistant MKN45 cell line of gastric cancer. Anticancer research 2008;28(4B) 2087-2092.

[75] Garnett MJ, Edelman EJ, Heidorn SJ, Greenman CD, Dastur A, Lau KW, Greninger P, Thompson IR, Luo X, Soares J *et al.* Systematic identification of genomic markers of drug sensitivity in cancer cells. Nature 2012;483(7391) 570-575.

[76] Barretina J, Caponigro G, Stransky N, Venkatesan K, Margolin AA, Kim S, Wilson CJ, Lehar J, Kryukov GV, Sonkin D *et al.* The Cancer Cell Line Encyclopedia enables predictive modelling of anticancer drug sensitivity. Nature 2012;483(7391) 603-607.

[77] Abreu RM, Ferreira IC, Calhelha RC, Lima RT, Vasconcelos MH, Adega F, Chaves R, Queiroz MJ. Anti-hepatocellular carcinoma activity using human HepG2 cells and hepatotoxicity of 6-substituted methyl 3-aminothieno[3,2-b]pyridine-2-carboxylate derivatives: in vitro evaluation, cell cycle analysis and QSAR studies. European journal of medicinal chemistry 2011;46(12) 5800-5806.

[78] Sinha R, Vidyarthi AS, Shankaracharya. A molecular docking study of anticancer drug paclitaxel and its analogues. Indian journal of biochemistry & biophysics 2011;48(2) 101-105.

[79] Stewart ZA, Pietenpol JA. Cell cycle checkpoints as therapeutic targets. Journal of mammary gland biology and neoplasia 1999;4(4) 389-400.

[80] Verdier-Pinard P, Wang F, Burd B, Angeletti RH, Horwitz SB, Orr GA. Direct analysis of tubulin expression in cancer cell lines by electrospray ionization mass spectrometry. Biochemistry 2003;42(41) 12019-12027.

[81] Spankuch B, Heim S, Kurunci-Csacsko E, Lindenau C, Yuan J, Kaufmann M, Strebhardt K. Down-regulation of Polo-like kinase 1 elevates drug sensitivity of breast cancer cells in vitro and in vivo. Cancer research 2006;66(11) 5836-5846.

[82] Strebhardt K, Ullrich A. Targeting polo-like kinase 1 for cancer therapy. Nature reviews Cancer 2006;6(4) 321-330.

[83] Tsuruo T, Naito M, Tomida A, Fujita N, Mashima T, Sakamoto H, Haga N. Molecular targeting therapy of cancer: drug resistance, apoptosis and survival signal. Cancer science 2003;94(1) 15-21.

[84] Arnold CN, Goel A, Boland CR. Role of hMLH1 promoter hypermethylation in drug resistance to 5-fluorouracil in colorectal cancer cell lines. International journal of cancer Journal international du cancer 2003;106(1) 66-73.

[85] Palii SS, Van Emburgh BO, Sankpal UT, Brown KD, Robertson KD. DNA methylation inhibitor 5-Aza-2'-deoxycytidine induces reversible genome-wide DNA damage that is

distinctly influenced by DNA methyltransferases 1 and 3B. Molecular and cellular biology 2008;28(2) 752-771.

[86] Segura-Pacheco B, Trejo-Becerril C, Perez-Cardenas E, Taja-Chayeb L, Mariscal I, Chavez A, Acuna C, Salazar AM, Lizano M, Duenas-Gonzalez A. Reactivation of tumor suppressor genes by the cardiovascular drugs hydralazine and procainamide and their potential use in cancer therapy. Clinical cancer research : an official journal of the American Association for Cancer Research 2003;9(5) 1596-1603.

[87] Goffin J, Eisenhauer E. DNA methyltransferase inhibitors-state of the art. Annals of oncology : official journal of the European Society for Medical Oncology / ESMO 2002;13(11) 1699-1716.

[88] Shen H, Sun T, Ferrari M. Nanovector delivery of siRNA for cancer therapy. Cancer gene therapy 2012;19(6) 367-373.

[89] Elbashir SM, Harborth J, Lendeckel W, Yalcin A, Weber K, Tuschl T. Duplexes of 21-nucleotide RNAs mediate RNA interference in cultured mammalian cells. Nature 2001;411(6836) 494-498.

[90] Davis ME, Zuckerman JE, Choi CH, Seligson D, Tolcher A, Alabi CA, Yen Y, Heidel JD, Ribas A. Evidence of RNAi in humans from systemically administered siRNA via targeted nanoparticles. Nature 2010;464(7291) 1067-1070.

[91] Heidel JD, Liu JY, Yen Y, Zhou B, Heale BS, Rossi JJ, Bartlett DW, Davis ME. Potent siRNA inhibitors of ribonucleotide reductase subunit RRM2 reduce cell proliferation in vitro and in vivo. Clinical cancer research : an official journal of the American Association for Cancer Research 2007;13(7) 2207-2215.

Section 2

Proteomic Expression Profiling in Cancer

Chapter 7

Oncoproteomic Approaches in Lung Cancer Research

Mª Dolores Pastor, Ana Nogal, Sonia Molina-Pinelo, Luis Paz-Ares and Amancio Carnero

Additional information is available at the end of the chapter

http://dx.doi.org/10.5772/53873

1. Introduction

With more than 1 million annual deaths, among both females and males, lung cancer is the world leading cause of cancer-related death (1). The most important risk factor for lung cancer is smoking, with smokers presenting a 10 fold risk increase compared to non-smokers. Lung cancers are usually divided into two categories: small-cell lung cancer (SCLC), representing approximately 15% of cases, and non-small cell lung cancer (NSCLC). This sub-division represents around 85% of all lung cancer cases and includes the histological sub-types adenocarcinoma, large-cell carcinoma and squamous cell carcinoma (2). The lung cancer 5-year survival rate is one of the lowest at 10-15% and treatment depends on the extent of the disease at the time of diagnosis (3). Approximately 30% of patients have early stage lung cancer when diagnosed and those tumours can be surgically removed, 20% have local and/or regionally advanced tumours and are treated with chemo and radiotherapy, and almost half of the patients have advanced metastatic disease when only palliative treatments are available (4). Consequently there is a pressing need for new screening and early diagnostic techniques that are specific and non-invasive, and also for tools that can predict prognosis, optimize treatments and identify new therapeutic targets. Genomic approaches have been used to that end in the last years. Nonetheless, given the importance of proteins to a cells' phenotype, post-translational modifications, and the poor correlation between mRNA and protein expression levels (5, 6), proteomic analyses may enlighten the pathogenesis of lung cancer. A variety of techniques such as two dimensional gel electrophoresis (2D-PAGE, 2D-DIGE), protein arrays, protein labelling and tagging (ICAT, iTRAQ, SILAC), are being used in cancer research (7, 8) and have the potential to aid clinical practice as a complement to histopathology, as a selection method for individualized therapy, and in the assessment of drug efficacy, resistance, and toxicity (9).

2. Lung cancer

In the beginning of the 20th century, lung cancer was a rare disease. Nowadays it has the highest incidence and mortality rates in the world with lifestyle and environmental factors thought to be the major contributors to the development of this disease (10). Epidemiological evidence has shown that two to three decades after a peak in smoking prevalence in a given population, there is a peak in lung cancer deaths, making tobacco smoking the main cause of lung cancer development. This relationship was established in the 1950's and 60's (10-12). Other causes include environmental tobacco smoking, air pollution, indoor radon, occupational exposure to respiratory carcinogens, asbestos, and fumes from cooking stoves and fires (10). Even though smoking is undeniably the major cause of lung cancer, making it the leading cause of preventable death in the world, it is important to recognize that the majority of smokers will not develop this neoplasia over time and that this is probably due to individual variation in the susceptibility to respiratory carcinogens and the existence of a previous lung disease (13, 14). Tobacco components can induce DNA damage through several mechanisms including gene point mutations, deletions, insertions, recombinations, rearrangements, and chromosomal alterations, which drive the development of the disease (15). Nonetheless, the current classification of lung cancer does not emphasize the important of specific molecular and genetic alterations that can differentiate between SCLC and NSCLC. This is also true for the NSCLC subtypes adenocarcinoma, large cell carcinoma, and squamous cell carcinoma, that were until recently, treated similarly, regardless of their biological heterogeneity (16). Lung cancer is characterized by genetic instability of the chromosomes, nucleotides, and the transcriptome. These abnormalities are usually targeted to proto-oncogenes, tumour suppressor genes, DNA repair genes, among others. The silencing of telomerase is present in normal cells, but in almost all SCLC and over 80% of NSCLC, telomerase is activated, promoting cell immortalization (17). The epidermal growth factor receptor (EGFR) is overexpressed or abnormally activated by mutation in 50-90% of all NSCLC, especially in squamous cell carcinomas, leading to increased cell proliferation and survival through the RAS/RAF/MEK/MAPK and PI3K/AKT pathways (18). Activating mutations of the *KRAS* gene from the RAS proto-oncogene family are present in 20% of all NSCLS and between 30-50% of lung adenocarcinomas (19). The fusion of the echinoderm microtubule-associated protein-like 4 (*EML4*) and the anaplastic lymphoma kinase (*ALK*) genes occurs in approximately 7% of NSCLC and is associated with a persistent mitogenic signal. The *EML4-ALK*, *EGFR*, and *KRAS* mutations are almost always mutually exclusive (19). Tumour suppressor genes are also affected in lung cancer. Mutations in *TP53* are the most common genetic alterations found in human cancers and occur in approximately 75% of SCLC and in 50% of NSCLC (17). Alterations in the PI3K/AKT pathway, the CDKN2A/RB1 pathway, *VEGF*, and epigenetic changes are also present in lung cancer (19). Several drugs have been developed to target these alterations and improve survival of lung cancer patients, such as tyrosine kinase inhibitors and monoclonal antibodies, revealing the importance of the molecular characterization of tumours in order to improve detection, diagnosis, treatment and prognosis of lung cancer.

Proteins are crucial operators in the majority of biological systems and a comprehensive knowledge of their expression, modifications, and function in the lung cancer setting, may be more informative than DNA and RNA studies alone. New technologies are being developed that allow the analysis of thousands of cancer cell proteins, possibly generating new therapeutic targets and biomarkers that will have an impact on early detection, therapy and prognostic evaluation of lung cancer patients.

3. Proteomic techniques in lung cancer research

The proteomic technologies which are being implemented in lung cancer research are mainly based on two dimensional gel electrophoresis, as seen on Figure 1 where the 2D-PAGE and 2D-DIGE workflows are represented, or proteomics based on isotope labelling methods as ICAT, iTRAQ, SILAC, followed by mass spectrometry (MS) analysis.

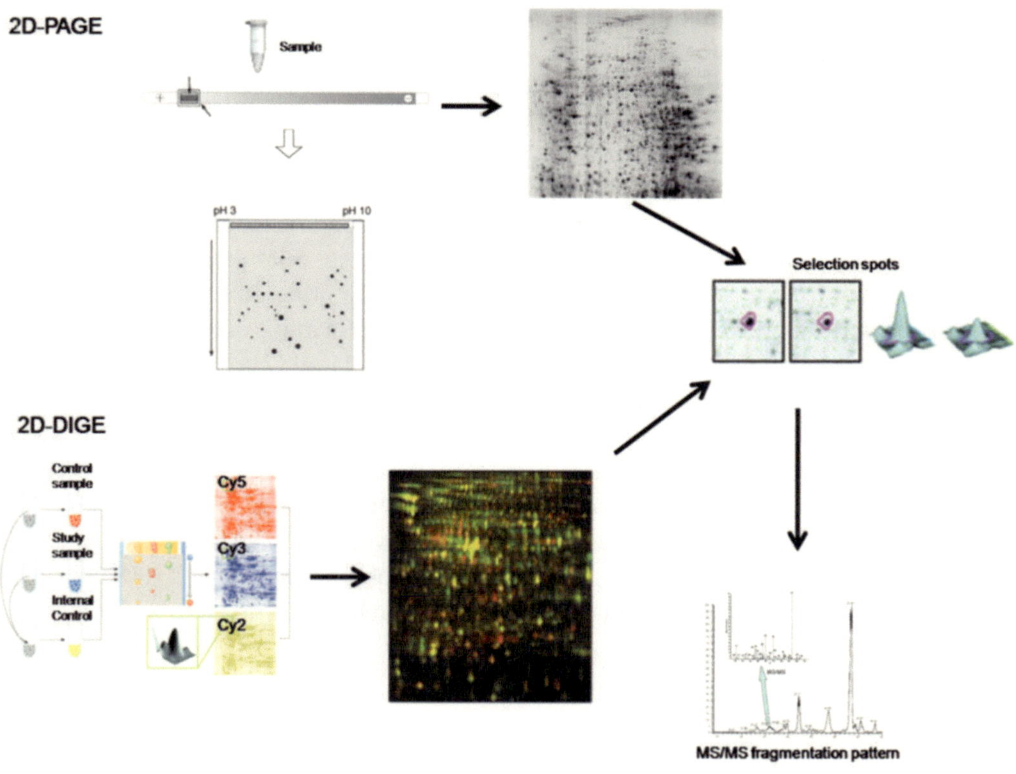

Figure 1. Basic workflow of gel-based proteomic approaches. In 2D-PAGE, protein samples are separated according to their isoelectric point in a process termed isoelectric focusing, using gel strips with a fixed pH range. Then, the focused strip is placed on top of a polyacrylamide gel to allow proteins to separate according to their molecular weight during electrophoresis, generating a gel with protein spots. In 2D-DIGE, proteins from up to three samples are labelled with fluorescent dyes prior to their isoelectric focusing and subsequent gel electrophoresis. Gels are scanned with different wavelengths revealing spots and differences in expression between analysed samples. Protein spots of interest in both techniques are then excised, digested, and identified by MS.

4. Two dimensional gel electrophoresis 2D-PAGE

2D-PAGE is the most used proteomic technique for studying the proteome as well as to search for cancer biomarkers (20, 21). In this methodology intact proteins are firstly separated by their isoelectric point (pI) and then according to their molecular weight. This procedure generates protein spots that are separated from the gel and digested into peptides for MS identification. Multidimensional separation of peptides may also be required given that, although the digestion step facilitates the identification process, it increases sample complexity, decreasing the sensitivity and coverage of the technique. Disadvantages of 2D-PAGE include the separation of low abundant proteins and of membrane proteins. The use of fractioning methods or higher protein concentrations for less detectable proteins and the use of mild detergents to increase the solubility of membrane proteins may be a solution for the aforementioned issues (22, 23). Other problems include co-migration of different proteins, the separation of a protein with different post-translational modifications, proteins with pI values below 4 or above 9, or the separation of very small or very large proteins. Differential gel electrophoresis (2D-DIGE), a modification of 2D-PAGE with fluorescent dyes (Cy3, Cy5 and Cy2), is able to increase reproducibility and throughput and also allows the accurate quantitation of protein expression difference (24). Differential analysis software can recognize the differentially expressed proteins and these can later be trypsin digested into peptides generating peptide mass fingerprints (PMF). The absolute masses of these peptides can be measured by matrix assisted laser desorption ionization time-of-flight mass spectrometry (MALDI-TOF MS), a technique that is both relatively easy to use and reasonably sensitive for identifying proteins. Additionally other MS techniques, such as electrospray ionization (ESI-MS/MS), are capable of providing amino acid sequence information on peptide fragments of the initial protein (25). Liquid chromatography coupled to tandem mass spectrometry workflow (LC-MS/MS) has become a standard method to identify proteins from complex biological samples. Also, direct MS analysis of tissue, known as MALDI imaging, is a method that has been used to elucidate proteome features characterizing histological differences in lung cancer between adenocarcinoma and squamous- cell carcinoma (26). Another example of a novel way to generate proteomic data is presented in the study of dynamic proteome changes on lung cancer cells (H1299) treated with the cytotoxic drug camptothecin using single-protein labelling on large scale (27).

5. Isotope-labelled mass spectrometry

Isotope-labelling methods, as seen on Figure 2, are gel-free procedures that introduce stable isotope tags to proteins through chemical reactions using isotope-coded affinity tags (ICAT) (28) and isobaric tag for relative and absolute quantitation (iTRAQ) (29), or through metabolic labelling with isotope labelled amino acids in cell culture (SILAC) (30).

ICAT is used to analyse pairs of protein samples, such as a treated sample and its control. Extracted proteins from both samples are labelled with a light or heavy ICAT reagent by reacting with a specific amino acid (cysteine). Samples are then mixed, trypsin digested, fractioned, and analysed by LC-MS/MS (31). Isotope peak ratios for each peptide determine the differential protein expression. The drawback of this technique is that it can only analyse cysteine containing proteins, two samples, and it can only identify 300-400 peptides.

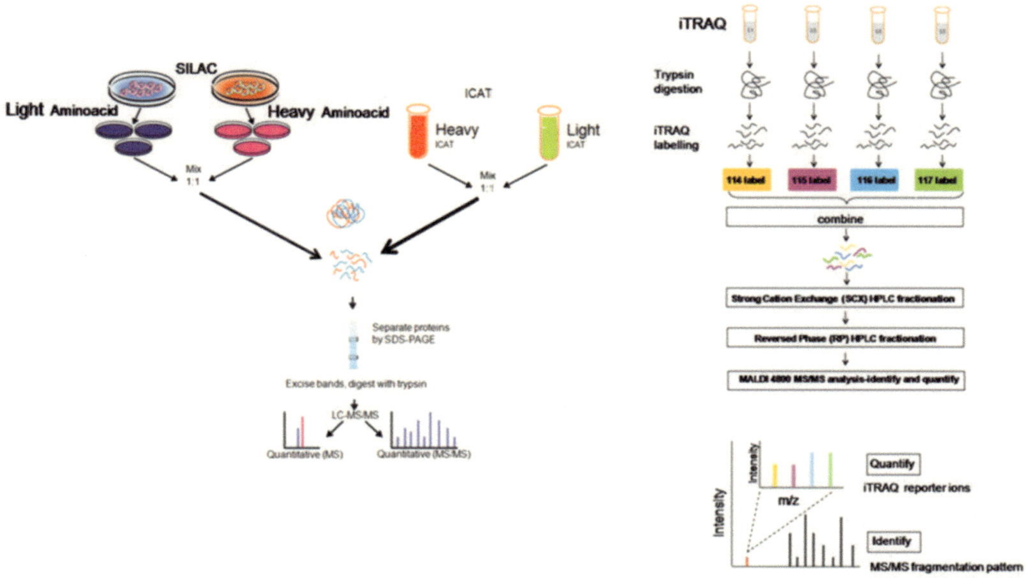

Figure 2. Basic workflow of gel-free quantitative approaches in proteomics. In SILAC, one cellular culture is grown in normal medium and the other with a growth medium with heavy labelled amino-acids. In ICAT, one protein extract is labelled with a light ICAT reagent and the other with a heavy ICAT reagent. In both techniques, samples are mixed, digested, separated and analysed by MS to determine protein identity and differential expression. In iTRAQ, special isobaric tags are applied in 4 to 8 samples up for comparison. They are then pooled together, fractionated and analysed by MS, allowing protein identification and quantitation among studied samples.

iTRAQ is another labelling technique first developed by Ross and co-workers (32) which uses isobaric tags to label and compare proteins extracted from samples. iTRAQ contains a set of four or eight isobaric reagents and therefore can analyse up to four or eight protein samples at one time. After trypsin digestion samples are labelled with four or eight (4-plex or 8-plex) independent iTRAQ reagents. The reporter groups of the iTRAQ reagents separate from the peptides and generate small fragments for each sample with mass-to-charge (m/z) of 114, 115, 116, and 117 for 4-plex, plus 113, 118, 119, and 121 for 8-plex. The intensity of each peak correlates with the quantity of each reporter group and thus with the quantity of the peptide. This method allows the analysis of various samples at a time and also, given that most peptides are suitable to be labelled by iTRAQ, it minimizes information loss and allows the identification of proteins with different post-translational modifications. Disadvantages of iTRAQ include a separate lengthy sample processing, that increases the chances of experimental errors, and the generation of chemical side products during the labelling process that can reduce the sensitivity of the method (33).

SILAC, first developed by Mann and co-workers, is based on the metabolic incorporation of "heavy" and "light" forms of amino acids into the proteins of living cultured cells (34) .

Typically, heavy (13C or 15N) arginine or lysine are used in the culture medium of a cell culture while the other cell culture is supplied with regular amino acids. After several division rounds, these amino acids are incorporated into the newly synthesized proteins. Following trypsin digestion, peptides are analysed by MS and the light and heavy peptides appear in two distinct peaks and, by comparing the signal intensities differences, relative quantitation can be performed. This technique has been widely used for cancer biomarker discovery (35), and cell signalling dynamics (36).

6. Label-free mass spectrometry

Multidimensional Protein Identification Technology (MudPIT) is a generic label-free LC-MS shotgun screening method (36). It separates peptides according to two independent physicochemical properties using liquid chromatography (LC/LC) online with the ion source of a mass spectrometer, allowing the separation and identification of peptides without labelling. The success of this technique depends on the experimental workflow, from protein extraction to sample stability, given that the reproducibility of technical replicates is better than that of experimental replicates. Drawbacks of this method include the fact that not all peptides are equally detectable given the competition between ions, dynamic range limitations and MS sensitivity (37). With time and improvements, label-free MS could be widely used for biomarker discovery and validation.

7. Detection of post-translational modifications (PTMs)

PTMs are the chemical alterations that occur to a protein after translation. They include proteolytic cleavage, glycosylation, phosphorylation, acetylation, ubiquitination, farnesylation, methylation, sialylation, oxidation, prolyl isomerization and hydroxylation (38). Glycosylation and phosphorylation are two of the most biologically relevant PTMs and appear to be key processes in tumour progression in many types of cancers including lung cancer (39, 40)

Glycosylation, the process of adding saccharides to proteins, plays a fundamental role in protein stabilization, molecular and cellular recognition, growth and cellular communication, and can also be a part of immune responses and cancer progression (41). The comparative study of the carbohydrate chains of glycoproteins may provide useful information for the diagnosis, prognosis, and immunotherapy of tumours (42). The proteomic analysis of glycoproteins starts with the enrichment of these molecules from a complex protein sample by the use lectins. This step is followed by a separation of glycoproteins by procedures such as 2D-PAGE and 2D-DIGE coupled with glycoprotein staining methods, for example Pro-Q Emerald 488 glycoprotein stain (43), lectin fluorescence stain (44), and isotope labelling (45). Identification of separated glycoproteins and their glycan structures can be accomplished by chromatographic methods (nano-LC with hydrophilic columns, nano-LC with graphitized carbon packing, anion-exchange chromatography), electromigration approaches (capillary electrophoresis, capillary electrochromatography), capillary LC/MALDI-TOF/TOF MS & tandem MS (MS/MS), and chip-based approaches (46). Although there are some difficulties when analysing lung tumours, one study has identified 34 glycoproteins with significant differences between lung adenocarcinomas and healthy controls. The α1,6-fucosylation levels were incremented in the lung cancer group in comparison with healthy group (47).

Phosphorylation is the addition of a phosphate group to a protein and is a key regulatory mechanism of cellular signalling processes. Phosphoproteomics and the characterization of phosphorylation sites, which less than 2% are currently known, are some of the most challenging tasks in current proteomic research (48). To isolate and identify phosphorylated proteins one must use immunoaffinity or immunoprecipitation with a specific antibody, chromatofocusing, ion exchange chromatography and affinity chromatography, such as immobilized metal ion affinity chromatography (IMAC) (49). Separation methods include electrophoresis, 2D-PAGE or 2D-DIGE coupled with phosphoprotein staining (Pro-Q Diamond phosphoprotein gel stain) or isotope labelling (ICAT, SILAC) (50, 51). Analysis and identification methods of phosphoproteins and phosphopeptides are mass spectrometry-based approaches, such MALDI-TOF MS, LC-ESI-MS and MS/MS (52). Given that the key regulators of signalling cascades are kinases and phosphatases, lung cancer phosphoproteomics might reveal the correlation between phosphorylation and cancer mechanisms.

8. Samples in lung cancer proteomics

The lung is a heterogeneous organ composed by several highly differentiated cells (bronchial, alveolar, inflammatory) and vascular structures. Its main function is to perform gas exchanges between the atmosphere and the bloodstream. When studying lung cancer with proteomic tools, several different samples can be used: tumour tissue, blood, pleural effusions, among others (53). The accessibility of blood makes for a great sample for oncoproteomic studies. Moreover, it contains many circulating molecules secreted by the tumour that can be used as biomarkers. Nonetheless, due to the abundance of plasma proteins, depletion of these proteins is necessary to reveal the presence of less abundant ones. Tumour tissue samples, fresh-frozen or formalin-fixed and paraffin-embedded, are the ideal for any oncoproteomic study. However, adjacent normal tissue, inflammatory cells, stromal components, and others might also be present. This will result in non-tumour derived protein contamination. To compensate tumour heterogeneity careful sample cell content analysis and the increase of sample numbers is required to obtain relevant results. The pleura is a thin double-layered tissue that surrounds the lung and it is filled with pleural fluid. This liquid is constantly produced and reabsorbed, and its main function is to facilitate respiratory movements and reduce attrition between the lungs and the thorax wall. Pleural effusion is the pathological accumulation of fluid that occurs in inflammatory conditions and lung cancer. In the latter case, pleural effusion is often drained to search for cancer cell infiltration. Its protein composition is similar to plasma, but its proximity to tumour cells makes it useful for lung cancer biomarker detection by proteomic techniques.

9. Proteomics in the discovery and validation of lung cancer biomarkers

9.1. Diagnostic biomarkers

To discover a lung cancer diagnostic biomarker, a molecule that is specific and directly correlates with the presence of this disease, the majority of studies perform a comparison between the protein profiles of tumour samples and normal lung tissue. The ideal would be to study the development of the carcinogenic process from normal tissue, to metaplasia, to dysplasia, and finally to invasive cancer, in order to discover early markers of disease before the onset of clinical features.

In response to inflammation, a cancer enabling characteristic, acute-phase reactant proteins (APRPs) are produced. Recent proteomic studies have shown that APRPs haptoglobin (Hp) β chain (54), serum amyloid A (SAA) (55), and apolipoprotein A-1 (Apo A-1) (56) proteins are potential lung cancer diagnostic biomarkers. SAA proteins are involved in the transport of cholesterol to the liver, the recruitment of immune cells, and the induction extracellular matrix degrading enzymes. SAA1 and SAA2, which are synthesised in response to activated monocytes/macrophages, were recently identified, by LC-MS/MS, ELISA and immunohistochemistry analyses, as lung cancer biomarkers given their higher expression levels in blood and tissue from lung cancer patients when compared to healthy subjects and patients with other cancers and respiratory diseases (55). In another related study, serum and pleural effusions from NSCLC patients were compared by 2D-DIGE to those from patients with benign lung diseases. Gelsolin, possibly involved in cancer invasion, metalloproteinase inhibitor 2 (TIMP2), involved in lung parenchyma disorganization, and pigment epithelium derived factor (PEDF), an angiogenesis inhibitor, were among the candidate biomarkers (57). A study by Patz and co-workers, that aimed to test the diagnostic performance of four lung cancer biomarkers (carcinoembryonic antigen and squamous-cell carcinoma antigen, and 2D-PAGE and MALDI-MS discovered retinol binding protein – RBP - and α-1 antitrypsin), demonstrated that the four markers have inadequate diagnostic power when tested independently but proved useful when used in combination (58). A glycoproteomic study revealed plasma kallikrein (KLKB1), pleural effusion periostin, multimerin-2, CD166 and lysosome-associated membrane glycoprotein-2 (LAMP-2) as potential lung cancer biomarkers (59).

9.2. Prognostic biomarkers

Prognostic biomarkers, those that have expression levels correlating with the natural history of the disease, have the potential to influence survival by identifying high-risk patients and thus improve their management. The study of prognostic biomarkers in lung cancer has been made by correlating the expression of a molecule to the patient survival. An alternative approach is to compare groups of patients with different clinical stages of disease, based on the assumption that a more advanced tumour is more aggressive and may express proteins that drive the metastatic process. Proteomic studies have aimed at discovering altered protein levels and subsequently validating those differences using immunohistochemistry on archive samples. Using 2D-PAGE, Chen and co-workers associated 11 components of the glycolysis pathway to poor survival in lung adenocarcinoma (39) and also demonstrated their prognostic role in lung cancer at the mRNA level. Nonetheless, glycolysis involved enzyme phosphoglycerate kinase 1 was found to limit tumour growth in mice subcutaneously injected with the Lewis lung carcinoma cell line, by promoting antitumor immunity (60). A study using 2D-DIGE, MS, western blot, and immunohistochemistry correlated the up-regulation of annexin A3, a protein associated with cancer metastasis by angiogenic promotion, with advanced clinical stage, lymph node metastasis, increased relapse time, and overall decreased survival in lung adenocarcinoma, indicating that annexin A3 might be a prognostic lung cancer biomarker (61). The involvement of S100A11, a small calcium-binding protein implicated in the prognosis and metastasis in several tumours, has also been evaluated in lung cancer. Comparative proteomic analysis of two NSCLC cell lines, the non-metastatic CL1-0 and highly metastatic CL1-5, revealed that S100A11 was up-regulated in metastatic CL1-5 cells (62). Moreover, immunohistochemical analyses in NSCLC tissues showed that the up-regulation of S100A11 was significantly associated with a higher TNM stage and a positive lymph node status, indicating its importance in promoting invasion and metastasis of NSCLC. Altered expression of S100A6 was also implicated in NSCLC progression: elevated levels of this protein were associated with longer survival compared to S100A6-negative cases (63). Cytoskeletal reorganization is a central process regulating cell migration and metastasis and cytokeratins (CKs), a family of cytoskeletal intermediate filaments, have been suggested to play a role in carcinogenesis, by promoting cellular architecture reorganization during tumour development and progression. A 2D-PAGE and MS analysis has revealed that isoforms of CK7, 8, 18, and 19 were found in higher levels in adenocarcinoma samples than in adjacent tissues (64). Specific isoforms of the CKs were associated with unfavourable prognosis, CYFRA21-1 was a more accurate diagnostic marker, and CK18 was a stronger prognostic factor (65). Other cytoskeletal proteins found to be correlated with a poor prognosis in lung adenocarcinoma are non-muscle myosin IIA and vimentin proteins, involved in epithelial-mesenchymal transition, a process at the basis of invasive and metastatic behaviour (66). Phosphohistidine phosphatase (PHP14) was proposed to be another lung cancer prognostic biomarker, regulating cell migration and invasion by cytoskeleton rearrangement. Indeed, it has been shown that PHP14 knockdown in highly metastatic lung cancer cells (CL1-5) inhibited migration and invasion, whereas its over-expression in NCI H1299 cells enhanced these processes (67). Calmodulin, a protein implicated in cytoskeletal alterations during cell death, thymosin β4, a regulator of actin polymerization whose over-expression seems to stimulate lung tumour metastasis, thymosin β10 and cofilin proteins, regulators of actin dynamics, were identified and their expression and prognostic role validated on cohort of 188 lung cancer cases (68).

9.3. Predictive biomarkers

The discovery of predictive biomarkers, those on which the efficacy of a specific treatment can be foreseen, has been based on studying clinical samples from responding and non-responding patients and then validating results on selected cohorts. This type of biomarker aims at individualizing therapies in lung cancer but relies on extremely well characterized samples from cohorts of patients receiving a uniform treatment and closely monitored therapeutic responses. A recent MALDI-TOF-MS study that profiled serum from patients treated with cisplatin-gemcitabine in combination with the proteasome inhibitor bortezomib, revealed a 13-peptide signature that was able to distinguish with high accuracy, sensitivity, and specificity, patients with short and long progression-free survival (69). The epidermal growth factor receptor (EGFR) tyrosine kinase is an important target for treatment of NSCLC, and EGFR-inhibitor-based therapies have showed promising results. The serum MALDI-MS study conducted by Taguchi and co-workers in NSCLC patients

Type of Biomarker	Proteins	Techniques
Diagnostic	Hp β chain (54)	LC-ESI-MS/MS, ELISA
	SAA1 SAA2 (55)	LC-MS/MS, ELISA, IHC
	Apo A1 (56)	2D-PAGE, MALDI-TOF
	Gelsolin TIMP2 PEDF (57)	2D-DIGE
	RBP α-1 antitrypsin (58)	2D-DIGE, MALDI-TOF-MS
	KLKB1 Periostin Multimerin-2 CD166 LAMP-2 (59)	LC-MS/MS
Prognostic	Glycolysis (11 components) (39)	2D-PAGE
	Annexin A3 (61)	2D-DIGE, MS, IHC*
	S100A11 (62)	2D-PAGE, MALDI-TOF-MS/MS, IHC
	S100A6 (63)	SELDI-TOF-MS
	CK 7, 8, 9 and 19 (64)	2D-PAGE, MS
	CYFRA21-1 CK18 (65)	ELISA
	Myosin IIA Vimentin (66)	LC-MS/MS
	PHP14 (67)	2D-PAGE, ESI-TOF-MS/MS
	Calmodulin Thymosin β4 Thymosin β10 (68)	MALDI-MS, IHC
Predictive	13-peptide signature (69)	MALDI-TOF-MS
	8-peak signature (70)	MALDI-MS

* Immunohistochemistry

Table 1. Potential lung cancer biomarkers discovered by the use of proteomic tools

treated with gefitinib and erlotinib revealed an 8-peak profile predictive of outcome (70). This 8-peak signature was commercially launched as a commercial product (Veristrat ®, Biodesix, Broom field, CO, US) and its clinical relevance is being validated in the context of a randomized phase III clinical trial where patients with advanced NSCLC progressing after first-line treatment, stratified according to serum MALDI-MS profiling, are subsequently randomly allocated to receive either erlotinib or chemotherapy as second-line therapy (PROSE, Proteomics Stratified Erlotinib trial). To the best of our knowledge, this is the only clinical trial investigating the predictive role of a proteomics biomarker in lung cancer patients. A summary of all mentioned biomarkers can be found on Table 1.

10. Conclusions

Proteomic approaches are improving rapidly and the development of high-throughput platforms is showing promising results as the list of candidate biomarkers for lung cancer is continuously growing. However, there is a great need for careful interpretation of this intricate data in order to generate biologically relevant hypotheses. The proteome is highly complex and current tools cannot yet provide a definitive solution for its exploration. In addition, cancer is a multifactorial disease so diverse that a great deal of time and effort will be necessary to define its associated proteome modifications and to translate these into practical clinical applications. In fact for many of the identified proteins, their functional role in lung cancer development is not yet known and a solid clinical validation is still lacking. Nonetheless, it is likely that some of these candidate biomarkers will serve to identify new possible therapeutic strategies.

Author details

Mª Dolores Pastor, Ana Nogal, Sonia Molina-Pinelo, Luis Paz-Ares and Amancio Carnero
Institute of Biomedicine of Seville (HUVR/CSIC/University of Seville), Spain

Ana Nogal
Biomedical Sciences Institute of Abel Salazar (University of Porto), Portugal

Amancio Carnero
Consejo Superior de Investigaciones Científicas (CSIC), Spain

11. References

[1] Jemal A, Siegel R, Xu J, Ward E. Cancer statistics, 2010. CA A Cancer Journal for Clinicians. 2010 Sep-Oct;60(5):277-300.
[2] Lehtio J, De Petris L. Lung cancer proteomics, clinical and technological considerations. Journal of Proteomics. 2010 Sep 10;73(10):1851-63.
[3] Jemal A, Siegel R, Ward E, Hao Y, Xu J, Thun MJ. Cancer statistics, 2009. CA A Cancer Journal for Clinicians. 2009 Jul-Aug;59(4):225-49.

[4] Groome PA, Bolejack V, Crowley JJ, Kennedy C, Krasnik M, Sobin LH, et al. The IASLC Lung Cancer Staging Project: validation of the proposals for revision of the T, N, and M descriptors and consequent stage groupings in the forthcoming (seventh) edition of the TNM classification of malignant tumours. Journal of Thoracic Oncology. 2007 Aug;2(8):694-705.

[5] Chen G, Gharib TG, Wang H, Huang CC, Kuick R, Thomas DG, et al. Protein profiles associated with survival in lung adenocarcinoma. Proceedings of the National Academy of Sciences of the United States of America. 2003 Nov 11;100(23):13537-42.

[6] Ocak S, Chaurand P, Massion PP. Mass spectrometry-based proteomic profiling of lung cancer. Proceedings of the American Thoracic Society. 2009 Apr 15;6(2):159-70.

[7] Cho WC, Cheng CH. Oncoproteomics: current trends and future perspectives. Expert Review of Proteomics. 2007 Jun;4(3):401-10.

[8] van der Merwe DE, Oikonomopoulou K, Marshall J, Diamandis EP. Mass spectrometry: uncovering the cancer proteome for diagnostics. Advances in Cancer Research. 2007;96:23-50.

[9] Au JS, Cho WC, Yip TT, Law SC. Proteomic approach to biomarker discovery in cancer tissue from lung adenocarcinoma among nonsmoking Chinese women in Hong Kong. Cancer Investigation. 2008 Mar;26(2):128-35.

[10] Alberg AJ, Ford JG, Samet JM. Epidemiology of lung cancer: ACCP evidence-based clinical practice guidelines (2nd edition). Chest. 2007 Sep;132(3 Suppl):29S-55S.

[11] Doll R, Hill AB. Smoking and carcinoma of the lung; preliminary report. British Medical Journal. 1950 Sep 30;2(4682):739-48.

[12] Mills CA, Porter MM. Tobacco smoking habits and cancer of the mouth and respiratory system. Cancer Research. 1950 Sep;10(9):539-42.

[13] Alberg AJ, Samet JM. Epidemiology of lung cancer. Chest. 2003 Jan;123(1 Suppl):21S-49S.

[14] Brody JS, Spira A. State of the art. Chronic obstructive pulmonary disease, inflammation, and lung cancer. Proceedings of the American Thoracic Society. 2006 Aug;3(6):535-8.

[15] Adcock IM, Caramori G, Barnes PJ. Chronic obstructive pulmonary disease and lung cancer: new molecular insights. Respiration. 2011;81(4):265-84.

[16] Borczuk AC, Toonkel RL, Powell CA. Genomics of lung cancer. Proceedings of the American Thoracic Society. 2009 Apr 15;6(2):152-8.

[17] Meyerson M, Franklin WA, Kelley MJ. Molecular classification and molecular genetics of human lung cancers. Seminars in Oncology. 2004 Feb;31(1 Suppl 1):4-19.

[18] Breuer RH, Postmus PE, Smit EF. Molecular pathology of non-small-cell lung cancer. Respiration. 2005 May-Jun;72(3):313-30.

[19] West L, Vidwans SJ, Campbell NP, Shrager J, Simon GR, Bueno R, et al. A novel classification of lung cancer into molecular subtypes. PLoS One. 2012;7(2):e31906.

[20] Lilley KS, Razzaq A, Dupree P. Two-dimensional gel electrophoresis: recent advances in sample preparation, detection and quantitation. Current Opinion in Chemical Biology. 2002 Feb;6(1):46-50.

[21] Yu KH, Rustgi AK, Blair IA. Characterization of proteins in human pancreatic cancer serum using differential gel electrophoresis and tandem mass spectrometry. Journal of Proteome Research. 2005 Sep-Oct;4(5):1742-51.

[22] Qin S, Ferdinand AS, Richie JP, O'Leary MP, Mok SC, Liu BC. Chromatofocusing fractionation and two-dimensional difference gel electrophoresis for low abundance serum proteins. Proteomics. 2005 Aug;5(12):3183-92.

[23] Luche S, Santoni V, Rabilloud T. Evaluation of nonionic and zwitterionic detergents as membrane protein solubilizers in two-dimensional electrophoresis. Proteomics. 2003 Mar;3(3):249-53.

[24] Unlu M, Morgan ME, Minden JS. Difference gel electrophoresis: a single gel method for detecting changes in protein extracts. Electrophoresis. 1997 Oct;18(11):2071-7.

[25] Mann M, Hendrickson RC, Pandey A. Analysis of proteins and proteomes by mass spectrometry. Annual Review of Biochemistry. 2001;70:437-73.

[26] Gygi SP, Corthals GL, Zhang Y, Rochon Y, Aebersold R. Evaluation of two-dimensional gel electrophoresis-based proteome analysis technology. Proceedings of the National Academy of Sciences of the United States of America. 2000 Aug 15;97(17):9390-5.

[27] Kameshita I, Ishida A, Fujisawa H. Analysis of protein-protein interaction by two-dimensional affinity electrophoresis. Analytical Biochemistry. 1998 Aug 15;262(1):90-2.

[28] Haqqani AS, Nesic M, Preston E, Baumann E, Kelly J, Stanimirovic D. Characterization of vascular protein expression patterns in cerebral ischemia/reperfusion using laser capture microdissection and ICAT-nanoLC-MS/MS. FASEB Journal. 2005 Nov;19(13):1809-21.

[29] Shadforth IP, Dunkley TP, Lilley KS, Bessant C. i-Tracker: for quantitative proteomics using iTRAQ. BMC Genomics. 2005;6:145.

[30] Ong SE, Blagoev B, Kratchmarova I, Kristensen DB, Steen H, Pandey A, et al. Stable isotope labeling by amino acids in cell culture, SILAC, as a simple and accurate approach to expression proteomics. Molecular & Cellular Proteomics. 2002 May;1(5):376-86.

[31] Graves PR, Haystead TA. Molecular biologist's guide to proteomics. Microbiology and Molecular Biology Reviews. 2002 Mar;66(1):39-63; table of contents.

[32] Ross PL, Huang YN, Marchese JN, Williamson B, Parker K, Hattan S, et al. Multiplexed protein quantitation in Saccharomyces cerevisiae using amine-reactive isobaric tagging reagents. Molecular & Cellular Proteomics. 2004 Dec;3(12):1154-69.

[33] DeSouza L, Diehl G, Rodrigues MJ, Guo J, Romaschin AD, Colgan TJ, et al. Search for cancer markers from endometrial tissues using differentially labeled tags iTRAQ and cICAT with multidimensional liquid chromatography and tandem mass spectrometry. Journal of Proteome Research. 2005 Mar-Apr;4(2):377-86.

[34] Mann M. Functional and quantitative proteomics using SILAC. Nature Reviews Molecular Cell Biology. 2006 Dec;7(12):952-8.

[35] Gronborg M, Kristiansen TZ, Iwahori A, Chang R, Reddy R, Sato N, et al. Biomarker discovery from pancreatic cancer secretome using a differential proteomic approach. Molecular & Cellular Proteomics. 2006 Jan;5(1):157-71.

[36] Guerrera IC, Keep NH, Godovac-Zimmermann J. Proteomics study reveals cross-talk between Rho guanidine nucleotide dissociation inhibitor 1 post-translational modifications in epidermal growth factor stimulated fibroblasts. Journal of Proteome Research. 2007 Jul;6(7):2623-30.

[37] Zhang B, VerBerkmoes NC, Langston MA, Uberbacher E, Hettich RL, Samatova NF. Detecting differential and correlated protein expression in label-free shotgun proteomics. Journal of Proteome Research. 2006 Nov;5(11):2909-18.

[38] Krueger KE, Srivastava S. Posttranslational protein modifications: current implications for cancer detection, prevention, and therapeutics. Molecular & Cellular Proteomics. 2006 Oct;5(10):1799-810.

[39] Chen G, Gharib TG, Huang CC, Thomas DG, Shedden KA, Taylor JM, et al. Proteomic analysis of lung adenocarcinoma: identification of a highly expressed set of proteins in tumors. Clinical Cancer Research. 2002 Jul;8(7):2298-305.

[40] Okano T, Kondo T, Kakisaka T, Fujii K, Yamada M, Kato H, et al. Plasma proteomics of lung cancer by a linkage of multi-dimensional liquid chromatography and two-dimensional difference gel electrophoresis. Proteomics. 2006 Jul;6(13):3938-48.

[41] Dennis JW, Granovsky M, Warren CE. Glycoprotein glycosylation and cancer progression. Biochimica et Biophysica Acta. 1999 Dec 6;1473(1):21-34.

[42] Lowe JB. Glycosylation, immunity, and autoimmunity. Cell. 2001 Mar 23;104(6):809-12.

[43] Hart C, Schulenberg B, Steinberg TH, Leung WY, Patton WF. Detection of glycoproteins in polyacrylamide gels and on electroblots using Pro-Q Emerald 488 dye, a fluorescent periodate Schiff-base stain. Electrophoresis. 2003 Feb;24(4):588-98.

[44] Patwa TH, Zhao J, Anderson MA, Simeone DM, Lubman DM. Screening of glycosylation patterns in serum using natural glycoprotein microarrays and multi-lectin fluorescence detection. Analytical Chemistry. 2006 Sep 15;78(18):6411-21.

[45] Ueda K, Katagiri T, Shimada T, Irie S, Sato TA, Nakamura Y, et al. Comparative profiling of serum glycoproteome by sequential purification of glycoproteins and 2-nitrobenzensulfenyl (NBS) stable isotope labeling: a new approach for the novel biomarker discovery for cancer. Journal of Proteome Research. 2007 Sep;6(9):3475-83.

[46] Mechref Y, Novotny MV. Miniaturized separation techniques in glycomic investigations. Journal of Chromatography B Analytical Technologies in the Biomedical and Life Sciences. 2006 Sep 1;841(1-2):65-78.

[47] Yang Z, Hancock WS, Chew TR, Bonilla L. A study of glycoproteins in human serum and plasma reference standards (HUPO) using multilectin affinity chromatography coupled with RPLC-MS/MS. Proteomics. 2005 Aug;5(13):3353-66.

[48] Mukherji M. Phosphoproteomics in analyzing signaling pathways. Expert Review of Proteomics. 2005 Jan;2(1):117-28.

[49] Schmidt SR, Schweikart F, Andersson ME. Current methods for phosphoprotein isolation and enrichment. Journal of Chromatography B Analytical Technologies in the Biomedical and Life Sciences. 2007 Apr 15;849(1-2):154-62.

[50] Goshe MB, Veenstra TD, Panisko EA, Conrads TP, Angell NH, Smith RD. Phosphoprotein isotope-coded affinity tags: application to the enrichment and

identification of low-abundance phosphoproteins. Analytical Chemistry. 2002 Feb 1;74(3):607-16.
[51] Raggiaschi R, Gotta S, Terstappen GC. Phosphoproteome analysis. Bioscience Reports. 2005 Feb-Apr;25(1-2):33-44.
[52] Carr SA, Annan RS, Huddleston MJ. Mapping posttranslational modifications of proteins by MS-based selective detection: application to phosphoproteomics. Methods in Enzymology. 2005;405:82-115.
[53] De Petris L, Pernemalm M, Elmberger G, Bergman P, Orre L, Lewensohn R, et al. A novel method for sample preparation of fresh lung cancer tissue for proteomics analysis by tumor cell enrichment and removal of blood contaminants. Proteome Science. 2010;8:9.
[54] Kang SM, Sung HJ, Ahn JM, Park JY, Lee SY, Park CS, et al. The Haptoglobin beta chain as a supportive biomarker for human lung cancers. Molecular BioSystems. 2011 Apr;7(4):1167-75.
[55] Sung HJ, Ahn JM, Yoon YH, Rhim TY, Park CS, Park JY, et al. Identification and validation of SAA as a potential lung cancer biomarker and its involvement in metastatic pathogenesis of lung cancer. Journal of Proteome Research. 2011 Mar 4;10(3):1383-95.
[56] Maciel CM, Junqueira M, Paschoal ME, Kawamura MT, Duarte RL, Carvalho Mda G, et al. Differential proteomic serum pattern of low molecular weight proteins expressed by adenocarcinoma lung cancer patients. Journal of Experimental Therapeutics and Oncology. 2005;5(1):31-8.
[57] Rodriguez-Pineiro AM, Blanco-Prieto S, Sanchez-Otero N, Rodriguez-Berrocal FJ, de la Cadena MP. On the identification of biomarkers for non-small cell lung cancer in serum and pleural effusion. Journal of Proteomics. 2010 Jun 16;73(8):1511-22.
[58] Patz EF, Jr., Campa MJ, Gottlin EB, Kusmartseva I, Guan XR, Herndon JE, 2nd. Panel of serum biomarkers for the diagnosis of lung cancer. Journal of Clinical Oncology. 2007 Dec 10;25(35):5578-83.
[59] Soltermann A, Ossola R, Kilgus-Hawelski S, von Eckardstein A, Suter T, Aebersold R, et al. N-glycoprotein profiling of lung adenocarcinoma pleural effusions by shotgun proteomics. Cancer. 2008 Apr 25;114(2):124-33.
[60] Tang SJ, Ho MY, Cho HC, Lin YC, Sun GH, Chi KH, et al. Phosphoglycerate kinase 1-overexpressing lung cancer cells reduce cyclooxygenase 2 expression and promote anti-tumor immunity in vivo. International Journal of Cancer. 2008 Dec 15;123(12):2840-8.
[61] Liu YF, Xiao ZQ, Li MX, Li MY, Zhang PF, Li C, et al. Quantitative proteome analysis reveals annexin A3 as a novel biomarker in lung adenocarcinoma. Journal of Pathology. 2009 Jan;217(1):54-64.
[62] Tian T, Hao J, Xu A, Luo C, Liu C, Huang L, et al. Determination of metastasis-associated proteins in non-small cell lung cancer by comparative proteomic analysis. Cancer Science. 2007 Aug;98(8):1265-74.
[63] De Petris L, Orre LM, Kanter L, Pernemalm M, Koyi H, Lewensohn R, et al. Tumor expression of S100A6 correlates with survival of patients with stage I non-small-cell lung cancer. Lung Cancer. 2009 Mar;63(3):410-7.

[64] Gharib TG, Chen G, Wang H, Huang CC, Prescott MS, Shedden K, et al. Proteomic analysis of cytokeratin isoforms uncovers association with survival in lung adenocarcinoma. Neoplasia. 2002 Sep-Oct;4(5):440-8.

[65] De Petris L, Branden E, Herrmann R, Sanchez BC, Koyi H, Linderholm B, et al. Diagnostic and prognostic role of plasma levels of two forms of cytokeratin 18 in patients with non-small-cell lung cancer. European Journal of Cancer. 2011 Jan;47(1):131-7.

[66] Maeda J, Hirano T, Ogiwara A, Akimoto S, Kawakami T, Fukui Y, et al. Proteomic analysis of stage I primary lung adenocarcinoma aimed at individualisation of postoperative therapy. British Medical Journal. 2008 Feb 12;98(3):596-603.

[67] Xu A, Hao J, Zhang Z, Tian T, Jiang S, Liu C, et al. 14-kDa phosphohistidine phosphatase and its role in human lung cancer cell migration and invasion. Lung Cancer. 2010 Jan;67(1):48-56.

[68] Xu BJ, Gonzalez AL, Kikuchi T, Yanagisawa K, Massion PP, Wu H, et al. MALDI-MS derived prognostic protein markers for resected non-small cell lung cancer. Proteomics - Clinical Applications. 2008 Oct;2(10-11):1508-17.

[69] Voortman J, Pham TV, Knol JC, Giaccone G, Jimenez CR. Prediction of outcome of non-small cell lung cancer patients treated with chemotherapy and bortezomib by time-course MALDI-TOF-MS serum peptide profiling. Proteome Science. 2009;7:34.

[70] Taguchi F, Solomon B, Gregorc V, Roder H, Gray R, Kasahara K, et al. Mass spectrometry to classify non-small-cell lung cancer patients for clinical outcome after treatment with epidermal growth factor receptor tyrosine kinase inhibitors: a multicohort cross-institutional study. Journal of the National Cancer Institute. 2007 Jun 6;99(11):838-46.

Chapter 8

Phosphoproteomics-Based Characterization of Cancer Cell Signaling Networks

Hiroko Kozuka-Hata, Yumi Goto and Masaaki Oyama

Additional information is available at the end of the chapter

http://dx.doi.org/10.5772/52915

1. Introduction

Signal transduction systems regulate complex biological events such as cell proliferation and differentiation via phosphorylation/dephosphorylation kinetic reactions. Therefore, dysregulation of these systems lead to a variety of diseases such as diabetes, abnormal bone metabolism, autoimmune disease and cancer [1-4]. Above all, cancer is well-known to be caused by aberrant regulation of signaling pathways. Although a large number of studies regarding phosphorylation events in cancer cell networks were performed, a global view of these complex systems has not been fully elucidated. Recent technological advances in mass spectrometry-based proteomics have enabled us to identify thousands of proteins in a single project [5-7] and, in combination with relative quantitation techniques such as Stable Isotope Labeling by Amino acids in Cell culture (SILAC), quantitative analysis regarding signaling-related molecules can also be performed [8,9]. Recently, establishment of phosphorylation-directed peptide/protein enrichment technology has led us to capture the comprehensive status of phosphorylated cellular signaling molecules in a time-resolved manner [10-12]. Tyrosine-phosphoproteome analysis conducted by utilizing anti-phosphotyrosine antibodies unveils key regulatory signaling dynamics triggered by tyrosine kinases such as epidermal growth factor receptor (EGFR) in various contexts of cancer cell signaling. Furthermore, chemistry-based phosphopeptide enrichment technologies such as immobilized metal affinity chromatography (IMAC) [13,14] and metal oxide chromatography (MOC) including titanium dioxide (TiO_2) allows us to describe a serine/threonine/tyrosine-phosphorylation dependent global landscape of cellular signaling at the network level [15,16]. In this chapter, we introduce recent technological development regarding quantitative phosphoproteomics and discuss the future direction of cancer research toward exploration of drug targets in complex signaling networks from a system-level point of view.

2. Shotgun proteomics technology

2.1. Mass spectrometry-based proteomics methodology

Recent progress in mass spectrometry-based proteomics technique has greatly contributed to elucidation of the regulatory networks constituted by a small amount of signaling-related molecules [17]. Especially, modern mass spectrometers termed linear ion trap (LTQ) Orbitrap instrument coupled to nano-flow liquid chromatography (nanoLC) enables us to identify and quantify thousands of signaling factors, leading to characterize diverse aspects of biological processes [18,19]. This system is made up of LTQ [20] and Orbitrap [21], which permits reliable peptide identification with high sensitivity, high mass resolution and high mass accuracy. In principle, there are two methodologies (in-gel digestion and in-solution digestion) for mass spectrometric sample preparation (Figure 1). Recently, liquid-fractionation entrapment technology has also been developed to improve comprehensiveness as well as sensitivity.

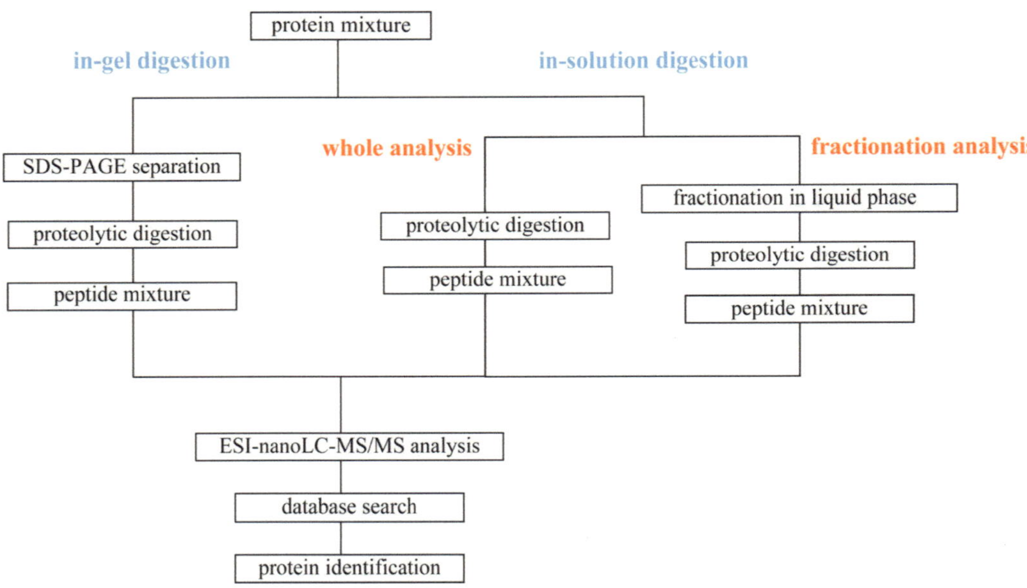

Figure 1. Experimental workflow for advanced mass spectrometry-based proteomics. Two standard methodologies (in-gel digestion and in-solution digestion) are usually applied to sample preparation.

2.2. In-solution fractionation techniques

In order to achieve peptide identification more comprehensively, in-solution fractionation techniques including two dimensional (2D) nanoLC system, Gelfree 8100 Fractionation System (Protein Discovery) [22] and 3100 OFFGEL Fractionator (Agilent) [23] have been developed for further sample separation. 2D nanoLC system consists of on-line strong cation exchange (SCX) and reversed-phase (RP) columns (Figure 2A), whereas off-line fractionation systems such as Gelfree 8100 Fractionation System and 3100 OFFGEL Fractionator separate proteins by molecular weight and isoelectric point, respectively

(Figure 2B, 2C). These systems enable us not only to reduce the complexity of samples but also to minimize the amount of starting materials compared with in-gel digestion.

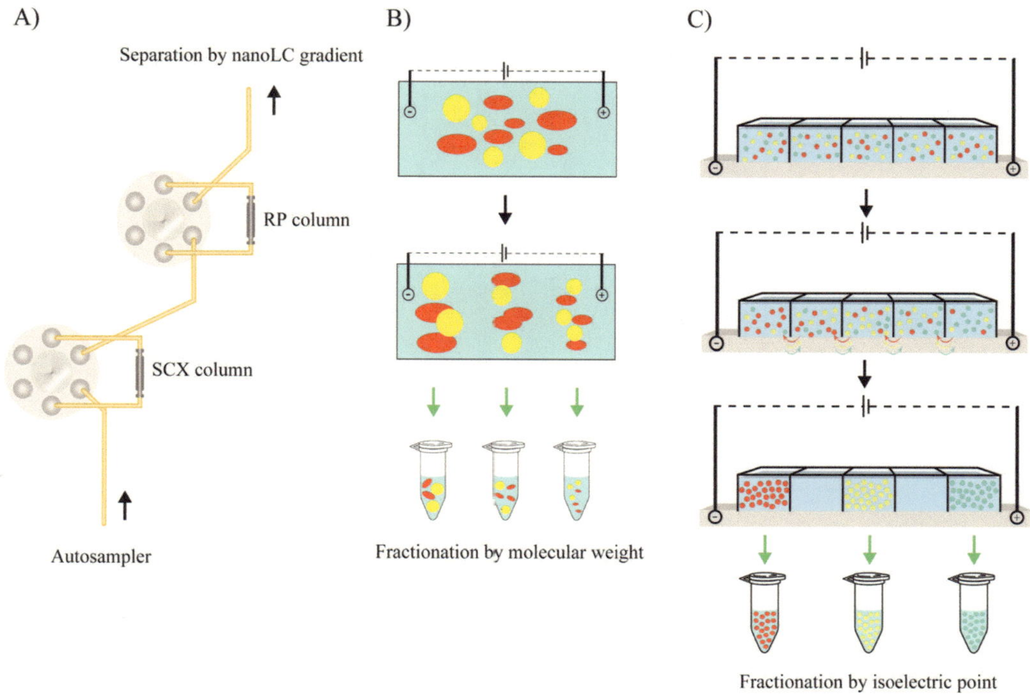

Figure 2. Schematic illustrations for in-solution protein/peptide separation techniques based on fractionation A) using SCX and RP columns (2D nanoLC system), B) by molecular weight (Gelfree 8100 Fractionation System) and C) by isoelectric point (3100 OFFGEL Fractionator).

3. Quantitative proteomics

Quantitative description based on mass spectrometry is not readily available because of the principle that ionization efficiency for mass spectrometric detection depends on the chemical property of each peptide. In recent years, several methods have been intensively developed for absolute and relative quantification [24]. The former methodology enables us to determine the absolute amount of proteins using standard peptides or proteins that are labeled by stable isotopes [25-27]. Meanwhile, the latter can provide information on the relative change in protein/peptide amount. There are two major approaches for relative quantification termed label-free and stable isotope-based methods.

3.1. Label-free methods

The label-free methods that utilize spectral counting or signal intensity for relative quantitation (Figure 3) are simple and economical but less accurate than isotope-based methods [28,29].

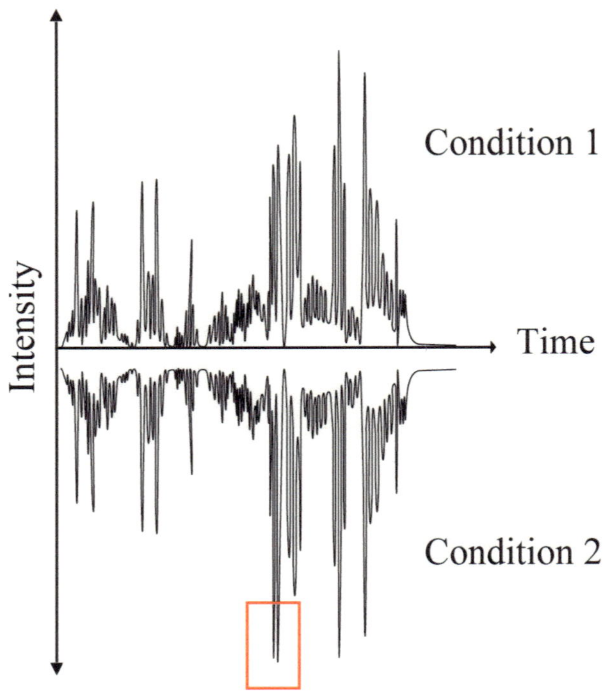

Figure 3. Representative chromatograms acquired under two different conditions. Relative quantitation can be performed by comparing these chromatograms. The red rectangle indicates the peak intensities increased in condition 2 compared with condition 1.

3.2. Stable isotope-based methods

Stable isotope-based methods allow us to distinguish the status of protein/peptide amount of even post translational modifications (PTMs) in a more accurate manner. Stable isotope-labeled reagents were incorporated into specific amino acids by chemical derivatization or metabolic labeling. Isotope-Coded Affinity Tag (ICAT) [30,31], isobaric Tag for Relative and Absolute Quantitation (iTRAQ) [32-34] and Tandem Mass Tag (TMT) [35,36] belong to the former chemical derivatization techniques. As for metabolic labeling strategies, Stable Isotope Labeling by Amino acids in Cell culture (SILAC) technique [37,38] is known as the most useful and accurate for relative quantitation.

3.2.1. ICAT

The chemical structure of the ICAT reagent consists of three regions: a reactive group with cysteine, an isotopically coded linker and a biotin tag (Figure 4). In order to perform a quantitative analysis, the cellular proteomes in two different conditions are labeled with light and heavy ICAT reagents, respectively. After the two samples are combined, they are proteolytically digested and purified with avidin affinity chromatography. The differential analyses are sequentially performed by detecting mass shift using liquid chromatography combined with tandem mass spectrometry (LC-MS/MS).

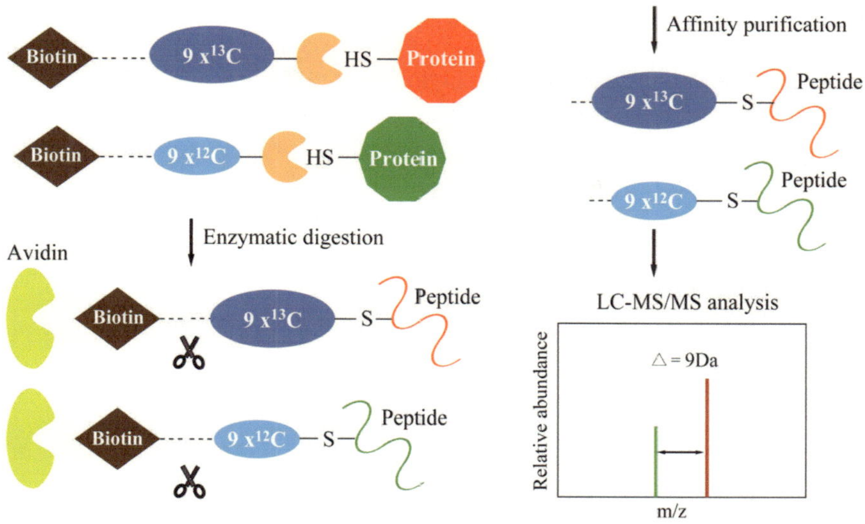

Figure 4. Peptide quantitation using cleavable ICAT. Differentially labeled peptides with ICAT tag at cysteine residues are preferentially enriched and analysed by LC-MS/MS. The ratio of heavy (red peak) to light (green peak) area indicates relative abundance of each peptide.

3.2.2. Isobaric reagents (iTRAQ and TMT)

The isobaric reagents such as iTRAQ and TMT contain an isobaric tag and an amine specific peptide reactive group. This strategy enables us to label all peptides derived from samples. Relative quantification of the mixed sample is performed at the MS/MS fragmentation stage (Figure 5).

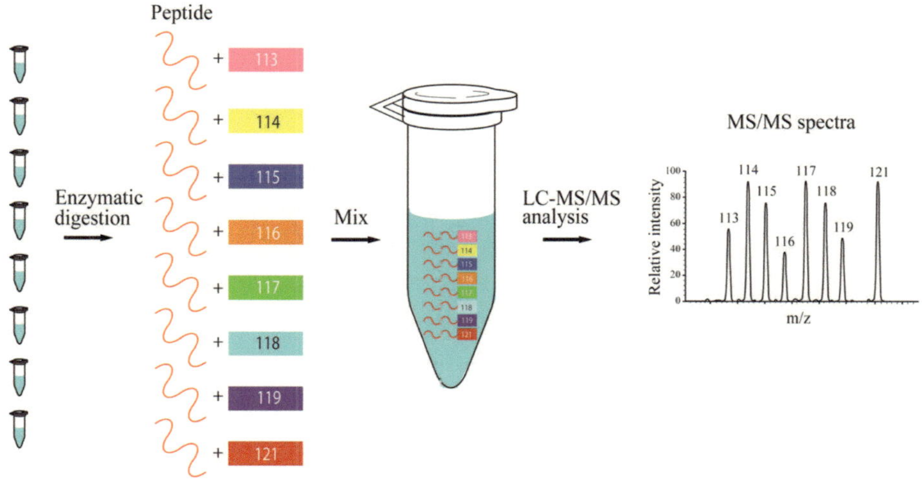

Figure 5. Peptide quantitation using iTRAQ. Peptides labeled by isobaric tags on the N-termini and lysine side chains are mixed and analyzed by LC-MS/MS. After fragmentation, MS/MS spectra of reporter ions are observed in the low mass region. The ratio of these peaks represents a relative amount of each peptide.

3.2.3. SILAC

As for metabolic labeling, Stable Isotope Labeling by Amino acids in Cell culture (SILAC) technique has widely been used to quantify protein abundance or PTM status in different conditions (Figure 6). Two cell populations are grown in different culture media including light or heavy stable isotopes of arginine and/or lysine. The lysates from these cell populations are equally combined, proteolytically digested and analyzed by LC-MS/MS. Regarding each mass pair detected, the ratio of the peak intensities corresponds to the relative peptide abundance.

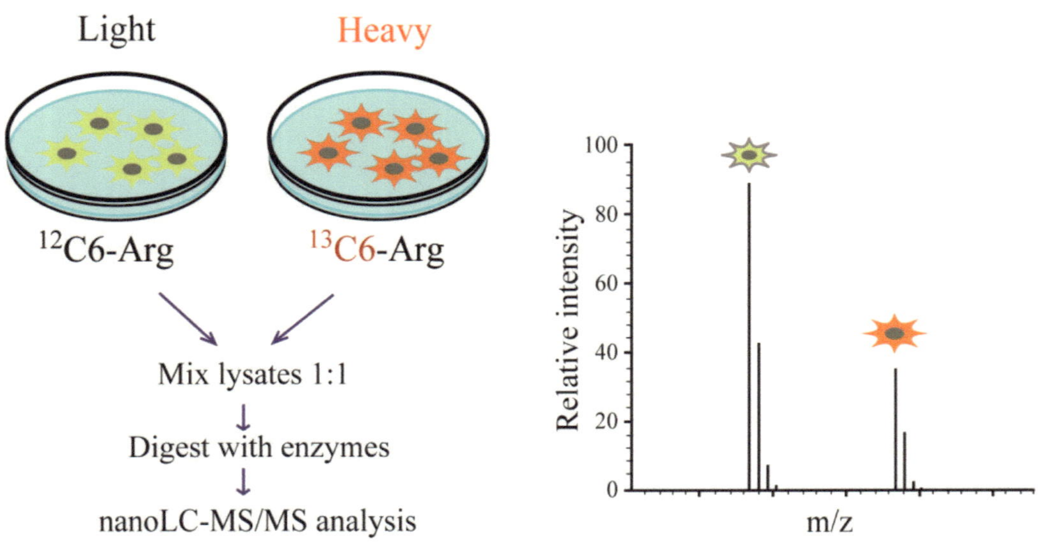

Figure 6. Peptide quantitation using SILAC. Proteins metabolically labeled by differential stable isotopes are combined, proteolytically digested and subjected to nanoLC-MS/MS analysis. The ratio of heavy to light peak area accounts for a relative amount of each peptide.

4. Analytical methodologies for enrichment of phosphorylated molecules

The mechanistic principles for transmitting signals within cellular networks rely greatly on PTMs such as phosphorylation, ubiquitination and acetylation. Although reversible phosphorylation events are well-studied in signal transduction research, a global landscape of phosphorylation-dependent signaling networks remains almost unclear. Here we introduce several phosphoprotein/phosphopeptide enrichment methods for mass spectrometry-based global phosphoproteome analysis.

4.1. Immunoprecipitation using anti-phosphotyrosine antibodies

Anti-phosphotyrosine antibodies are frequently used to enrich tyrosine-phosphorylated proteins (Figure 7A) for analyzing phosphotyrosine-based biological networks using mass spectrometry. These are some previous studies in which this methodology was successfully applied for phosphotyrosine-related signaling networks in leukemia cells [39] and human HeLa cells [10]. Salomon et al. identified 64 phosphorylation sites on 32 distinct proteins in leukemia cells by treatment with STI571 (Gleevec) [39]. Blagoev et al. showed that 81 signaling related molecules including 31 novel effectors were activated in response to epidermal growth factor (EGF) stimulation in a time-dependent manner [10]. These researches provided the key aspects of cellular regulation in each signaling context.

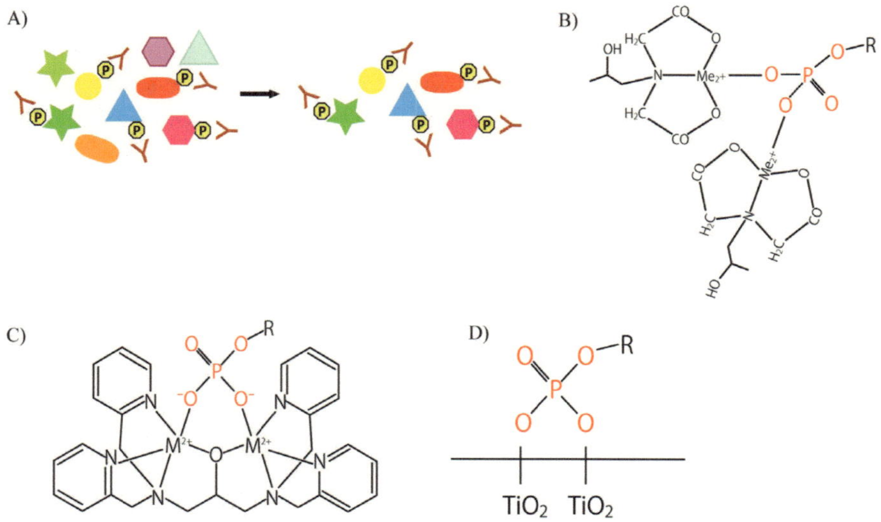

Figure 7. Overview of the affinity status of phosphorylated molecules with A) anti-phosphotyrosine antibody, B) IMAC, C) Phos-Tag and D) TiO_2

4.2. IMAC

Immobilized Metal Affinity Chromatography (IMAC) is based on the notion that phosphate groups can chelate with metal ions such as iron, zinc or gallium (Figure 7B). Stensballe et al. showed that some phosphopeptides could be unambiguously identified using only low-picomole of samples by Fe(III)-IMAC technique [13]. This approach is also known to be suitable for identification of multiply phosphorylated peptides rather than singly modified ones.

4.3. Phos-Tag

Phos-Tag has a vacancy on two metal ions that is accessible for phosphomonoester dianion (Figure 7C). The peptides with phosphorylated serine, threonine and tyrosine residues can be all captured by the chemical structure [40,41].

4.4. TiO_2

Titanium dioxide (TiO_2)-based method is one of the most frequently used technique for phosphopeptide enrichment (Figure 7D) [15,16]. Olsen et al. detected 6,600 phosphorylation sites on 2,244 proteins in human HeLa cells and showed that 14 % of the identified phosphorylation sites were altered by at least 2-fold in response to EGF stimulation [16]. The unbiased large-scale phosphoproteome data provided more extensive insights regarding phosphorylation-dependent cellular processes.

5. Proteomics-driven computational analysis

In recent years, several functional annotation and network analysis tools have been developed to understand cellular processes from a system-level point of view. Here we introduce two representative computational tools for analyzing large-scale proteome data. Database for Annotation, Visualization and Integrated Discovery (DAVID) [42] (http://david.abcc.ncifcrf.gov/home.jsp), which consists of an integrated biological knowledgebase and some analytical tools, enables extraction of the related information from the functional annotation databases (Figure 8).

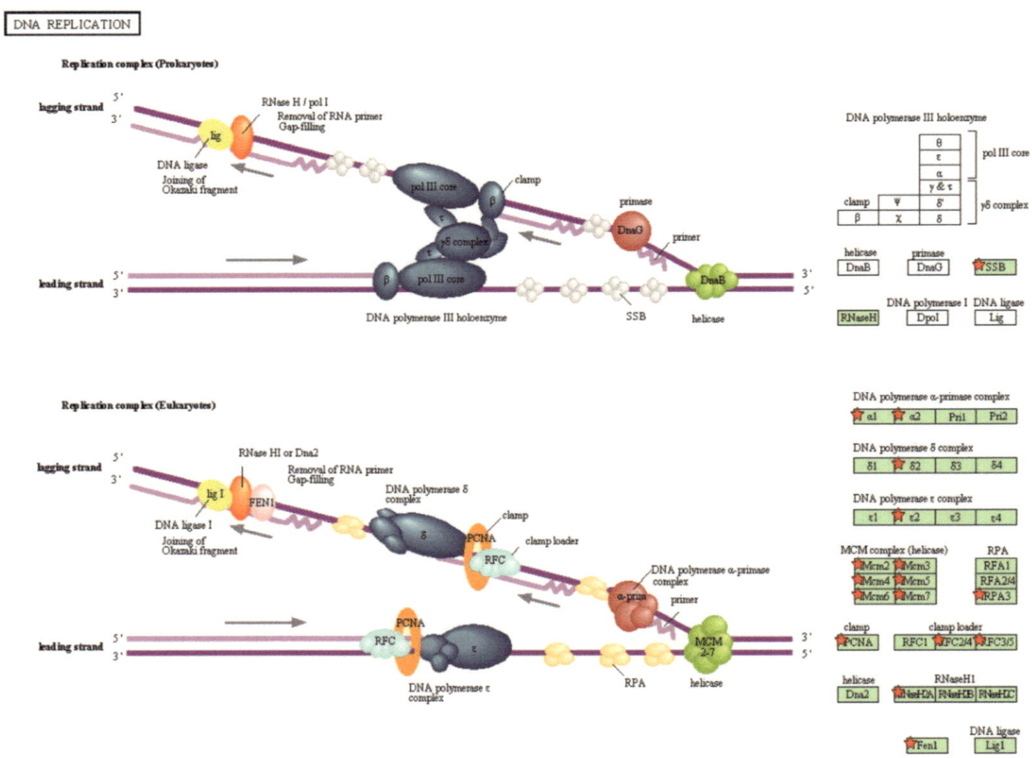

Figure 8. DAVID-based functional description of DNA replication (KEGG pathway). Red symbols indicate the molecules detected by the shotgun proteome analysis of glioblastoma stem cells [43].

Ingenuity Pathways Analysis (IPA) software (http://www.ingenuity.com) (Ingenuity Systems) is used to find networks in relation to experimental proteome data using the Ingenuity Knowledge Base derived from thousands of peer-reviewed journals (Figure 9).

A)

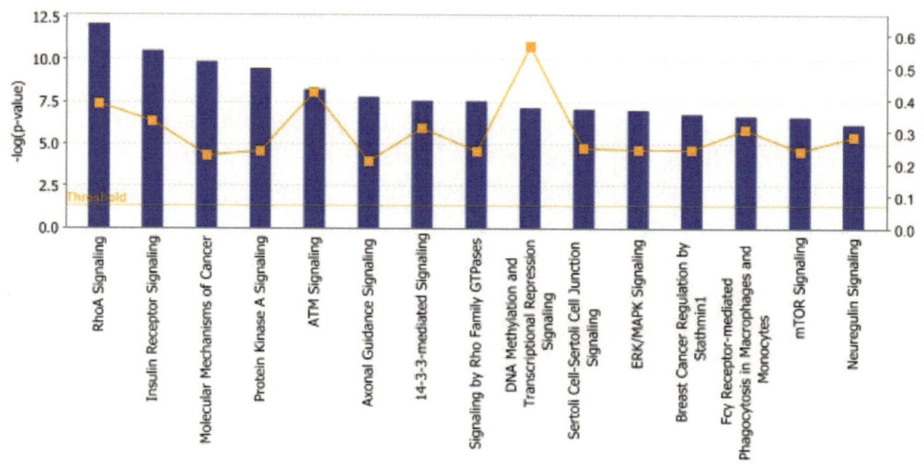

B)

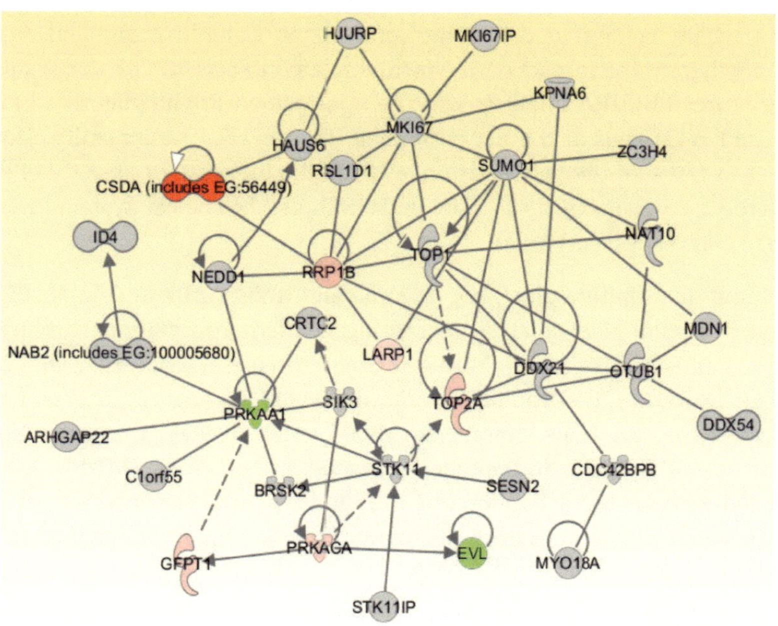

Figure 9. Representative description using IPA software. A) Statistical classification of canonical pathways extracted from experimental data. B) Pathway analysis based on quantitative proteome data.

6. Proteomics-based description of cancer signaling networks

6.1. Phosphoproteome dynamics in cancer cells

Signal transduction systems regulated by tyrosine phosphorylation events are widely known to play a crucial role in fundamental biological processes such as cell proliferation, differentiation and migration. Thus, phosphoproteomics-based approaches have first been applied to reveal the molecular mechanisms governed by tyrosine phosphorylation in response to external growth factors such as EGF [10,11,44,45], fibroblast growth factor (FGF) [46] or heregulin (HRG) [47]. Schulze et al. identified interaction partners of the four members belonging to the ErbB receptor family (EGFR, ErbB2, ErbB3 and ErbB4) using the corresponding synthetic peptides as baits in an unbiased proteomic manner [45]. They revealed that most interaction partners to tyrosine residues were located at the C-terminal end outside the kinase domain of each ErbB family member. Hinsby et al. demonstrated that 28 components were induced by basic fibroblast growth factor (bFGF) stimulation in FGFR-1 expressing cells [46]. The effect of EGF stimulation on human epithelial carcinoma A431 cells was also examined in a time-resolved manner [11] (Figure 10A). Among a total of 136 proteins identified, 56 molecules were quantified by more than 1.5-fold changes upon EGF stimulation. Moreover, the temporal perturbation effects of the Src-family kinase inhibitor, PP2, on the prolonged activation phase were also evaluated regarding various cellular proteins including Src-family kinase substrates. Consequently, the effect of PP2 on the molecules which belong to cell adhesion such as Catenin δ showed significant down-regulation, whereas the impact on the factors related to classical cascades such as EGFR was modest (Figure 10B). IPA analysis was then performed to elucidate the PP2 effects on the EGF-induced A431 cells at the network level (Figure 11). These results clearly showed the differences in tyrosine-phosphorylation levels in the presence or absence of PP2. Thus, these data provide further insight into how such complex biological systems would function in response to external perturbation.

By combining quantitative phosphoproteome and transcriptome data *in silico*, Oyama et al. performed a system-level analysis regarding cellular information networks in wild-type (WT) and tamoxifen-resistant (TamR) human breast adenocarcinoma MCF-7 cells in response to HRG and 17β-estradiol (E2) stimulation [47] (Figure 12). The integrative analysis of phosphoproteome and transcriptome in MCF-7 cells revealed that activation of glycogen-synthase kinase 3β (GSK3β) and mitogen-activated protein kinase (MAPK) 1/3 signaling might be associated with altered activation of CREB and AP-1 transcription factors in TamR MCF-7 cells, which potentially defines drug-resistance properties against tamoxifen (Figure 13).

6.2. Large-scale proteomic characterization of cancer stem/initiating cells

Cancer cells are widely known to be heterogeneous, even though they were derived from a single transformed cell [48]. Some of them show resistance to anti-cancer drugs and radiation therapies [49,50] and recent studies also demonstrated the existence of cancer stem cells (CSCs) in various types of cancer cells including leukemia [51], breast cancer [52], glioma [53,54] and colon cancer [55,56]. Moreover, it has been getting clear that CSCs have

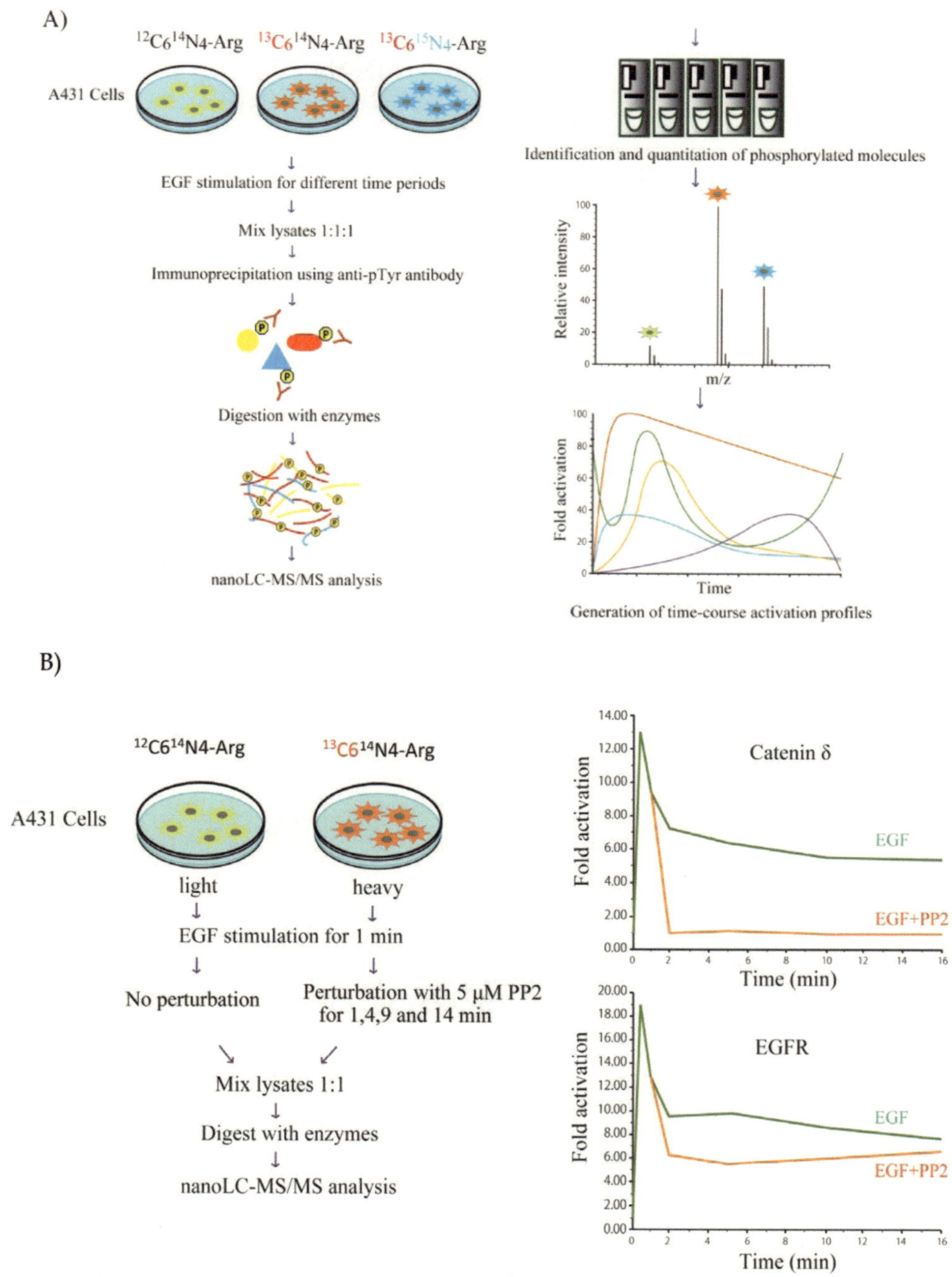

Figure 10. Schematic procedures for identification and SILAC-based quantitation of tyrosine-phosphoproteome in A431 cells [11]. A) The experimental procedure using three different SILAC media to describe tyrosine-phosphoproteome dynamics in response to EGF stimulation. B) Comparative analysis using two distinct SILAC media for evaluation of the perturbation effects by Src-family kinase inhibitor, PP2. Green lines show EGF activation profiles ,whereas red ones indicate temporal perturbation effects by PP2.

A)

B)

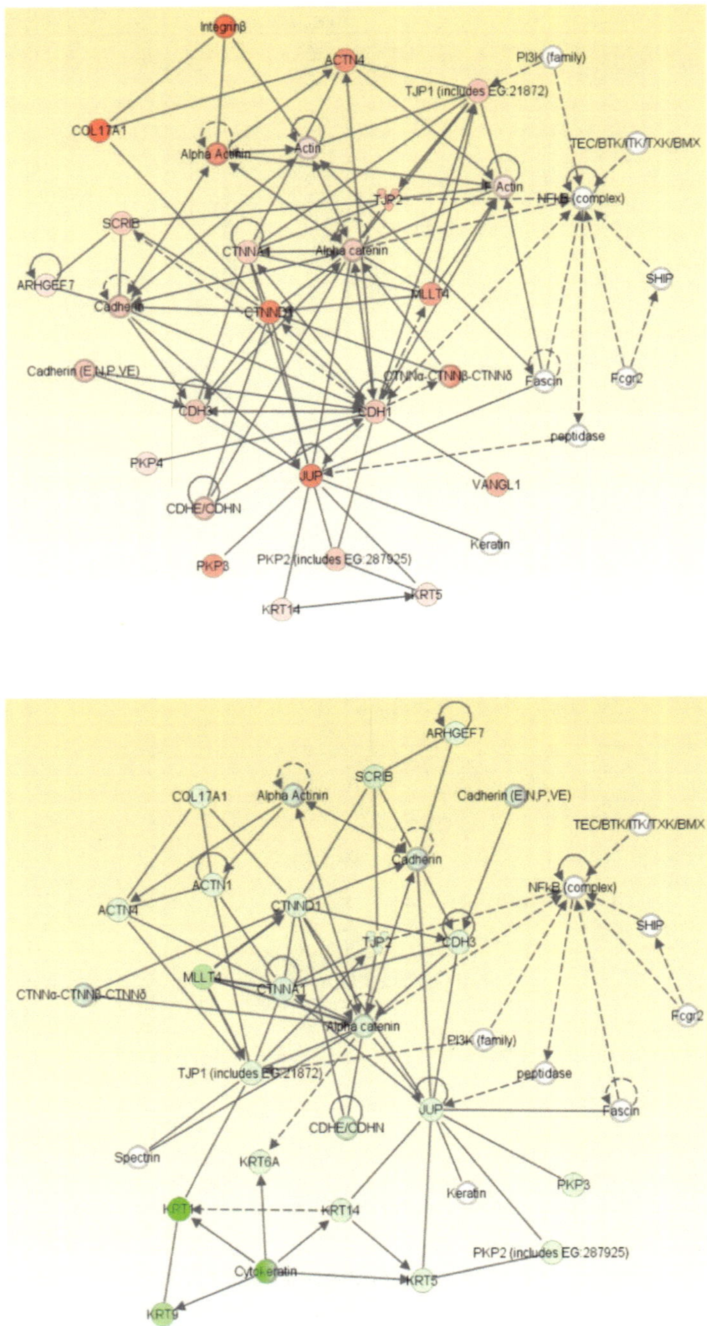

Figure 11. Network analysis of the quantitative phosphoproteome data on A431 cells A) upon EGF stimulation and B) subsequently perturbed by PP2, respectively. Red and green nodes indicate up- and down-regulated signalling molecules, respectively.

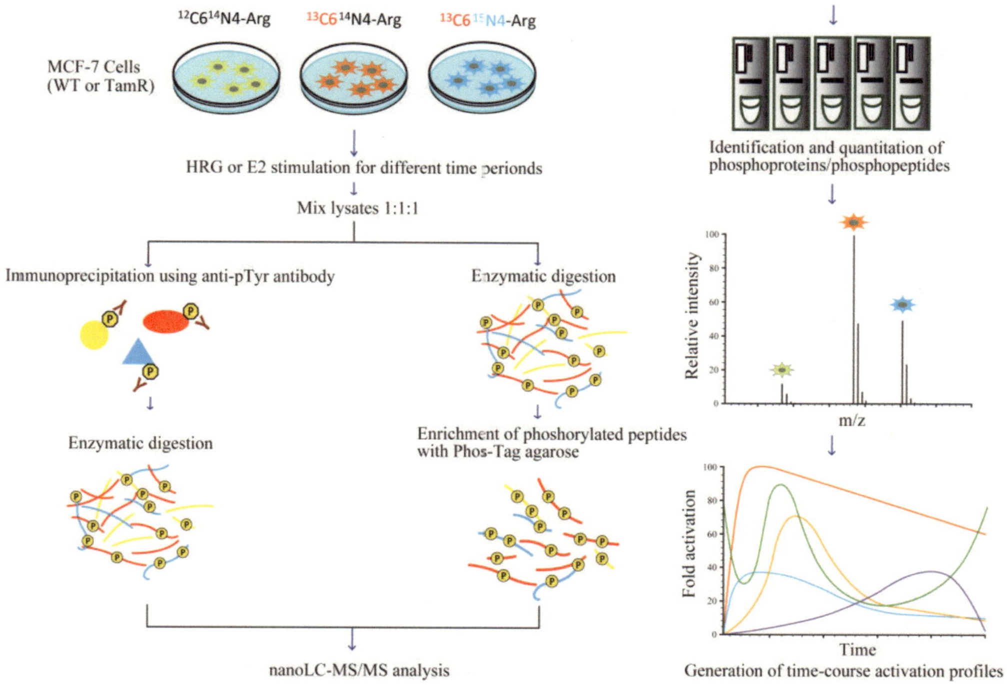

Figure 12. A schematic procedure for identification and quantitation of large-scale phosphoproteome in ligand-stimulated MCF7 cells [47]. The phosphorylated molecules captured by anti-pTyr antibodies or Phos-tag agarose were analysed by nanoLC-MS/MS.

the ability of treatment refractory [57-60] as well as biological properties similar to normal stem cells such as self-renewal and differentiation potency [61]. Recent studies also pointed out the possibility that CSCs were derived from normal stem cells and any non-CSCs might also convert to CSCs [62]. Therefore, comprehensive elucidation of signaling networks in CSCs is considered to be one of the most important steps in cancer research. Thus, we applied mass spectrometry-based shotgun proteomics technology to characterize protein expression profiles [43] and global phosphorylation-dependent signaling networks [63] in glioblastoma stem/initiating cells derived from brain tissues (Figure 14).

In order to gain a comprehensive overview of protein expression in glioblastoma stem/initiating cells, we conducted a shotgun proteome analysis, leading to identification of 2,089 proteins in total [43]. The DAVID-based pathway analysis showed the expressed proteome were enriched in ribosome (Figure 15), spliceosome and proteasome to a high degree. Thus, global protein expression analysis using advanced mass spectrometry offers novel viewpoints for characterization of key factors besides other methodologies such as fluorescence-activated cell sorting (FACS) and gene expression analyses.

The global phosphoproteome analysis of these glioblastoma stem cells also enabled us to determine 6,073 phosphopeptides derived from 2,282 proteins using two fragmentation methodologies of collision induced dissociation and higher energy C-trap dissociation [63]. The IPA analysis of the phosphoproteome data unveiled a variety of canonical pathways that have been reported to play a crucial role in cancer cells and normal stem cells (Figure 16). Among them, mTOR signaling, which is known to play an important part in stem cell regulation [64,65], was found to be one of the most highly enriched pathways. Very interestingly, the phosphorylation status of EIF4EBP1 and RPS6, which enhance mRNA translation, were up-regulated by EGF stimulation (Figure 17). The analysis also led to identification of various novel phosphorylation sites on the molecules with stem cell-like and glioma properties such as nestin and vimentin [66]. More intriguingly, some novel phosphopeptides derived from undefined regions within the human transcript sequences were also determined from the large-scale phosphoproteome data and the phosphorylation status of the peptide encoded by supervillin-like (LOC645954) was found to be altered upon EGF stimulation (Figure 18).

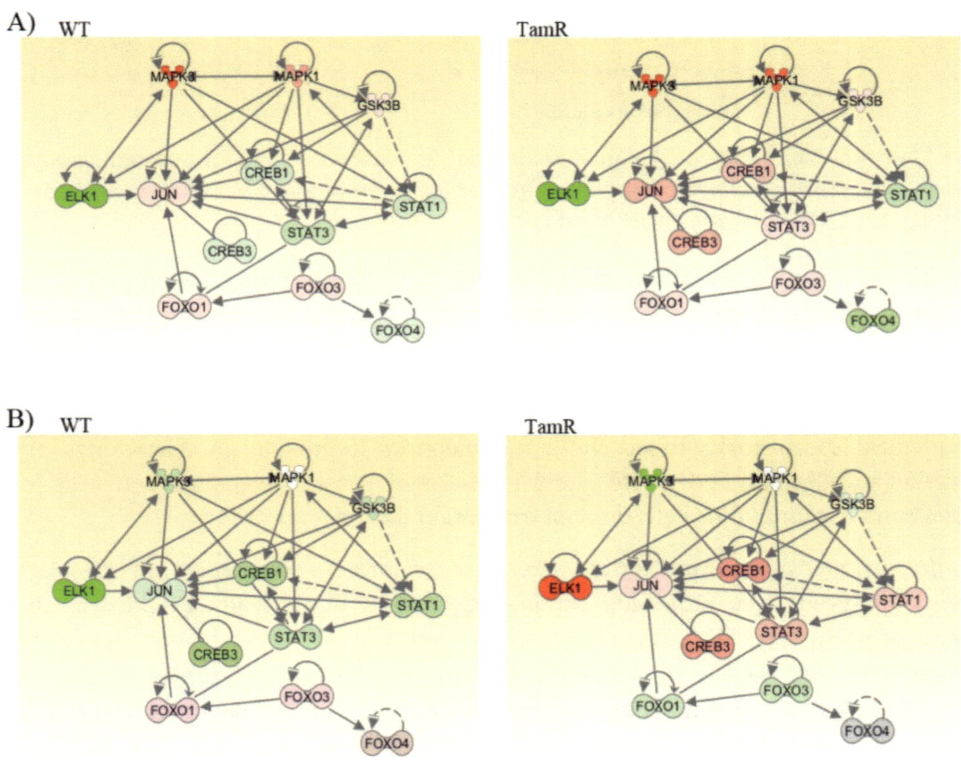

Figure 13. Integrative network analyses of quantitative phosphoproteome and transcriptome data obtained from MCF7 cells A) after HRG stimulation and B) after E2 stimulation. Red and green nodes indicate up- and down-regulated signaling molecules, respectively.

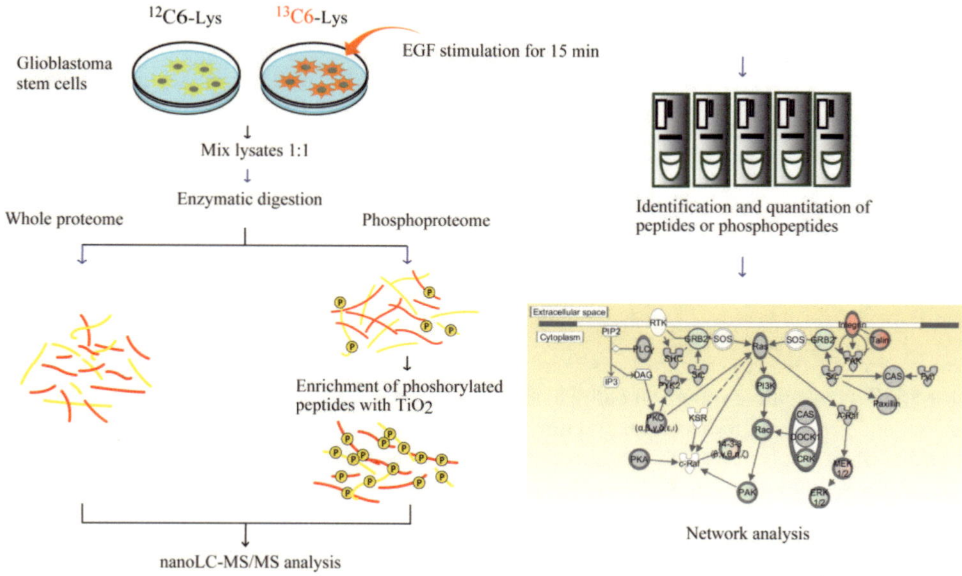

Figure 14. Schematic procedures for identification and quantitation of the expressed proteome and phosphoproteome in glioblastoma stem cells. The whole proteome and phosphoproteome were analysed by nanoLC-MS/MS.

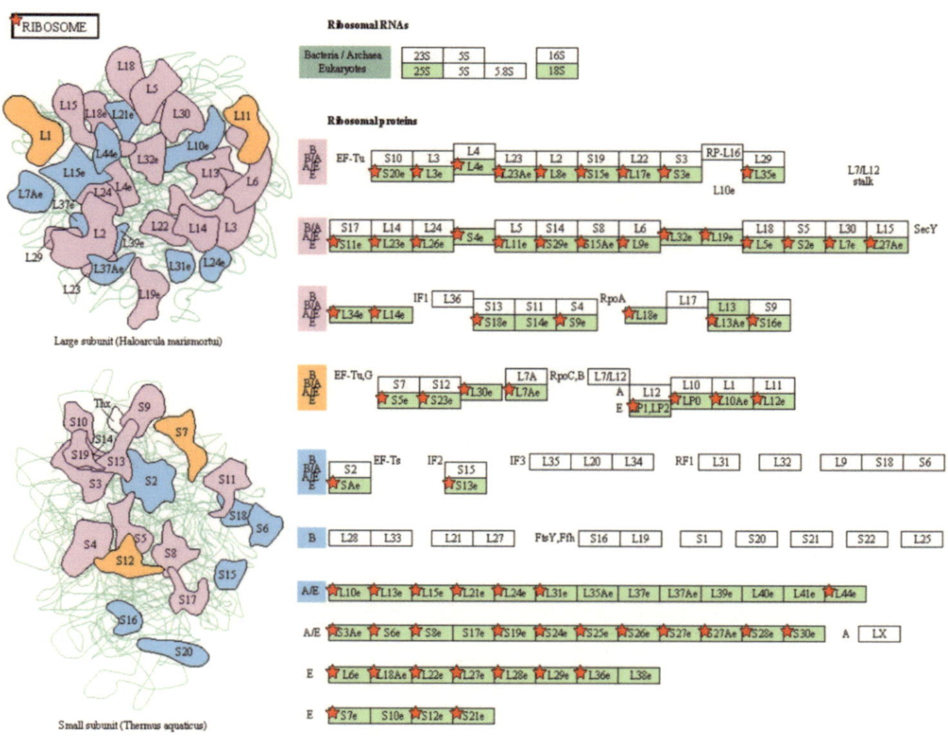

Figure 15. DAVID-based functional description of Ribosome pathway (KEGG pathway). Red symbols indicate the molecules detected in the proteomic analysis of glioblastoma stem cells [43].

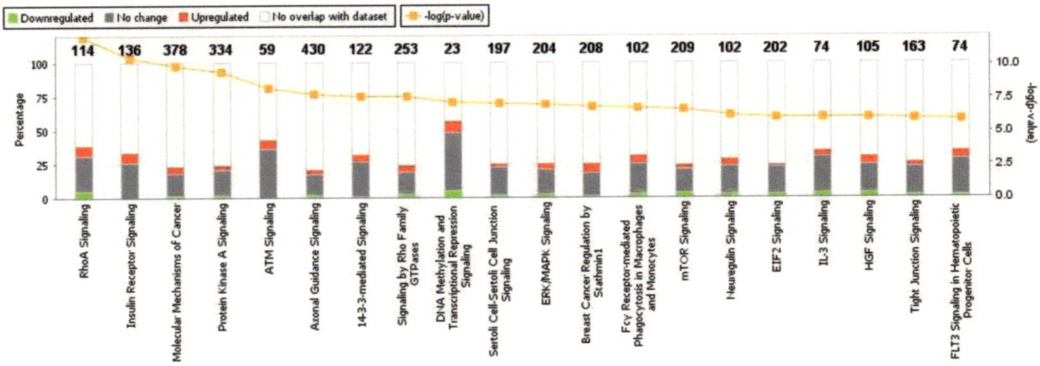

Figure 16. Representative canonical pathways enriched in the phophoproteome of glioblastoma stem cells. Red and green bars indicate up- and down-regulation of phosphorylation levels in response to EGF stimulation, respectively. Orange dots denote –log(p-value) by Fisher's Exact test, indicating the statistical significance of the molecules in each criterion.

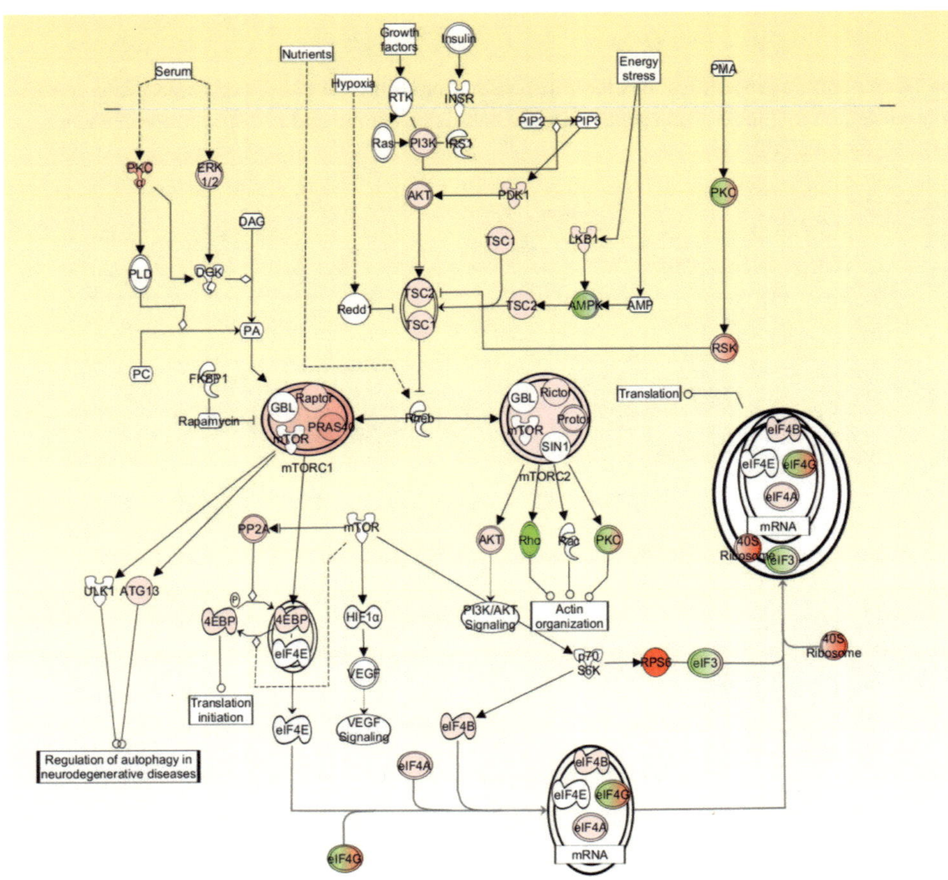

Figure 17. IPA-based network description of mTOR signaling extracted from the large-scale phosphoproteome data on glioblastoma stem cells. Red and green nodes indicate up- and down-regulated signaling effectors in response to EGF stimulation, respectively.

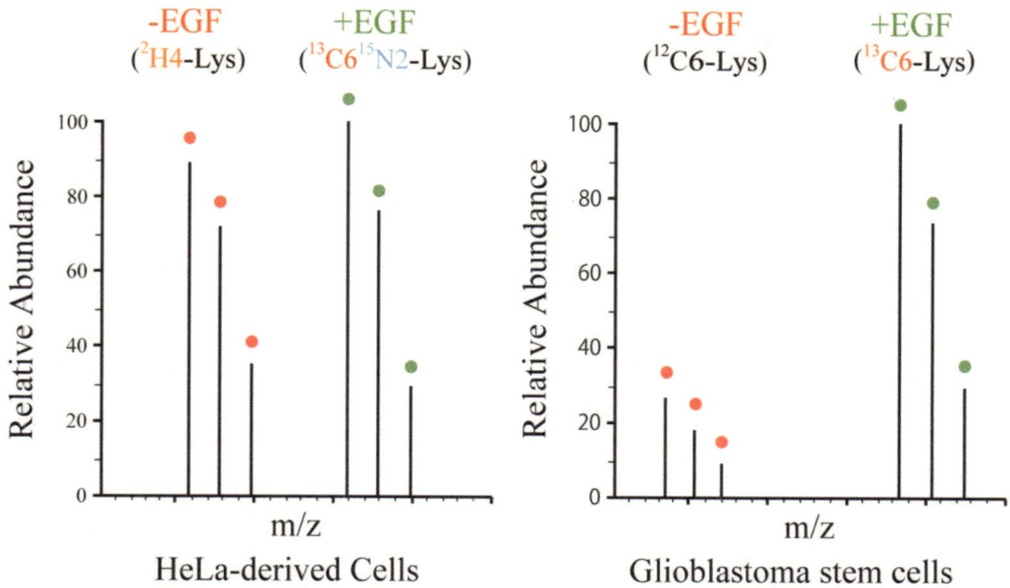

Figure 18. Mass spectra of the novel phosphopeptide encoded by supervillin-like (LOC645954) in HeLa-derived cells and glioblastoma stem cells upon EGF stimulation [63].

7. Conclusion

Advanced mass spectrometry-based proteomics has become a powerful tool for comprehensive understanding of signal transduction networks at the system level. In this chapter, we introduced recent proteomics technologies regarding relative quantitation and enrichment of phosphorylated proteins/peptides for large-scale description of signaling network dynamics. Utilizing these approaches, thousands of phosphorylation sites on diverse signaling-related molecules can now be identified in an unbiased fashion. Quantitative information on the effects of ligand stimulation and inhibitor perturbation also proved beneficial to understand the phosphorylation dynamics at the network level. Furthermore, extensive *in silico* analyses based on comprehensive proteome data enabled us to describe a system-level view of biological networks in a statistical manner. Consequently, mass-spectrometry-based proteomics will pave the way to evaluate molecular hubs in signaling systems and to develop novel targets for treatment of various diseases caused by signaling aberration [67,68].

Author details

Hiroko Kozuka-Hata, Yumi Goto and Masaaki Oyama
Medical Proteomics Laboratory, Institute of Medical Science, University of Tokyo, Shirokanedai, Minato-ku, Tokyo, Japan

Acknowledgement

We thank all the members of Medical Proteomics Laboratory, IMSUT. This work was supported by Genome Network Project and Cell Innovation Program, Ministry of Education, Culture, Sports, Science and Technology of Japan.

8. References

[1] Hunter T. Signaling—2000 and beyond. Cell 2000;100 (1): 113-27.

[2] Schlessinger J. Cell signaling by receptor tyrosine kinases. Cell 2000;103(2): 211-25.

[3] Cuesta N, Martín-Cófreces NB, Murga C, van Santen HM. Receptors, signaling networks, and disease. Sci Signal 2011;4(161): mr3.

[4] Cohen P. The twentieth century struggle to decipher insulin signalling. Nat Rev Mol Cell Biol 2006;7(11): 867-73.

[5] Aebersold R, Mann M. Mass spectrometry-based proteomics. Nature 2003;422 (6928): 198-207.

[6] Rikova K, Guo A, Zeng Q, Possemato A, Yu J, Haack H, Nardone J, Lee K, Reeves C, Li Y, Hu Y, Tan Z, Stokes M, Sullivan L, Mitchell J, Wetzel R, Macneill J, Ren JM, Yuan J, Bakalarski CE, Villen J, Kornhauser JM, Smith B, Li D, Zhou X, Gygi SP, Gu TL, Polakiewicz RD, Rush J, Comb MJ. Global survey of phosphotyrosine signaling identifies oncogenic kinases in lung cancer. Cell 2007;131(6): 1190-203.

[7] Stokes MP, Rush J, Macneill J, Ren JM, Sprott K, Nardone J, Yang V, Beausoleil SA, Gygi SP, Livingstone M, Zhang H, Polakiewicz RD, Comb MJ. Profiling of UV-induced ATM/ATR signaling pathways. Proc Natl Acad Sci U S A 2007;104(50): 19855-60.

[8] Mann M. Functional and quantitative proteomics using SILAC. Nat Rev Mol Cell Biol 2006;7(12): 952-8.

[9] Ong SE, Blagoev B, Kratchmarova I, Kristensen DB, Steen H, Pandey A, Mann M. Stable isotope labeling by amino acids in cell culture, SILAC, as a simple and accurate approach to expression proteomics. Mol Cell Proteomics 2002;1(5): 376-86.

[10] Blagoev B, Ong SE, Kratchmarova I, Mann M. Temporal analysis of phosphotyrosine-dependent signaling networks by quantitative proteomics. Nat Biotechnol 2004;22(9): 1139-45.

[11] Oyama M, Kozuka-Hata H, Tasaki S, Semba K, Hattori S, Sugano S, Inoue J, Yamamoto T. Temporal perturbation of tyrosine phosphoproteome dynamics reveals the system-wide regulatory networks. Mol Cell Proteomics 2009;8(2): 226-31.

[12] Hammond DE, Hyde R, Kratchmarova I, Beynon RJ, Blagoev B, Clague MJ. Quantitative analysis of HGF and EGF-dependent phosphotyrosine signaling networks. J Proteome Res 2010;9(5): 2734-42.

[13] Stensballe A, Andersen S, Jensen ON. Characterization of phosphoproteins from electrophoretic gels by nanoscale Fe(III) affinity chromatography with off-line mass spectrometry analysis. Proteomics 2001;1(2): 207-22.

[14] Ficarro SB, McCleland ML, Stukenberg PT, Burke DJ, Ross MM, Shabanowitz J, Hunt DF, White FM. Phosphoproteome analysis by mass spectrometry and its application to Saccharomyces cerevisiae. Nat Biotechnol 2002;20(3): 301-5.
[15] Larsen MR, Thingholm TE, Jensen ON, Roepstorff P, Jørgensen TJ. Highly selective enrichment of phosphorylated peptides from peptide mixtures using titanium dioxide microcolumns. Mol Cell Proteomics 2005;4(7): 873-86.
[16] Olsen J V, Blagoev B, Gnad F, Macek B, Kumar C, Mortensen P, Mann M. Global, in vivo, and site-specific phosphorylation dynamics in signaling networks. Cell 2006;127(3): 635-48.
[17] Walther TC, Mann M. Mass spectrometry-based proteomics in cell biology. J Cell Biol 2010;190(4): 491-500.
[18] Olsen JV, Schwartz JC, Griep-Raming J, Nielsen ML, Damoc E, Denisov E, Lange O, Remes P, Taylor D, Splendore M, Wouters ER, Senko M, Makarov A, Mann M, Horning S. A dual pressure linear ion trap Orbitrap instrument with very high sequencing speed. Mol Cell Proteomics 2009;8(12): 2759-69.
[19] Choudhary C, Mann M. Decoding signalling networks by mass spectrometry-based proteomics. Nat Rev Mol Cell Biol 2010;11(6): 427-39.
[20] Schwartz JC, Senko MW, Syka JE. A two-dimensional quadrupole ion trap mass spectrometer. J Am Soc Mass Spectrom 2002;13(6): 659-69.
[21] Hu Q, Noll RJ, Li H, Makarov A, Hardman M, Graham Cooks R. The Orbitrap: a new mass spectrometer. J Mass Spectrom 2005;40(4): 430-43.
[22] Tran JC, Doucette AA. Multiplexed size separation of intact proteins in solution phase for mass spectrometry. Anal Chem 2009;81(15): 6201-9.
[23] de Godoy LM, Olsen JV, Cox J, Nielsen ML, Hubner NC, Fröhlich F, Walther TC, Mann M. Comprehensive mass-spectrometry-based proteome quantification of haploid versus diploid yeast. Nature 2008;455(7217): 1251-4.
[24] Cox J, Mann M. Quantitative, high-resolution proteomics for data-driven systems biology. Annu Rev Biochem 2011;80: 273-99.
[25] Steen H, Jebanathirajah JA, Springer M, Kirschner MW. Stable isotope-free relative and absolute quantitation of protein phosphorylation stoichiometry by MS. Proc Natl Acad Sci U S A 2005;102(11): 3948-53.
[26] Hanke S, Besir H, Oesterhelt D, Mann M. Absolute SILAC for accurate quantitation of proteins in complex mixtures down to the attomole level. J Proteome Res 2008;7(3): 1118-30.
[27] Singh S, Springer M, Steen J, Kirschner MW, Steen H. FLEXIQuant: a novel tool for the absolute quantification of proteins, and the simultaneous identification and quantification of potentially modified peptides. J Proteome Res 2009;8(5): 2201-10.
[28] Liu B, Lin Y, Darwanto A, Song X, Xu G, Zhang K. Identification and characterization of propionylation at histone H3 lysine 23 in mammalian cells. J Biol Chem 2009;284(47): 32288-95.
[29] Sadygov R, Wohlschlegel J, Park SK, Xu T, Yates JR 3rd. Central limit theorem as an approximation for intensity-based scoring function. Anal Chem 2006;78(1): 89-95.

[30] Gygi SP, Rist B, Gerber SA, Turecek F, Gelb MH, Aebersold R. Quantitative analysis of complex protein mixtures using isotope-coded affinity tags. Nat Biotechnol 1999;17(10): 994–9.

[31] Yi EC, Li XJ, Cooke K, Lee H, Raught B, Page A, Aneliunas V, Hieter P, Goodlett DR, Aebersold R. Increased quantitative proteome coverage with (13)C/(12)C-based, acid-cleavable isotope-coded affinity tag reagent and modified data acquisition scheme. Proteomics 2005;5(2): 380-7.

[32] Ross PL, Huang YN, Marchese JN, Williamson B, Parker K, Hattan S, Khainovski N, Pillai S, Dey S, Daniels S, Purkayastha S, Juhasz P, Martin S, Bartlet-Jones M, He F, Jacobson A, Pappin DJ. Multiplexed protein quantitation in Saccharomyces cerevisiae using amine-reactive isobaric tagging reagents. Mol Cell Proteomics 2004;3(12): 1154–69.

[33] Zieske LR. A perspective on the use of iTRAQ reagent technology for protein complex and profiling studies. J Exp Bot 2006;57(7): 1501–8.

[34] Gafken PR, Lampe PD. Methodologies for characterizing phosphoproteins by mass spectrometry. Cell Commun Adhes 2006;13(5–6): 249–62.

[35] Thompson A, Schäfer J, Kuhn K, Kienle S, Schwarz J, Schmidt G, Neumann T, Johnstone R, Mohammed AK, Hamon C. Tandem mass tags: a novel quantification strategy for comparative analysis of complex protein mixtures by MS/MS. Anal Chem 2003;75(8): 1895–904.

[36] Dayon L, Hainard A, Licker V, Turck N, Kuhn K, Hochstrasser DF, Burkhard PR, Sanchez JC. Relative quantification of proteins in human cerebrospinal fluids by MS/MS using 6-plex isobaric tags. Anal Chem 2008;80(8): 2921–31.

[37] Ong SE, Blagoev B, Kratchmarova I, Kristensen DB, Steen H, Pandey A, Mann M. Stable isotope labeling by amino acids in cell culture, SILAC, as a simple and accurate approach to expression proteomics. Mol Cell Proteomics 2002;1(5): 376-86.

[38] Ong SE, Kratchmarova I, Mann M. Properties of 13C-substituted arginine in stable isotope labeling by amino acids in cell culture (SILAC). J Proteome Res 2003;2(2): 173-81.

[39] Salomon AR, Ficarro SB, Brill LM, Brinker A, Phung QT, Ericson C, Sauer K, Brock A, Horn DM, Schultz PG, Peters EC. Profiling of tyrosine phosphorylation pathways in human cells using mass spectrometry. Proc Natl Acad Sci U S A 2003;100(2): 443-8.

[40] Kinoshita E, Kinoshita-Kikuta E, Takiyama K, Koike T. Phosphate-binding tag, a new tool to visualize phosphorylated proteins. Mol Cell Proteomics 2006;5(4): 749-57.

[41] Nabetani T, Kim YJ, Watanabe M, Ohashi Y, Kamiguchi H, Hirabayashi Y. Improved method of phosphopeptides enrichment using biphasic phosphate-binding tag/C18 tip for versatile analysis of phosphorylation dynamics. Proteomics 2009;9(24): 5525-33.

[42] Dennis G Jr., Sherman BT, Hosack DA, Yang J, Gao W, Lane HC, Lempicki RA. DAVID: Database for Annotation, Visualization, and Integrated Discovery. Genome Biol 2003;4(5): P3.

[43] Kozuka-Hata H, Nasu-Nishimura Y, Koyama-Nasu Y, Ao-Kondo H, Tsumoto K, Akiyama T, Oyama M. Global proteome analysis of glioblastoma stem cells by high-

resolution mass spectrometry. Current Topics in Peptide & Protein Research 2012;13: 1-47.

[44] Tasaki S, Nagasaki M, Kozuka-Hata H, Semba K, Gotoh N, Hattori S, Inoue J, Yamamoto T, Miyano S, Sugano S, Oyama M. Phosphoproteomics-based modeling defines the regulatory mechanism underlying aberrant EGFR signaling. PLoS One 2010;5(11): e13926.

[45] Schulze WX, Deng L, Mann M. Phosphotyrosine interactome of the ErbB-receptor kinase family. Mol Syst Biol. 2005;1: 2005.0008.

[46] Hinsby AM, Olsen JV, Mann M. Tyrosine phosphoproteomics of fibroblast growth factor signaling: a role for insulin receptor substrate-4. J Biol Chem 2004;279(45): 46438-47.

[47] Oyama M, Nagashima T, Suzuki T, Kozuka-Hata H, Yumoto N, Shiraishi Y, Ikeda K, Kuroki Y, Gotoh N, Ishida T, Inoue S, Kitano H, Okada-Hatakeyama M. Integrated quantitative analysis of the phosphoproteome and transcriptome in tamoxifen-resistant breast cancer. J Biol Chem 2011;286(1): 818-29.

[48] Park CH, Bergsagel DE, McCulloch EA. Mouse myeloma tumor stem cells: a primary cell culture assay. J Natl Cancer Inst 1971;46(2): 411-22.

[49] Cho RW, Clarke MF. Recent advances in cancer stem cells. Curr Opin Genet Dev 2008;18(1): 48-53.

[50] Lobo NA, Shimono Y, Qian D, Clarke MF. The biology of cancer stem cells. Annu Rev Cell Dev Biol 2007;23: 675-99.

[51] Bonnet D, Dick JE. Human acute myeloid leukemia is organized as a hierarchy that originates from a primitive hematopoietic cell. Nat Med 1997;3(7): 730-7.

[52] Al-Hajj M, Wicha MS, Benito-Hernandez A, Morrison SJ, Clarke MF. Prospective identification of tumorigenic breast cancer cells. Proc Natl Acad Sci U S A 2003;100(7): 3983-8.

[53] Singh SK, Hawkins C, Clarke ID, Squire JA, Bayani J, Hide T, Henkelman RM, Cusimano MD, Dirks PB. Identification of human brain tumour initiating cells. Nature 2004;432(7015): 396-401.

[54] Lee J, Kotliarova S, Kotliarov Y, Li A, Su Q, Donin NM, Pastorino S, Purow BW, Christopher N, Zhang W, Park JK, Fine HA. Tumor stem cells derived from glioblastomas cultured in bFGF and EGF more closely mirror the phenotype and genotype of primary tumors than do serum-cultured cell lines. Cancer Cell 2006;9(5): 391-403.

[55] Dalerba P, Dylla SJ, Park IK, Liu R, Wang X, Cho RW, Hoey T, Gurney A, Huang EH, Simeone DM, Shelton AA, Parmiani G, Castelli C, Clarke MF. Phenotypic characterization of human colorectal cancer stem cells. Proc Natl Acad Sci U S A 2007;104(24): 10158-63.

[56] Ricci-Vitiani L, Lombardi DG, Pilozzi E, Biffoni M, Todaro M, Peschle C, De Maria R. Identification and expansion of human colon-cancer-initiating cells. Nature 2007;445(7123): 111-5.

[57] Diehn M, Cho RW, Lobo NA, Kalisky T, Dorie MJ, Kulp AN, Qian D, Lam JS, Ailles LE, Wong M, Joshua B, Kaplan MJ, Wapnir I, Dirbas FM, Somlo G, Garberoglio C, Paz B,

Shen J, Lau SK, Quake SR, Brown JM, Weissman IL, Clarke MF. Association of reactive oxygen species levels and radioresistance in cancer stem cells. Nature 2009;458(7239): 780-3.

[58] Phillips TM, McBride WH, Pajonk F. The response of CD24(-/low)/CD44+ breast cancer-initiating cells to radiation. J Natl Cancer Inst 2006;98(24): 1777-85.

[59] Liu G, Yuan X, Zeng Z, Tunici P, Ng H, Abdulkadir IR, Lu L, Irvin D, Black KL, Yu JS. Analysis of gene expression and chemoresistance of CD133+ cancer stem cells in glioblastoma. Mol Cancer 2006;5: 67.

[60] Bao S, Wu Q, McLendon RE, Hao Y, Shi Q, Hjelmeland AB, Dewhirst MW, Bigner DD, Rich JN. Glioma stem cells promote radioresistance by preferential activation of the DNA damage response. Nature 2006;444(7120): 756-60.

[61] Bianco P, Robey PG. Stem cells in tissue engineering. Nature 2001;414(6859): 118–21.

[62] Dontu G, Al-Hajj M, Abdallah WM, Clarke MF, Wicha MS. Stem cells in normal breast development and breast cancer. Cell Prolif 2003;36 Suppl 1: 59-72.

[63] Kozuka-Hata H, Nasu-Nishimura Y, Koyama-Nasu Y, Ao-Kondo H, Tsumoto K, Akiyama T, Oyama M. Phosphoproteome of human glioblastoma initiating cells reveals novel signaling regulators encoded by the transcriptome. PLoS ONE 2012;7(8): e43398.

[64] Murakami M, Ichisaka T, Maeda M, Oshiro N, Hara K, Edenhofer F, Kiyama H, Yonezawa K, Yamanaka S. mTOR is essential for growth and proliferation in early mouse embryos and embryonic stem cells. Mol Cell Biol 2004;24(15): 6710-8.

[65] Gangloff YG, Mueller M, Dann SG, Svoboda P, Sticker M, Spetz JF, Um SH, Brown EJ, Cereghini S, Thomas G, Kozma SC. Disruption of the mouse mTOR gene leads to early postimplantation lethality and prohibits embryonic stem cell development. Mol Cell Biol 2004;24(21): 9508-16.

[66] Mani SA, Guo W, Liao MJ, Eaton EN, Ayyanan A, Zhou AY, Brooks M, Reinhard F, Zhang CC, Shipitsin M, Campbell LL, Polyak K, Brisken C, Yang J, Weinberg RA. The epithelial-mesenchymal transition generates cells with properties of stem cells. Cell 2008;133(4): 704-15.

[67] Oyama M, Tasaki S, Kozuka-Hata H. Tyrosine-Phosphoproteome Dynamics. In: Choi S. (ed.) Systems Biology for Signaling Networks: Springer; 2010. p447-54.

[68] Kozuka-Hata H, Tasaki S, Oyama M. Phosphoproteomics-based systems analysis of signal transduction networks. Front Physiol 2011;2: 113.

Chapter 9

Phosphoproteomics for the Mapping of Altered Cell Signaling Networks in Breast Cancer

Olga Villamar-Cruz and Luis E. Arias-Romero

Additional information is available at the end of the chapter

http://dx.doi.org/10.5772/53109

1. Introduction

Breast cancer is the most commonly diagnosed cancer in women worldwide and consequently has been extensively investigated in terms of histopathology, immunochemistry and familial history [1]. Fortunately, technological advances have enabled characterization of the molecular subtypes of breast cancer [2, 3] and this in turn has facilitated the development of molecularly targeted therapeutics for this disease.

Profiling breast cancer with expression arrays has become common, and it has been suggested that the results from early studies will lead to understanding the molecular differences between clinical cases and allow individualization of care. Breast cancer may now be subclassified into luminal, basal, and ErbB2/HER2 subtypes with distinct differences in prognosis and response to therapy. These groups of tumors confirmed long-recognized clinical differences in phenotype, but added new knowledge regarding breast cancer biology. For example, the gene expression profiling revealed that within the estrogen receptor (ER)-positive tumors at least two subtypes, luminal A and luminal B, could be distinguished that vary markedly in gene expression and prognosis [3]. Conversely, hormone receptor–negative breast cancer comprised two distinct subtypes, the ErbB2 subtype and the basal-like subtype [3, 4]. These subtypes differ in biology and behavior, and both show a poor outcome. Importantly a very similar classification of breast cancers has now been characterized using immunohistochemistry to analyze patterns of protein expression in tumor sections and suggesting that a few protein biomarkers can be used to stratify breast cancers into different groups that can be mapped to the subtypes outlined below [5-8].

Luminal breast cancers are the most common subtype of breast cancer. The luminal subtypes make up the hormone receptor–expressing breast cancers, and have expression patterns reminiscent of the luminal epithelial component of the breast [2]. These patterns include expression of luminal cytokeratins 8/18, ER and genes associated with ER activation such as LIV1 and CCND1 (also known as cyclin D1) [2, 9]. Fewer than 20% of luminal tumors have mutations in TP53, and these tumors are often grade I [3, 9]. Within the luminal cluster there are at least two subtypes, luminal A and luminal B. Although both are hormone receptor expressing, these two luminal subtypes have distinguishing characteristics. Luminal A has, in general, higher expression of ER-related genes and lower expression of proliferative genes than luminal B [3, 4].

The basal-like subtype of breast cancer was so named because the expression pattern of this subtype mimicked that of the basal epithelial cells of other parts of the body and normal breast myoepithelial cells [2]. These similarities include lack of expression of ER and related genes; low expression of ErbB2; strong expression of basal cytokeratins 5, 6, and 17; and expression of proliferation-related genes [2, 9]. Immunohistochemical profiling using tissue microarrays has identified that a group of tumors characterized by basal cytokeratin expression are also characterized by low expression of BRCA1 *[10]*. Basal-like tumors are more likely to have aggressive features such as TP53 mutations and a markedly higher likelihood of being grade III ($P < 0.0001$) than luminal A breast cancers ($P < 0.0001$) [3].

Finally, the other breast cancer subtype that has been identified is distinguished by amplification of the gene encoding the human epidermal growth factor receptor 2 (ErbB2/HER2). The human ErbB/HER receptor family comprises four tyrosine kinase receptors (HER1/ErbB1, also termed the epidermal growth factor receptor (EGFR), HER2/ErbB2, HER3/ErbB3, and HER4/ErbB4) that play important roles in the progression of various types of cancers, including breast, prostate, and colon cancer [11]. Deregulation of ErbB receptor signaling leads to enhanced cell proliferation, migration, and malignant transformation. Overexpression, amplification, or mutation of the *ERBB2* gene occurs in approximately 20–30% of invasive breast cancers, and is associated with disease progression, poor prognosis, increased risk of metastases and shorter overall survival [12].

ErbB2-mediated signal transduction is believed to depend largely on heterodimerization with EGFR or ErbB3, and these heterodimers activate a signaling program that drives cell proliferation, resistance to apoptosis, loss of polarity, and increased motility and invasiveness [13, 14]. Trastuzumab is a humanized monoclonal antibody targeted against the extracellular portion of ErbB2. This is the first ErbB2-targeted agent to be approved by the United States Food and Drug Administration (FDA) for the treatment of both early stage and metastatic ErbB2-overexpressing (ErbB2 positive) breast cancers [15, 16]. Subsequently, lapatinib, an orally bioavailable small molecule dual ErbB2- and EGFR/HER1-specific tyrosine kinase inhibitor (TKI), received FDA approval in combination with capecitabine for patients with advanced ErbB2 positive breast cancer [17].

Although ErbB2-targeted therapies have had a significant impact on patient outcomes, resistance to these agents is common. In clinical trials, 74% of patients with ErbB2 positive metastatic breast cancer did not have a tumor response to first-line trastuzumab monotherapy [18] and 50% did not respond to trastuzumab in combination with chemotherapy [15]. These examples illustrate the problem that inherent (*de novo*) resistance to ErbB2-targeted agents poses for effective treatment of ErbB2 positive breast cancer. Moreover, only approximately one-quarter of patients with ErbB2 positive metastatic breast cancer who were previously treated with trastuzumab achieved a response with lapatinib plus capecitabine [17]. These limitations have led to efforts to better understand the underlying cellular networks that confer resistance to these agents in order to better select patients who are most likely to benefit from specific therapies and to develop new agents that can overcome resistance.

The goal of this review is to give a concise overview of current approaches in the field of phosphoproteomics and to show how a combination of several approaches can be used to obtain a more comprehensive understanding of a given signaling pathway. A number of proteomic approaches have been developed over the years to identify aberrantly activated kinases and their downstream substrates. Most often, phosphorylation is used as a surrogate for monitoring kinase activity in cells. In the past, kinases and their activities were generally studied on an individual basis using biochemical approaches. However, technological advances in the recent past have led to development of several high-throughput strategies to study the phosphoproteome. High-throughput technologies for monitoring phosphorylation events include array-based technologies such as peptide arrays [19-21], antibody arrays [22] and mass spectrometry [23, 24]. Quantitative phosphoproteomic profiling allows researchers to investigate aberrantly activated signaling pathways and therapeutic targets in cancers. Finally, phosphoproteomic approaches can not only assist in determining the appropriate therapeutic targets but also elucidate mechanisms such as off-target effects resulting from binding of inhibitors to unintended kinases/non-kinase proteins. Here, we will discuss some of the popular approaches to characterize the kinome and the phosphoproteome along with illustrative examples where such approaches have been employed for global analysis of breast cancer.

2. Challenges of phosphoproteomics

Phosphoproteomic analysis is plagued by the same challenges facing all proteomic experiments: complexity, dynamic range, and temporal dynamics. The true complexity of the phosphoproteome has yet to be determined, but the Phosphosite database (http://www.phosphosite.org) now lists 30 000 phosphorylation sites on 17 000 proteins, and this number is steadily increasing as each large-scale phosphorylation analysis continues to identify a large number of novel sites. With so many of the proteins in the cell being phosphorylated, the dynamic range of the phosphoproteome is similar to that of the proteome (i.e., $1x10^9$), but is further increased by substoichiometric modification. In addition, the temporal dynamics of protein phosphorylation regulate the rapid activation and deactivation of cellular signaling networks, further complicating analysis of the phosphoproteome. So the challenge is not simply to identify and catalog all of the phosphorylation sites, but rather to identify the site, quantify the stoichiometry, and monitor the temporal change in phosphorylation in response to a variety of cellular perturbations. Performing this task on a large number of phosphorylation sites across a broad swath of the signaling network is especially challenging, but is required to understand the mechanisms by which protein phosphorylation controls cell biology

3. Mass Spectometry (MS)-based approaches

Currently, the most powerful tool to interrogate the phosphoproteome is enrichment for phosphopeptides followed by reverse-phase liquid chromatography combined with tandem mass spectrometry (LC-MS/MS). When sample preparation and instrumentation are chosen appropriately, thousands of phosphorylation sites can be identified (**Figure 1**). Some research groups have already taken advantage of these methodologies for identifying proteins that could be useful therapeutic targets or novel molecular markers in breast cancer specimens. Many of these analyses have focused in tyrosine phosphorylation profiles due to the fact that approximately half of the tyrosine kinase complement of the human kinome is implicated in human cancers [4], and provides important targets for cancer treatment, as well as biomarkers for patient stratification. Recently, Chen et al. adapted LC-MS/MS technology to assess the tyrosine phosphorylation profile in the MCF10AT model of breast cancer progression [25]. This study identified and validated seven proteins, termed SPAG9, CYFIP1, RPS2, TOLLIP, SLC4A7, WBP2, and NSFLC1, to be authentic tyrosine kinase substrates. In addition, SPAG9, WBP2, TOLLIP, and NSFL1C were demonstrated to be authentic tyrosine phosphorylation targets of EGFR signaling, and differential expression of TOLLIP and SLC4A7 was subsequently validated in clinical breast cancer samples. Consistent with the MCF10AT model, more than 30% of the human breast cancer samples analyzed in this study displayed reduced expression of SLC4A7 compared with normal tissues. In contrast, only 25% of the samples showed increased levels of TOLLIP when normal cells become cancerous. Moreover detection of aberrant expression of TOLLIP and SLC4A7 in pre-neoplastic lesions suggests that they represent potential biomarkers that could complement mammography and histopathology for screening and early detection of breast cancer [25].

Most recently, a number of reports have demonstrated the importance of EGFR signaling in breast cancer [26-28]. Hochgrafe et al. characterized the tyrosine kinase signaling networks associated with different breast cancer subgroups [27]. By using this approach in a panel of 15 different breast cancer cell lines, the authors identified 544 phosphotyrosine sites in peptide sequences derived form 295 non redundant proteins, interestingly, 31 of these are novel tyrosine phosphorylation sites. Upon unsupervised hierarchical clustering using data for all tyrosine phosphorylated proteins, the 15 cell lines were clustered into two groups previously characterized as "basal" or "luminal" by transcript profiling [29]. Increased phosphorylation of several tyrosine kinases (i.e. Met, Lyn/Hck, EphA2, EGFR, and FAK) was characteristic of basal lines. In contrast, IGF1R/INSR, ErbB2, and ACK1 exhibited increased phosphorylation in luminal breast cancer cells. For all of the differentially phosphorylated kinases, increased phosphorylation was detected on sites that positively regulate kinase activity and downstream signaling. For example, Met Y1234, Lyn Y397, and FAK Y577 are activation loop sites [30], and phosphorylation of Y588 and Y594 in the juxtamembrane region of EphA2 is required for kinase activity [31]. In the case of EGFR and ErbB2, differential phosphorylation was predominantly on sites in the COOH-terminal tail that promote activation of the Ras/Raf/MEK/ERK pathway [32, 33]. A deeper analysis of the tyrosine phosphoproteome revealed a signature that characterizes the basal phenotype, and identified a prominent Src family kinase (SFK) signaling network in basal breast cancer cells that extends not only downstream to canonical SFK substrates regulating cell adhesion and migration but also upstream to specific RTKs such as EGFR, ErbB2 and Met among others. Subsequent functional analyses determined that SFKs transmit pro-proliferative, pro-survival and pro-mitogenic signals in these cells, and that Lyn is an important regulator of cell invasion. In addition, SFKs promoted tyrosine phosphorylation of specific RTKs in these cells, and this may attenuate cellular sensitivity to therapies directed against these receptors. Consequently, these findings provide important insights into the biology of basal breast cancers and have significant implications for the development of therapeutic strategies that target this subtype of breast cancer [27].

A very elegant study performed by Zhang et al. analyzed the EGF induced protein phosphorylation events in the Human Mammary Epithelial Cell (HMMC) 184A1 [26]. In this report, a time course phosphorylation profile of 78 tyrosine phosphorylation sites on 58 proteins was generated. For each phosphorylation site, a quantitative temporal phosphorylation profile was generated by comparing the relative ratios of peak areas for the iTRAQ marker ions in the MS/MS spectrum. Of the 58 proteins identified in this analysis, 52 have been already associated with the EGFR signaling network, whereas the other six proteins have not been previously identified in either proteomic or biochemical analyses of EGFR signaling. Contained in this group are phosphorylation sites on hypothetical protein FLJ00269, hypothetical protein FLJ21610, target of myb1-like 2 protein, and chromosome 3 open reading frame 6. In addition to the six proteins that had not been previously characterized in the EGFR signaling network, the authors also identified several novel phosphorylation sites on proteins known to be in the network. The bioinformatic analysis of the data generated by this method self-organize into clusters of phosphorylation sites that correlate with well known signaling nodes reported in the literature (i.e. the Ras/Raf/MEK/ERK and PI3K/AKT signaling pathways). In a related study, the same research group analyzed the EGF- and heregulin (HRG)-induced protein phosphorylation events that control cell migration and proliferation in the context of ErbB2 overexpression in HMMCs [34]. As a result of these analyses, 332 phosphorylated peptides from 175 proteins were identified, including 289 singly (tyrosine) phosphorylated peptides, 42 doubly phosphorylated peptides (21 tyrosine/tyrosine, 18 serine/tyrosine, and three threonine/tyrosine), and one triply phosphorylated peptide (tyrosine/tyrosine/tyrosine). A total of 20 phosphorylation sites were identified on EGFR, ErbB2, and ErbB3, including nine tyrosine and two serine sites on EGFR, eight tyrosine phosphorylation sites on ErbB2, and one tyrosine phosphorylation site on ErbB3. Of the 20 phosphorylation sites on EGFR family members, Y1114 on EGFR and Y1005 and Y1127 on ErbB2 represent novel sites that have not been previously described in the literature. To correlate signals with cell response, the authors also quantified proliferation and migration rates for these same cell states and stimulation conditions. Phenotypically, ErbB2 overexpression promoted increased cell migration, but had minimal effect on cell proliferation. More specifically, EGF stimulation of ErbB2-overexpressing cells promoted migration by the phosphorylation of proteins from multiple pathways (e.g., PI3K, MAPK, catenins, and FAK), whereas HRG stimulation of ErbB2-overexpressing cells activated only a very specific subset of proteins in the canonical migration pathway, in particular FAK, Src, paxillin, and p130Cas. In contrast, proliferation was primarily driven by EGF stimulation, and was not affected by ErbB2 expression levels [34]. Finally, Kumar et al. significantly extend their previous analysis of ErbB2-mediated signaling and cell function by using a model that predicts ErbB2 effects on HMMCs behavior by using MS phosphotyrosine data sets [28]. The results of this research showed that ErbB2 overexpression in the presence of EGF, as discussed above, produced interesting signal network changes and increased cell migration but did not affect cell proliferation [34]. These findings both highlight previously identified elements in the ErbB2 signaling network, and suggest new pathways and targets critically implicated in ErbB2-mediated signaling and its effect on migration and proliferation.

Although MS has proven to be an extraordinary tool for protein characterization, measurement of peptide intensities alone does not immediately provide quantitative information. There are several approaches to overcome this problem. Stable isotopes are incorporated either by metabolic labeling, as in the SILAC (stable isotope labeling with amino acids in cell culture) method, or by chemical derivatization **(Figure 1)** [35]. SILAC relies on metabolic incorporation of an isotopically labeled amino acid. Two groups of cells are grown in culture media that are identical except in one respect: the first media contains the "light" and the other a "heavy" form of a particular amino acid (for e.g. L-leucine or deuterated L-leucine). Through the use of special cell culture medium lacking the modified amino acids, the cells are forced to use the particular labeled or unlabeled form of the amino acid previously added to the medium. In each cell doubling, the cell population replaces at least half of the original form of the amino acid, eventually incorporating 100% of a given light or heavy form of the amino acid. A variety of amino acids are suitable in SILAC, including arginine, leucine, lysine, serine, methionine and tyrosine. The different cell line conditioned media can then be combined and run together in a single MS run. The advantages of SILAC include the fact that the labeling process is highly efficient, it does not require additional purifications to remove excess labeling reagent, nor does it involve multi-step labeling protocols and the sample preparation bias introduced by the comparison of two separate preparation steps is avoided. As well, SILAC allows the experimenter to use any method of protein or peptide purification (after enzymatic digestion) without introducing error into the final quantitative analysis. In one study, SILAC was utilized to examine differential membrane expression between normal and malignant breast cancer cells [36]. Approximately 1,000 proteins were identified with more than 800 of these proteins being classified as membrane or membrane-associated. Although the majority of the proteins remained unchanged when compared with the corresponding normal cells, a number of proteins were found upregulated or down-regulated by greater than 3-fold.

A few years ago, Bose et al. described a quantitative proteomic analysis to study ErbB2 signaling by using SILAC in 3T3 cells ectopically expressing ErbB2 [37]. By using this methodology, the authors identified a panel of 198 proteins that displayed increased phosphorylation levels and a group of 81 proteins that showed decreased phosphorylation levels merely by ErbB2 overexpression. The list of proteins that showed high phosphorylation levels included several well known ErbB2 downstream effectors and modulators of pro-survival, anti-apoptotic and proliferative pathways, such as PLCγ1, the regulatory and catalytic subunits of PI3K (p85β, p85α, and p110β), the Src family member Fyn, RasGAP, and HSP90. Importantly, several known EGFR signaling proteins, which had not been previously implicated in ErbB2 signaling, were also identified, including Stat1, Dok1, and δ-catenin. The 81 proteins that displayed decreased phosphorylation levels in 3T3-ErbB2 cells included FAK, p130-Cas/BCAR1, and caveolin 1 among others. In this study, the effect of the EGFR and ErbB2 selective tyrosine kinase inhibitor (TKI), PD168393, was also quantified, the results showed that 83 of the 198 proteins that displayed increased phosphorylation when ErbB2 was overexpressed were inhibited by 100 nM of PD168393 (>1.5-fold), and 27 proteins showed a smaller degree of inhibition (1.3- to 1.5-fold), suggesting that 110 of these 198 proteins are affected by this TKI. Under these conditions, 79 proteins were not affected by PD168393, including Fyn and three subunits of PI3K. This observation raises the question of whether different arms of the ErbB2 signaling pathway have differential inhibitor sensitivity. To validate the relevance of these proteins to ErbB2 signaling in a more realistic setting, the authors used the ErbB2 positive breast cancer cell line BT-474. As expected, PD168393 also inhibited the phosphorylation of PLCγ1 and Stat1 in BT-474 cells, supporting the idea that phosphoproteins identified by performing SILAC on 3T3-ErbB2 cells may be applicable to other ErbB2-overexpressing cell lines.

Although SILAC has proven to be a very powerful method to dissect signaling in tumor cell lines, metabolic labeling has a major limitation. Whereas proteins in cultured cells can be readily labeled, those in living organisms cannot. Approaches have been developed to metabolically label worms, flies [38] and even mice [39] and rats [40], but human tissues have to this day remained 'unlabelable'. When applying proteomics to tumor biology, it is imperative to quantify a representative number of proteins, to obtain reproducible results and to study cancer-relevant proteins of low abundance. Ishihama et al. have tried to solve this problem by adding labeled cultured cells to the tissue samples [41]. However the comparison of a single cell line with a whole tissue context has several limitations. More recently, Geiger et al. mixed labeled protein lysates from several previously established cancer-derived cell lines, which together are more representative of the full complexity of a tissue proteome than a single cell line, thereby increasing accuracy [42]. Initially, they SILAC-labeled the breast cancer cell line HCC1599 and mixed the lysate with the lysate of mammary carcinoma tissue from an individual with grade II lobular carcinoma. Although they were able to quantify 4,438 proteins at least once in triplicate analysis, the ratio distribution was broad and bimodal, containing 755 proteins with more than fourfold higher expression in the tumor compared to the cell line. Next, they selected four breast cancer cell lines differing in origin, stage, ER and ErbB2 expression; and this superset of SILAC-labeled cell lines that more accurately representing the tissue was used for further analysis. The comparison of the tumor proteome with this "super-SILAC" mix, drastically improved the quantification accuracy. The distribution was unimodal and 90% of quantified proteins were within a fourfold ratio between the tumor and the super-SILAC mix (3,837 of 4,286 quantified protein groups). Furthermore, the quantitative distribution was much narrower, with 76% of the proteins in the carcinoma and the super-SILAC mix differing by only twofold or less. Although super-SILAC has not been used to analyze the tumor phosphoproteome yet, the results of this research accurately quantified more than a hundred protein kinases despite their low abundance. Among them were ErbB2, EGFR, AKT, Pak1 and Pak2 and nine members of the MAPK cascade, all representing pathways central to malignancy. At first view, this new method has great potential to expand the use of accurate relative proteomic quantitation methods to study molecular aspects of tumor biology and perhaps as a tool for candidate biomarker discovery, so it is conceivable that it will likely become a valuable tool for understanding the molecular and mechanistic aspects of phosphorylation in tumor samples.

As described above, quantitative MS-based phosphoproteomics has been applied to identify oncogenic kinases which may serve as potential drug targets. To validate this hypothesis, cells are often treated with selected kinase inhibitors with the goal of altering cellular phenotype, but it is often difficult to establish whether the effect was due to on or off-target effects of the compound. In order to determine the mechanism of action, it may be necessary to quantify the specificity of the inhibitor. Two groups have pioneered the use of immobilized kinase inhibitors with broad specificity to enrich a substantial subset of protein kinases from total cell lysates followed by quantitative mass spectrometry. Daub et al. developed a kinase inhibitor pull-down technique in combination with phosphoproteomics to map and quantify more than one thousand phosphorylation sites on human protein kinases arrested in S- and M-phase of the cell cycle [43]. Researchers at Cellzome employed Kinobeads™ to enrich protein kinases and then performed competition-based assays using specific kinase inhibitor drugs such as imatinib (Gleevec), dasatinib (Sprycel) and bosutinib in BCR-Abl positive K562 cells [44]. Recently, Zhang et al. modified this approach in order to develop more potent inhibitors of the kinase AXL, which has an important role in mediating breast cancer cell motility and invasivity [45]. In this study, the authors used a chemical library of kinase inhibitors in order to identify small molecular inhibitors with selective activity on the AXL tyrosine kinase, the chemical compound NA80x1which has previously been reported to have inhibitory activity against Src kinase [46], inhibited AXL kinase activity in a dose-dependent manner, with an IC50 of 12.67 ± 0.45 μmol/L. Then, NA80x1 and a structurally similar, but much more potent inhibitor of Src and Abl kinases termed SKI-606, were chemically modified and attached to an affinity purification resin. To identify the specific targets (and some other off-targets) of these inhibitor derivatives, SILAC labeled proteins from the breast cancer cell line Hs578T were used for in vitro association experiments with the immobilized chemical compounds. The protein eluates from the respective affinity purifications were mixed and digested, and the resulting peptide fractions were analyzed by MS. In total, 146 different proteins were identified with at least two unique peptides in the MS experiments. Among them, 43 proteins were found to specifically bind to the immobilized compounds and 32 were kinases. In addition to known targets such as Src/Abl family kinases Src, Lyn, Arg, and the RTK AXL, which was functionally characterized as a cellular target in this study, a variety of other inhibitor-interacting proteins were identified, including eight more tyrosine kinases (such as FAK and four Eph receptor kinase family members) as well as nine members from the STE group of kinases involved in mitogen-activated protein kinase (MAPK) signaling (including six MAP4K/STE20 kinase family members and two MAP2K family members). This study is a clear example of how MS can help to identify off-targets of small molecular kinase inhibitors in order to develop more specific and potent chemicals for cancer therapies.

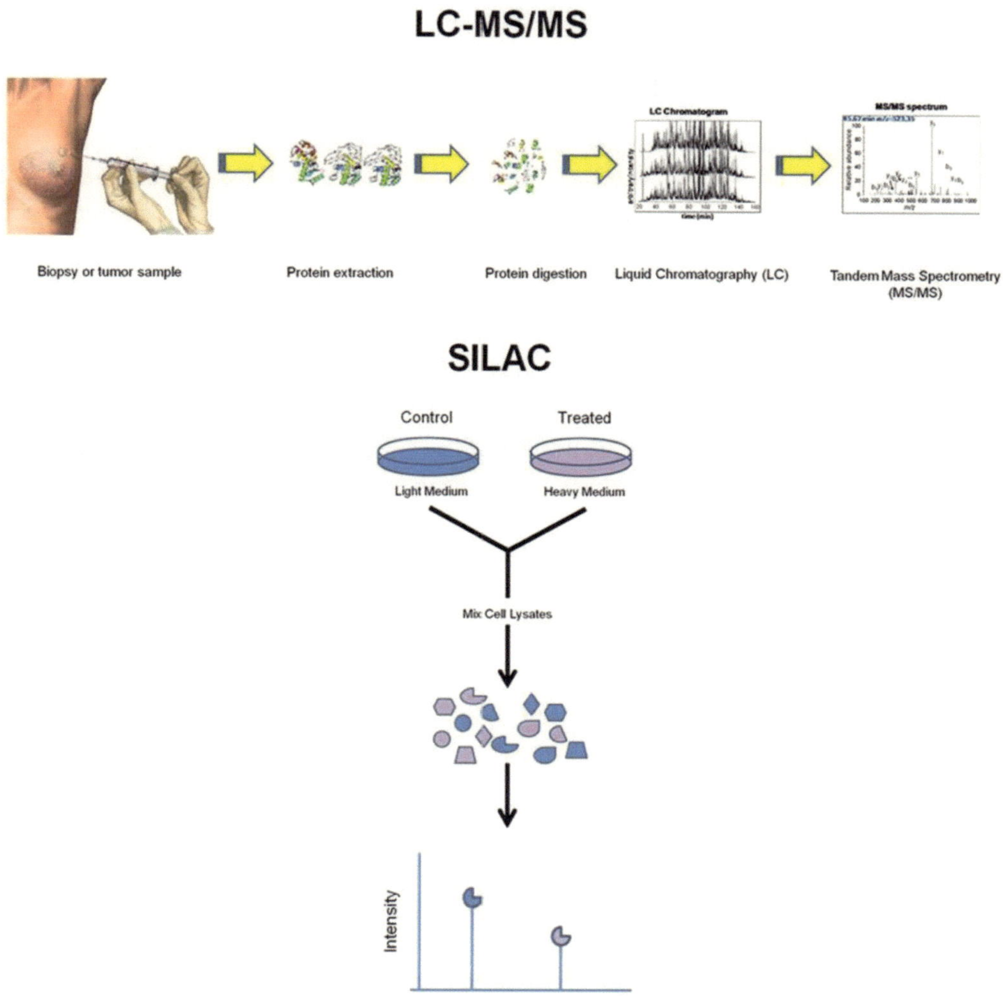

Figure 1. Mass Spectometry based approaches. The upper panel shows the pipelines of a prototypical proteomics experiment. Proteins are extracted from a biopsy or tumor sample and digested with trypsin to obtain peptides. The resulting peptides are resolved by reverse phase liquid chromatography (*LC*) and subsequently, analyzed by tandem mass spectrometry (MS/MS). Finally, the matched peptides allow the identification of the proteins using databases. The lower panel shows the schematic outline of the SILAC method. Separate cultures of cells are grown in normal medium (^{12}C6-arginine) or in medium containing arginine labeled at all six carbons with ^{13}C (^{13}C6-arginine). The cells in normal medium are left unstimulated whereas cells in the 13C-arginine medium are stimulated with an agent that activates signaling. The cells are harvested and equal amounts of lysate protein mixed together. In most cases, steps to enrich phosphoproteins and/or phosphopeptides after trypsin digestion are needed to detect low-abundance phosphopeptides. The peptides are resolved by LC-MS/MS and the data are used for automated database searching to identify peptides (and their corresponding protein) and to detect phosphopeptides.

4. Protein microarray approaches (non-MS)

To monitor previously identified phosphorylation sites, the combination of phosphospecific antibodies and western blotting has been the gold standard. However, until recently the limited throughput of this approach, with only one phosphorylation site investigated at a time, has driven the development of other, high-throughput approaches.

Arrays using phosphospecific antibodies to investigate phosphorylation sites have been developed [47, 48] and used to interrogate dozens of phosphorylation sites simultaneously [49]. As this technology requires antibodies with high-affinity and specificity, currently only a limited number of phosphorylation sites can be analyzed [50]. However, further development might lead to an even broader application of microarray technology for phosphoprotein studies.

Protein microarray formats can be divided into two major classes: forward phase arrays and reverse phase arrays **(Figure 2)** [51]. In a forward phase array, each spot contains one type of immobilized capture molecule, usually an antibody. Each array is incubated with one test

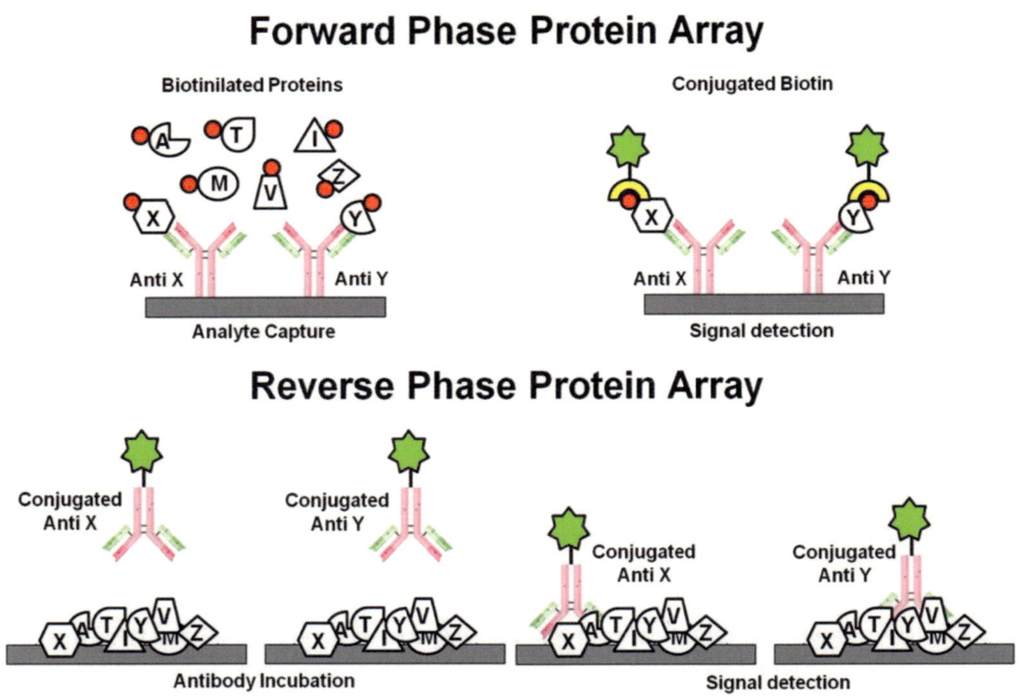

Figure 2. Protein microarray platforms. Forward phase arrays (top) immobilize a bait molecule such as an antibody designed to capture specific biotynilated proteins representing a specific treatment or condition. In this specific case, the bound analytes are detected by fluorescently labeled biotin. Reverse phase arrays immobilize the test sample analytes on the solid phase. An analyte specific labeled ligand (e.g., antibody; lower left) is applied in solution phase. Bound antibodies are detected by signal amplification (lower right).

sample such as a cellular lysate or serum sample representing a specific treatment condition, and multiple analytes from that sample are measured simultaneously. In contrast, the reverse phase array format immobilizes an individual test sample in each array spot, in a way that this array is comprised of hundreds of different patient samples or cellular lysates. In the reverse phase array format, each array is incubated with one detection protein (e.g., antibody), and a single analyte endpoint is measured and directly compared across multiple samples [47, 51-55].

5. Forward phase protein arrays

The most popular class of forward phase protein arrays in cancer research is the antibody array. A common application of antibody arrays is the identification of biomarkers or molecules that are potentially valuable for diagnosis or prognosis or as surrogate markers of drug response. The multiplex capability of antibody arrays allows the efficient screening of many marker candidates to reveal associations between proteins and disease states or experimental conditions. Multiplexed measurements also allow the evaluation of the use of multiple markers in combination. The use of combinations of proteins for disease diagnostics may produce fewer false positive and false negative results as compared with tests based on single proteins. Antibody microarrays, by increasing the number of proteins that can be conveniently measured in clinical samples, could more significantly take advantage of the benefit of using combined markers in diagnostics. Other example applications of antibody microarrays in cancer research are to evaluate the coordinated changes of members of signaling pathways or to measure changes in expression levels of a class of proteins, such as angiogenesis factors.

Only a few studies using antibody arrays for breast cancer research have been reported. One of the first studies was performed by Hudelist et al., who employed a high-throughput protein microarray system which contains 378 well characterized monoclonal antibodies printed at high density on a glass slide in duplicate in order to compare the gene expression pattern of malignant and adjacent normal breast tissue in a patient with primary breast cancer [56]. Using this technique, the authors identified a number of proteins that show increased expression levels in malignant breast tissues such as casein kinase Iε, p53, annexin XI, CDC25C, eIF-4E and MAP kinase 7. The expression of other proteins, such as the multifunctional regulator 14-3-3e was found to be decreased in malignant breast tissue, whereas the majority of proteins remained unchanged when compared to the corresponding non-malignant samples. Moreover, the protein expression pattern was corroborated by immunohistochemistry, in which antibodies against 8 representative proteins known to be involved in carcinogenesis were employed in paraffin-embedded normal and malignant tissue sections deriving from the same patient. In each case, the results obtained by IHC matched the data obtained by antibody microarray system. In another report [57], 224 antibodies revealed proteins that are related to doxorubicin therapy resistance in breast cancer cell lines. A decrease in the expression of MAP kinase-activated monophosphotyrosine, cyclin D2, cytokeratin 18, cyclin B1 and heterogeneous nuclear ribonucleoprotein m3-m4 was found to be associated with doxorubicin resistance. Other recent investigations helped identify a marker involved in invasion (interleukin (IL)-8) [58]. Studying the serum proteome from metastatic breast cancer patients and healthy controls with recombinant single-chain variable fragment (scFv) microarrays [59], breast cancer was identified with a specificity and sensitivity of 85% on the basis of 129 serum analytes.

Although a number of companies have already developed phospho-antibody arrays for breast cancer research, there are only a few reports of the use of this technology in breast cancer. In 2008, Eckestein et al. [60], studied the cellular mechanisms of resistance to cisplatin using MCF-7 cells as a model system. Cisplatin-resistant MCF-7 breast cancer cells were selected by exposure to sequential cycles of cisplatin that mimic the way the drug is used in the clinic. To investigate the phosphorylation status of the EGFR receptor family, a phosphoreceptor tyrosine kinase (phospho-RTK) array was used. In this assay, monoclonal capture antibodies, specific for a variety of RTKs, were spotted in an array format, and phosphorylation of EGFR family members was subsequently detected by a pan anti-phosphotyrosine antibody conjugated to horseradish peroxidase. In nonresistant cells the EGFR was phosphorylated at a low level. In contrast, in cisplatin resistant MCF-7 cells both the EGFR and ERBB2 receptors were strongly phosphorylated. The phospho-RTK array detected very low ErbB3 and ErbB4 phosphorylation in both MCF-7 and cisplatin resistant MCF-7 cells, suggesting, that these receptor subtypes are not activated in cisplatin-resistant breast cancer cells. By using similar arrays, the authors examined the Ras/Raf/MEK/ERK, PI3K/AKT, JNK and p38 signaling pathways, which are downstream effectors of EGFR in a number of cell systems. The analysis of these pathways showed that the Ras/Raf/MEK/ERK and PI3K/AKT pathways are hyperactive in the cisplatin-resistant breast cancer cells, whereas the JNK and p38 pathways were not affected. Similarly, this study shows that cisplatin-resistant breast cancer cells have an inactivation of the p53 pathway and display high levels of BCL-2. A transcriptional profile of the cisplatin-resistant breast cancer cells also showed that these cells have an upregulation of the amphiregulin gene, the expression and secretion of this protein is also elevated and this mechanism creates an autocrine loop that confers resistance to cisplatin.

A more recent study using this technology showed that activation of the PI3K-AKT pathway in tumors is modulated by negative feedback, including mTORC1-mediated inhibition of upstream signaling [61]. The authors clearly demonstrate that AKT inhibition induces the expression and phosphorylation of multiple receptor tyrosine kinases in a panel of different breast cancer cell lines. The results of this research suggest that receptor activation of PI3K-AKT causes AKT-dependent phosphorylation of FOXO proteins, which downregulate the expression of some of the receptors that are tightly coupled to PI3K, including ErbB3, IGF1R, and IR. In addition, AKT activation leads to activation of TORC1 and S6K, which feedback inhibits IRS1 expression and other non defined regulators of receptor signaling, resulting in down modulation of the signaling pathway. Thus, AKT inhibition will result in activation of FOXO-dependent transcription of receptors and inhibition of S6K-dependent inhibition of signaling with resultant activation of multiple receptors. The downstream effects of AKT will be suppressed, but other RTK-driven signaling pathways will be activated. In contrast, TORC1 inhibition blocks S6K-dependent feedback, activates IGF and ErbB kinases, but not their expression, and, thus, activates both AKT and ERK signaling. These findings have important basic and therapeutic implications.

6. Reverse phase protein arrays

Probing multiple arrays spotted with the same lysate concomitantly with different phosphospecific antibodies provides the effect of generating a multiplex readout. The utility of reverse phase protein microarrays lies in their ability to provide a map of known cell signaling proteins. Identification of critical nodes, or interactions, within the network is a potential starting point for drug development and/or the design of individual therapy regimens [62, 63]. The array format is also amenable to extremely sensitive analyte detection with detection levels approaching attogram amounts of a given protein and variances of less than 10% [51, 64]. Detection ranges could be substantially lower in a complex mixture such as a cellular lysate; however, the sensitivity of the reverse phase arrays is such that low abundance phosphorylated isoforms can still be measured from a spotted lysate amount of less than 10 cell equivalents. This level of sensitivity combined with analytical robustness is critical if the starting input material is only a few hundred cells from a biopsy specimen. Due to all this advantages, the reverse phase protein array has demonstrated a unique ability to analyze signaling pathways using small numbers of cultured cells or cells isolated by laser capture microdissection from human tissue procured during clinical trials [47, 53, 54, 65].

In a landmark study, Boyd et al. investigated how signaling pathways are differentially activated in different breast cancer subtypes [66]. In this study, the phosphorylation status of 100 proteins was examined in a panel of 30 different breast cancer cell lines. These cell lines have previously been classified into the three major molecular subtypes using a combination of gene expression data and ErbB2 status [67]. Briefly, cell lines were assigned to luminal or basal-like classes using gene expression data, and ErbB2 amplification status was assigned by means of quantitative reverse transcription to identify cell lines with more than four copies of the 17q12-q21 locus. Then, the phosphorylated protein status from the 30 breast cancer cell lines was analyzed by reverse phase protein arrays. In order to reduce dimensionality of the data and find patterns that might be related to the differential activity of signaling pathways in particular subtypes of breast cancer, the principle component analysis (or PCA, which convert a set of observations of possibly correlated variables into a set of values of linearly uncorrelated variables called principal components) was used. The results of this analysis showed that the global proteomic signature determined by this method largely separates basal-like cell lines from ErbB2 amplified and luminal cell lines along the second principal component. Also, with the exception of the ErbB2-amplified line BT474, the majority of the luminal lines are separated from the ErbB2 lines. This analysis suggests that the phosphorylated protein end points in this analysis are significantly correlated because the first three principal components can account for 61% of the variance in the data and also that distinct pathways may be activated in the different subtypes. Moreover, this analysis suggests that specific pathway activation events may be present in the different molecular subtypes. In particular, basal-like lines were found to be distinct from luminal and ErbB2-amplified lines in having low levels of pPTEN and high levels of total EGFR, pPyk2 Y402, and pPKC-α S567. ErbB2-amplified cell lines were distinct from the other subtypes in having high levels of pERBB3, pFAK, and pEGFR Y1173, and luminal cell lines were distinct in having higher levels of phosphorylation of p70S6K S371 and A-RAF S299. In addition, this analysis revealed patterns of pathway activation that are not obvious from published gene expression analyses. In particular, basal-like cell lines were found to have high levels of phosphorylation of non-receptor tyrosine kinases, such as c-Abl and Pyk2, and in addition showed generally high levels of ERK1/2 phosphorylation and high total EGFR expression. In contrast, ErbB2-amplified cell lines were found to have high levels of phosphorylation of components of the EGFR pathway (e.g., Shc, ErbB3, EGFR), as well as other receptor tyrosine kinases (e.g., c-MET). Finally, luminal cell lines that do not have apparent amplification of ErbB2 showed generally higher levels of activation of downstream signaling pathway components in the AKT/mTOR pathway (e.g., p70S6K).

A potentially important application of reverse phase protein array technology is the more personalized administration of targeted therapies based on the signaling status of a given patient's tumor. The assumption is that if a patient's tumor is addicted to the continued activation of a particular pathway for continued growth and survival [68], then phosphorylation at key nodes in that pathway may serve as hallmarks, indicating the presence of an activated pathway and the potential for therapeutic intervention with inhibitors targeting that pathway. Similarly, PI3K is a key transducer of growth factor signals from receptor tyrosine kinases, as well as a frequently mutated oncogene, suggesting that PI3K inhibitors might have beneficial effects in treating cancers driven by pathologic alterations of this pathway [69]. The results reported by Boyd et al., suggest that activation of these pathway modules occur in a subtype-specific manner and can provide the basis for therapeutic intervention. If this is true, basal tumors, which display high levels of EGFR, activated ERK1/2, and phosphorylation of Src-activated effector kinases, such as c-Abl and Pyk2 would be potential candidates for combined therapies with antibodies and/or small molecule inhibitors used in clinical trials. These findings also highlight the potential utility of reverse phase protein arrays in confirming pathway modulation upon therapeutic intervention and applications in examining pharmacodynamic biomarkers of drug response. For example, it is well documented that an inhibitor of all isoforms of the class I catalytic subunit of PI3K, GDC-0941, results in potent and selective inhibition of multiple nodes in the PI3K/AKT pathway and, thus, that reverse phase protein arrays might have utility monitoring surrogate markers of compound activity. Conversely, the results of this study also showed that a selective MEK inhibitor results in potent down-regulation of pERK1/2 and actually increases signaling through the PI3K/AKT axis. This result highlights the fact that signaling pathways are dynamically linked networks and that perturbations in one pathway may have unforeseen consequences on interacting pathways that may affect response to therapeutic agents [70].

In a more recent study, Iadevaia et al. used a reverse-phase protein array to measure the transient response of the MDA-MB-231 breast cancer cell line after stimulation by insulin-like growth factor (IGF-1) [71]. The experimental results showed that when active, IGFR propagates the signal downstream through the Ras/Raf/MEK/ERK (MAPK) and phosphoinositide-3-kinase/AKT (PI3K) signaling pathways. The signals from the MAPK and PI3K cascades are routed to the mTOR pathway through tuberous sclerosis (TSC2) inactivation. Phosphorylated mTOR activates p70S6K, which inactivates the insulin receptor substrate (IRS-1) through a negative feedback loop.

The experimental results indicate that combined inhibition of the MAPK and PI3K/AKT pathways optimally inhibited the signaling networks and decreased cell viability. In contrast, combined inhibition of the MAPK and mTOR cascades led to significant activation of p-AKT and increased cell viability. Although several other kinases and pathways may potentially regulate the viability of the MDA-MB-231 cells, the experimental results indicated that simultaneous inhibition of the MAPK and PI3K/AKT pathways was sufficient to significantly reduce cell proliferation. The procedure is currently being used to identify and validate drug combinations that can inhibit aberrant networks in a panel of human cancer cell lines. **Figure 3** summarizes some of the deregulated signaling pathways described by the use of Phosphoproteomics.

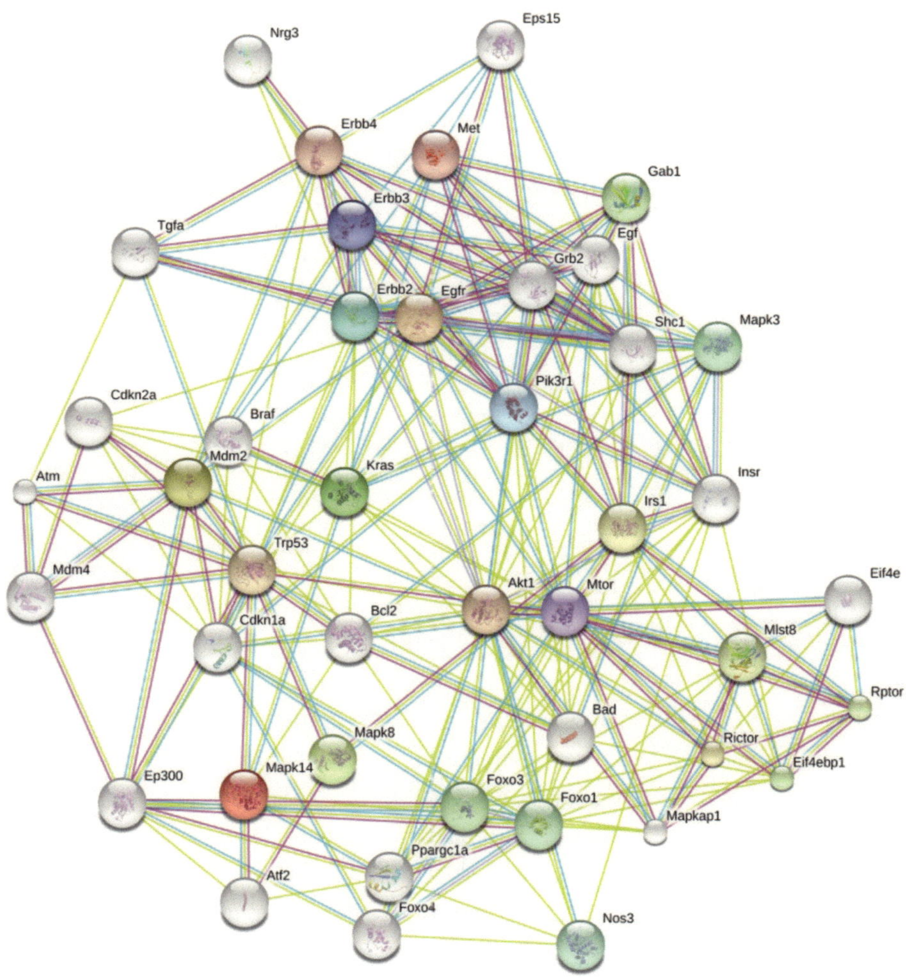

Figure 3. Altered signaling pathways in breast cancer. This interaction map was created in the String 9.0 program (http://string-db.org) and summarizes some of the most commonly affected signaling pathways in breast cancer. Predicted functional links, consist of different colored lines: one color for each type of evidence. In this specific case, pink lines represent experimental evidence, blue lines represent interactions already published in databases and green lines text data mining.

7. Clinical implications

Cancer is among the leading causes of death worldwide. Therefore, the design of effective strategies to successfully implement personalized cancer medicine in clinical practice needs to face substantial challenges in the future. One of the biggest challenges in cancer research is the fact there is currently an insufficient number of effective rationally targeted drugs to implement this strategy broadly, at the time of this review, at least 50 distinct selective kinase inhibitors had been developed to the level of a phase I clinical trial, some of them have already been tested in breast cancer patients and it is expected that many more will be developed as cancer phosphoproteome analysis efforts continue to identify additional potential targets (**Table 1**).

Kinase	Alteration	Therapeutic Agent	Reference
Receptor Tyrosine Kinases			
EGFR	Amplification, mutations	gefitinib, erlotinib	[72]
ErbB2/Her2	Amplification	lapatinib, trastuzumab	[73]
MET	Amplification	PF2341066, XL184, SU11274	[74]
FGFR2	Amplification, mutations	PKC412, BIF1120	[75]
AXL	Increased activation	R428	[76]
IGF1R/INSR	Overexpression	BMS-754807	[77]
EphA2	Overexpression	None available	
Non Receptor Tyrosine Kinases			
Ack1	Increased activation	None available	
FAK	Overexpression	None available	
Src/Lyn/Hck	Overexpression	dasatinib, AZD05030	[78]
Serine/Threonine Kinases			
PI3K	Mutations	BEZ235	[79]
mTOR	Increased activation	everolimus	[80]
PLK	Overexpression	GSK461364	[81]
Aurora Kinases A and B	Overexpression	MK5108	[82]
Raf	Increased activation	sorafenib	[83]
MEK	Increased activation	PD0325901	[84]
ERK1/2	Increased activation	None available	
Pak1	Amplification, overexpression	None available	

Table 1. Oncogenic Kinases as Therapeutic Targets in Breast Cancer.

The current phosphoproteomic goals imply the identification of phosphoproteins, mapping of phosphorylation sites, quantitation of phosphorylation under different conditions, and the determination of the stoichiometry of the phosphorylation. In addition, knowing when a protein is phosphorylated, which kinase/s is-are involved, and how each phosphorylation fits into the signaling network, are also important challenges for researchers in order to understand the significance of different biological events. The new phosphoproteomic technologies are fundamental for cataloguing all this information, and it is heading towards the collection of accurate data on phosphopeptides on a global scale. In addition, the possible difficulties to get sufficient amount of specific phosphorylated proteins of specific low abundant protein-kinases in vivo which might limit the usability of the phosphoproteome analysis, must be pointed out. The concept of personalized cancer medicine also has significant implications for the drug development industry, which is beginning to recognize and appreciate the need to alter the current business model for drug development and clinical testing. Moreover, the clinical success of such kinase inhibitors as imatinib, erlotinib, and lapatinib has validated this strategy and has prompted a virtual explosion in the development of additional kinase inhibitors for cancer therapy. Importantly, though, with these successes has also come the realization that these agents are generally effective for a relatively small subset of treated patients, often defined by a common genomic, proteomic and/or phosphoproteomic denominator present within the tumor cells. Such findings have highlighted the potential importance of identifying defined patient subpopulations before treatment with kinase inhibitors to optimize clinical outcomes.

Finally, it is important to state that to develop clinical proteomic applications using the identified proteins and phosphoproteins, collaboration between research scientists, clinicians and diagnostic companies, and proteomic experts is essential, particularly in the early phases of the biomarker development projects. The proteomics modalities currently available have the potential to lead to the development of clinical applications, and channeling the wealth of the information produced towards concrete and specific clinical purposes is urgent.

8. Concluding remarks

Cancer has been described as both a proteomic and a genomic disease [66]. Only those genetic defects creating a survival advantage increase the tumorigenic potential and are reflected in an altered functional state [19, 67]. Thus, the current challenges of cancer treatment, e.g. why do some patients respond to cancer drugs, while others do not, can only be answered with comprehensive efforts and by integrating knowledge on genetic and chromosomal aberrations, clinical data, IHC, and quantitative protein profiling.

Phosphoproteomics has played a significant role in our ability to understand molecular mechanisms that govern human cancers. Various technological platforms are now available for phosphoproteomic studies enabling us to address different aspects of tumor biology governed by phosphorylation-mediated signaling pathways. These studies have clearly taken us beyond looking at mutations or other genetic variations commonly observed in cancers and are providing us insights into functional consequences of these changes in conferring survival advantages to cancer cells. Such studies are already being used as the basis for determining therapeutic options. With an ever increasing list of kinase inhibitors being developed by pharmaceutical companies, such strategies have become vital not only to determine the targets of these inhibitors but also to study their off-target effects. We foresee phosphoproteomics emerging as a vital technique in clinical research to assist in diagnosis, prognosis and treatment of cancers. The major challenge ahead is to develop this technology further to make it amenable for use in the clinic with as few sample processing steps as possible.

There are several issues, however, that must be carefully and promptly addressed if we are going to fulfill the dream of bringing individualized cancer care closer to reality. First of all, we must acknowledge the value of long-term research and provide the appropriate legal and ethical framework to encourage the collaboration among all the stakeholders in the cancer ordeal. Bridging the gap between basic and clinical research, facilitating the engagement of the industry, creating new infrastructures and bio banks, as well as the creation of innovative clinical trials are among the items that require urgent action. The aim of cancer research is to improve the life expectancy and quality of life of patients and we must make every effort to coordinate current activities in order to achieve this goal.

Author details

Olga Villamar-Cruz and Luis E. Arias-Romero*
Cancer Biology Program, Fox Chase Cancer Center, Philadelphia, PA, USA

Acknowledgement

We gratefully acknowledge the helpful comments from E. Arechaga-Ocampo, C. Perez-Plasencia and our anonymous reviewers.

9. References

[1] Jemal, A., et al., Global cancer statistics. CA Cancer J Clin, 2011;61(2) 69-90.
[2] Perou, C.M., et al., Molecular portraits of human breast tumours. Nature, 2000;406(6797) 747-752.
[3] Sorlie, T., et al., Gene expression patterns of breast carcinomas distinguish tumor subclasses with clinical implications. Proc Natl Acad Sci U S A, 2001;98(19) 10869-10874.
[4] Sorlie, T., et al., Repeated observation of breast tumor subtypes in independent gene expression data sets. Proc Natl Acad Sci U S A, 2003;100(14) 8418-8423.
[5] Callagy, G., et al., Molecular classification of breast carcinomas using tissue microarrays. Diagn Mol Pathol, 2003;12(1) 27-34.
[6] Abd El-Rehim, D.M., et al., Expression of luminal and basal cytokeratins in human breast carcinoma. J Pathol, 2004;203(2) 661-671.

* Corresponding Author

[7] Jacquemier, J., et al., Protein expression profiling identifies subclasses of breast cancer and predicts prognosis. Cancer Res, 2005;65(3) 767-779.

[8] Nielsen, T.O., et al., Immunohistochemical and clinical characterization of the basal-like subtype of invasive breast carcinoma. Clin Cancer Res, 2004;10(16) 5367-5374.

[9] Sotiriou, C., et al., Breast cancer classification and prognosis based on gene expression profiles from a population-based study. Proc Natl Acad Sci U S A, 2003;100(18) 10393-10398.

[10] Abd El-Rehim, D.M., et al., High-throughput protein expression analysis using tissue microarray technology of a large well-characterised series identifies biologically distinct classes of breast cancer confirming recent cDNA expression analyses. Int J Cancer, 2005;116(3) 340-350.

[11] Hynes, N.E. and H.A. Lane, ERBB receptors and cancer: the complexity of targeted inhibitors. Nat Rev Cancer, 2005;5(5) 341-354.

[12] Slamon, D.J., et al., Studies of the HER-2/neu proto-oncogene in human breast and ovarian cancer. Science, 1989;244(4905) 707-712.

[13] Yarden, Y. and M.X. Sliwkowski, Untangling the ErbB signalling network. Nat Rev Mol Cell Biol, 2001;2(2) 127-137.

[14] Moasser, M.M., The oncogene HER2: its signaling and transforming functions and its role in human cancer pathogenesis. Oncogene, 2007;26(45) 6469-6487.

[15] Slamon, D.J., et al., Use of chemotherapy plus a monoclonal antibody against HER2 for metastatic breast cancer that overexpresses HER2. N Engl J Med, 2001;344(11) 783-792.

[16] Romond, E.H., et al., Trastuzumab plus adjuvant chemotherapy for operable HER2-positive breast cancer. N Engl J Med, 2005;353(16) 1673-1684.

[17] Geyer, C.E., et al., Lapatinib plus capecitabine for HER2-positive advanced breast cancer. N Engl J Med, 2006;355(26) 2733-2743.

[18] Vogel, C.L., et al., Efficacy and safety of trastuzumab as a single agent in first-line treatment of HER2-overexpressing metastatic breast cancer. J Clin Oncol, 2002;20(3) 719-726.

[19] Amanchy, R., et al., Identification of c-Src tyrosine kinase substrates using mass spectrometry and peptide microarrays. J Proteome Res, 2008;7(9) 3900-3910.

[20] Diks, S.H., et al., Kinome profiling for studying lipopolysaccharide signal transduction in human peripheral blood mononuclear cells. J Biol Chem, 2004;279(47) 49206-49213.

[21] Versele, M., et al., Response prediction to a multitargeted kinase inhibitor in cancer cell lines and xenograft tumors using high-content tyrosine peptide arrays with a kinetic readout. Mol Cancer Ther, 2009;8(7) 1846-1855.

[22] Gulmann, C., et al., Quantitative cell signalling analysis reveals down-regulation of MAPK pathway activation in colorectal cancer. J Pathol, 2009;218(4) 514-519.

[23] Chen, E.I. and J.R. Yates, 3rd, Cancer proteomics by quantitative shotgun proteomics. Mol Oncol, 2007;1(2) 144-159.

[24] Choudhary, C., et al., Mislocalized activation of oncogenic RTKs switches downstream signaling outcomes. Mol Cell, 2009;36(2) 326-339.

[25] Chen, Y., et al., Differential expression of novel tyrosine kinase substrates during breast cancer development. Mol Cell Proteomics, 2007;6(12) 2072-2087.

[26] Zhang, Y., et al., Time-resolved mass spectrometry of tyrosine phosphorylation sites in the epidermal growth factor receptor signaling network reveals dynamic modules. Mol Cell Proteomics, 2005;4(9) 1240-1250.

[27] Hochgrafe, F., et al., Tyrosine phosphorylation profiling reveals the signaling network characteristics of Basal breast cancer cells. Cancer Res, 2010;70(22) 9391-9401.

[28] Kumar, N., et al., Modeling HER2 effects on cell behavior from mass spectrometry phosphotyrosine data. PLoS Comput Biol, 2007;3(1) e4.

[29] Neve, R.M., et al., A collection of breast cancer cell lines for the study of functionally distinct cancer subtypes. Cancer Cell, 2006;10(6) 515-527.

[30] Hubbard, S.R., Juxtamembrane autoinhibition in receptor tyrosine kinases. Nat Rev Mol Cell Biol, 2004;5(6) 464-471.

[31] Fang, W.B., et al., Identification and functional analysis of phosphorylated tyrosine residues within EphA2 receptor tyrosine kinase. J Biol Chem, 2008;283(23) 16017-16026.

[32] Batzer, A.G., et al., Hierarchy of binding sites for Grb2 and Shc on the epidermal growth factor receptor. Mol Cell Biol, 1994;14(8) 5192-5201.

[33] Ricci, A., et al., Analysis of protein-protein interactions involved in the activation of the Shc/Grb-2 pathway by the ErbB-2 kinase. Oncogene, 1995;11(8) 1519-1529.

[34] Wolf-Yadlin, A., et al., Effects of HER2 overexpression on cell signaling networks governing proliferation and migration. Mol Syst Biol, 2006;2 54.

[35] Ong, S.E. and M. Mann, Mass spectrometry-based proteomics turns quantitative. Nat Chem Biol, 2005;1(5) 252-262.

[36] Liang, X., et al., Quantification of membrane and membrane-bound proteins in normal and malignant breast cancer cells isolated from the same patient with primary breast carcinoma. J Proteome Res, 2006;5(10) 2632-2641.

[37] Bose, R., et al., Phosphoproteomic analysis of Her2/neu signaling and inhibition. Proc Natl Acad Sci U S A, 2006;103(26) 9773-9778.

[38] Houtman, R., et al., Lung proteome alterations in a mouse model for nonallergic asthma. Proteomics, 2003;3(10) 2008-2018.

[39] Kruger, M., et al., SILAC mouse for quantitative proteomics uncovers kindlin-3 as an essential factor for red blood cell function. Cell, 2008;134(2) 353-364.

[40] McClatchy, D.B., et al., Quantification of the synaptosomal proteome of the rat cerebellum during post-natal development. Genome Res, 2007;17(9) 1378-1388.

[41] Ishihama, Y., et al., Quantitative mouse brain proteomics using culture-derived isotope tags as internal standards. Nat Biotechnol, 2005;23(5) 617-621.

[42] Geiger, T., et al., Super-SILAC mix for quantitative proteomics of human tumor tissue. Nat Methods, 2010;7(5) 383-385.

[43] Daub, H., et al., Kinase-selective enrichment enables quantitative phosphoproteomics of the kinome across the cell cycle. Mol Cell, 2008;31(3) 438-448.

[44] Bantscheff, M., et al., Quantitative chemical proteomics reveals mechanisms of action of clinical ABL kinase inhibitors. Nat Biotechnol, 2007;25(9) 1035-1044.

[45] Zhang, Y.X., et al., AXL is a potential target for therapeutic intervention in breast cancer progression. Cancer Res, 2008;68(6) 1905-1915.

[46] Boschelli, D.H., et al., Synthesis and Src kinase inhibitory activity of a series of 4-phenylamino-3-quinolinecarbonitriles. J Med Chem, 2001;44(5) 822-833.

[47] Paweletz, C.P., et al., Reverse phase protein microarrays which capture disease progression show activation of pro-survival pathways at the cancer invasion front. Oncogene, 2001;20(16) 1981-1989.

[48] Nielsen, U.B., et al., Profiling receptor tyrosine kinase activation by using Ab microarrays. Proc Natl Acad Sci U S A, 2003;100(16) 9330-9335.

[49] Sheehan, K.M., et al., Use of reverse phase protein microarrays and reference standard development for molecular network analysis of metastatic ovarian carcinoma. Mol Cell Proteomics, 2005;4(4) 346-355.

[50] Gulmann, C., et al., Array-based proteomics: mapping of protein circuitries for diagnostics, prognostics, and therapy guidance in cancer. J Pathol, 2006;208(5) 595-606.

[51] Liotta, L.A., et al., Protein microarrays: meeting analytical challenges for clinical applications. Cancer Cell, 2003;3(4) 317-325.

[52] Pavlickova, P., E.M. Schneider, and H. Hug, Advances in recombinant antibody microarrays. Clin Chim Acta, 2004;343(1-2) 17-35.

[53] Zha, H., et al., Similarities of prosurvival signals in Bcl-2-positive and Bcl-2-negative follicular lymphomas identified by reverse phase protein microarray. Lab Invest, 2004;84(2) 235-244.

[54] Grubb, R.L., et al., Signal pathway profiling of prostate cancer using reverse phase protein arrays. Proteomics, 2003;3(11) 2142-2146.

[55] Nishizuka, S., et al., Proteomic profiling of the NCI-60 cancer cell lines using new high-density reverse-phase lysate microarrays. Proc Natl Acad Sci U S A, 2003;100(24) 14229-14234.

[56] Hudelist, G., et al., Use of high-throughput protein array for profiling of differentially expressed proteins in normal and malignant breast tissue. Breast Cancer Res Treat, 2004;86(3) 281-291.

[57] Smith, L., et al., The analysis of doxorubicin resistance in human breast cancer cells using antibody microarrays. Mol Cancer Ther, 2006;5(8) 2115-2120.

[58] Lin, Y., et al., Identification of interleukin-8 as estrogen receptor-regulated factor involved in breast cancer invasion and angiogenesis by protein arrays. Int J Cancer, 2004;109(4) 507-515.

[59] Carlsson, A., et al., Serum proteome profiling of metastatic breast cancer using recombinant antibody microarrays. Eur J Cancer, 2008;44(3) 472-480.

[60] Eckstein, N., et al., Epidermal growth factor receptor pathway analysis identifies amphiregulin as a key factor for cisplatin resistance of human breast cancer cells. J Biol Chem, 2008;283(2) 739-750.

[61] Chandarlapaty, S., et al., AKT inhibition relieves feedback suppression of receptor tyrosine kinase expression and activity. Cancer Cell, 2011;19(1) 58-71.

[62] Liotta, L.A., E.C. Kohn, and E.F. Petricoin, Clinical proteomics: personalized molecular medicine. JAMA, 2001;286(18) 2211-2214.

[63] Petricoin, E.F., et al., Clinical proteomics: translating benchside promise into bedside reality. Nat Rev Drug Discov, 2002;1(9) 683-695.

[64] Espina, V., et al., Protein microarray detection strategies: focus on direct detection technologies. J Immunol Methods, 2004;290(1-2) 121-133.

[65] Wulfkuhle, J.D., et al., Signal pathway profiling of ovarian cancer from human tissue specimens using reverse-phase protein microarrays. Proteomics, 2003;3(11) 2085-2090.

[66] Boyd, Z.S., et al., Proteomic analysis of breast cancer molecular subtypes and biomarkers of response to targeted kinase inhibitors using reverse-phase protein microarrays. Mol Cancer Ther, 2008;7(12) 3695-3706.

[67] O'Brien, C., et al., Functional genomics identifies ABCC3 as a mediator of taxane resistance in HER2-amplified breast cancer. Cancer Res, 2008;68(13) 5380-5389.
[68] Weinstein, I.B. and A. Joe, Oncogene addiction. Cancer Res, 2008;68(9) 3077-3080; discussion 3080.
[69] Workman, P., et al., Drugging the PI3 kinome. Nat Biotechnol, 2006;24(7) 794-796.
[70] Araujo, R.P., L.A. Liotta, and E.F. Petricoin, Proteins, drug targets and the mechanisms they control: the simple truth about complex networks. Nat Rev Drug Discov, 2007;6(11) 871-880.
[71] Iadevaia, S., et al., Identification of Optimal Drug Combinations Targeting Cellular Networks: Integrating Phospho-Proteomics and Computational Network Analysis. Cancer Res, 2010;70(17) 6704-6714.
[72] Lynch, T.J., et al., Activating mutations in the epidermal growth factor receptor underlying responsiveness of non-small-cell lung cancer to gefitinib. N Engl J Med, 2004;350(21) 2129-2139.
[73] Gomez, H.L., et al., Efficacy and safety of lapatinib as first-line therapy for ErbB2-amplified locally advanced or metastatic breast cancer. J Clin Oncol, 2008;26(18) 2999-3005.
[74] Zou, H.Y., et al., An orally available small-molecule inhibitor of c-Met, PF-2341066, exhibits cytoreductive antitumor efficacy through antiproliferative and antiangiogenic mechanisms. Cancer Res, 2007;67(9) 4408-4417.
[75] Hilberg, F., et al., BIBF 1120: triple angiokinase inhibitor with sustained receptor blockade and good antitumor efficacy. Cancer Res, 2008;68(12) 4774-4782.
[76] Holland, S.J., et al., R428, a selective small molecule inhibitor of Axl kinase, blocks tumor spread and prolongs survival in models of metastatic breast cancer. Cancer Res, 2010;70(4) 1544-1554.
[77] Hou, X., et al., Dual IGF-1R/InsR inhibitor BMS-754807 synergizes with hormonal agents in treatment of estrogen-dependent breast cancer. Cancer Res, 2011;71(24) 7597-7607.
[78] Blume-Jensen, P. and T. Hunter, Oncogenic kinase signalling. Nature, 2001;411(6835) 355-365.
[79] Maira, S.M., et al., Identification and characterization of NVP-BEZ235, a new orally available dual phosphatidylinositol 3-kinase/mammalian target of rapamycin inhibitor with potent in vivo antitumor activity. Mol Cancer Ther, 2008;7(7) 1851-1863.
[80] Schwarzlose-Schwarck, S., et al., The mTOR Inhibitor Everolimus in Combination with Carboplatin in Metastatic Breast Cancer - a Phase I Trial. Anticancer Res, 2012;32(8) 3435-3441.
[81] Warner, S.L., B.J. Stephens, and D.D. Von Hoff, Tubulin-associated proteins: Aurora and Polo-like kinases as therapeutic targets in cancer. Curr Oncol Rep, 2008;10(2) 122-129.
[82] Shimomura, T., et al., MK-5108, a highly selective Aurora-A kinase inhibitor, shows antitumor activity alone and in combination with docetaxel. Mol Cancer Ther, 2010;9(1) 157-166.
[83] Clark, J.W., et al., Safety and pharmacokinetics of the dual action Raf kinase and vascular endothelial growth factor receptor inhibitor, BAY 43-9006, in patients with advanced, refractory solid tumors. Clin Cancer Res, 2005;11(15) 5472-5480.
[84] Sebolt-Leopold, J.S., MEK inhibitors: a therapeutic approach to targeting the Ras-MAP kinase pathway in tumors. Curr Pharm Des, 2004;10(16) 1907-1914.